Lecture Notes on Respiratory Disease

Written and illustrated by

R.A.L. BREWIS MD FRCP
Consultant Physician,
Royal Victoria Infirmary,
Newcastle upon Tyne
Senior Lecturer in Medicine,
University of Newcastle upon Tyne

FOURTH EDITION

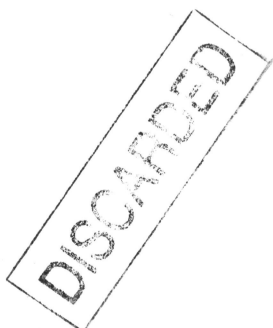

OXFORD

BLACKWELL SCIENTIFIC PUBLICATIONS

LONDON EDINBURGH BOSTON

MELBOURNE PARIS BERLIN VIENNA

ok

© 1975, 1980, 1985, 1991 by
Blackwell Scientific Publications
Editorial offices:
Osney Mead, Oxford OX2 0EL
25 John Street, London WC1N 2BL
23 Ainslie Place, Edinburgh EH3 6AJ
238 Main Street, Cambridge
    Massachusetts 02142, USA
54 University Street, Carlton
    Victoria 3053, Australia

Other Editorial Offices:
Librairie Arnette SA
2, rue Casimir-Delavigne
75006 Paris
France

Blackwell Wissenschafts-Verlag
Meinekestrasse 4
D-1000 Berlin 15
Germany

Blackwell MZV
Feldgasse 13
A-1238 Wien
Austria

First published 1975
Revised reprint 1976
Reprinted 1977, 1978
Second edition 1980
Spanish edition 1980
Third edition 1985
Fourth edition 1991
Reprinted 1992
Four Dragons edition 1992

Set by Semantic Graphics, Singapore
Printed and bound in Great Britain by
Hartnolls Ltd, Bodmin, Cornwall

DISTRIBUTORS

Marston Book Services Ltd
PO Box 87
Oxford OX2 0DT
(*Orders:* Tel: 0865 791155
        Fax: 0865 791927
        Telex: 837515)

USA
Blackwell Scientific Publications, Inc.
238 Main Street,
Cambridge, MA 02142
(*Orders:* Tel: 800 759-6102
            617 876-7000)

Canada
Times Mirror Professional Publishing, Ltd
5240 Finch Avenue East
Scarborough, Ontario M1S 5A2
(*Orders:* Tel: 800 268-4178
            416 298-1588)

Australia
Blackwell Scientific Publications
(Australia) Pty Ltd
54 University Street
Carlton, Victoria 3053
(*Orders:* Tel: 03 347-0300)

British Library
Cataloguing in Publication Data

Brewis, R. A. L. (Robert Alistair Livingston)
    Lecture notes on respiratory disease.–
    4th ed
    1. Humans. Respiratory system. Diseases
    I. Title
    616.2

ISBN 0–632–02777–0
    0–632–03568–4 BSP Four Dragons

Contents

Preface to the Fourth Edition

The aims and structure remain the same as in the previous editions, but the whole text has been reviewed and updated. There are over twenty new figures. There are new chapters on lung disease in AIDS and in severely immuno-compromised patients, smoking, adult respiratory distress syndrome (ARDS) and ventilatory failure and sleep apnoea. There has been revision and expansion elsewhere, notably to take into account computerized tomography (CT). Throughout the book I have tried to keep in mind the needs of the students and junior doctors that I regularly come into contact with. I am grateful to the students and young doctors and to many others for stimulation and encouragement.

R.A.L.B.
Newcastle upon Tyne

Preface to the First Edition

The aim of this book is to present a concise review of respiratory disease. In addition to offering the medical student an alternative to attending lectures, it is hoped that this book might provide the MRCP candidate with his basic minimum requirements in the respiratory field, and the more mature general medical reader with a painless refresher course.

The emphasis throughout is on information which is useful and relevant to everyday clinical medicine. In reviewing pulmonary physiology and the assessment of pulmonary function, all unnecessary complexities, symbols and equations have been avoided and attention has been focused on concepts and investigations which are in everyday use. A number of rare conditions receive little or no mention, but the practical aspects of management of the more common disorders are dealt with in some detail.

Numerous teachers, colleagues, students and patients have played a part in the development of my interest in respiratory disease, but I owe a particular debt to Professsor Jack Howell for opening my eyes to some of the special fascinations of the subject. I am grateful to Miss Veronica Downey for help with typing; without her watchful eye on my other commitments it would have been impossible to attend to the business of writing. I am grateful to Dr Martin Farebrother for reading parts of the manuscript and to Mr Per Saugman for his encouragement and courtesy. I hope to express my gratitude to my wife and family by seeing a little more of them.

R.A.L.B.

Newcastle upon Tyne, 1974

Chapter 1
Review of Anatomy of the Lung

The essential function of the lung is exchange of oxygen and carbon dioxide between the blood and the atmosphere. This takes place by a process of molecular diffusion across the alveolar membrane. A very large surface area is necessary to achieve this gaseous exchange—in an adult man it is estimated that the surface area of the alveoli is about 60 m². The structure of the lung represents an evolutionary solution to the problems of accommodating this huge membrane, moving air and blood to and from its surfaces and protecting it from external insults.

Surface anatomy

The position of the lungs and some useful external landmarks are indicated in Fig. 1.1. A few points are worthy of special mention.

1 The apices of the lungs extend well above the clavicles.

2 The posterior surface of the lungs extends further downwards than the anterior surface.

3 The upper lobes are situated *in front of* the lower lobes so that the lung immediately below the anterior chest wall is largely derived from the upper lobe and that beneath the posterior chest wall is mainly lower lobe.

4 The diaphragm, in its resting position, rises quite high into the thorax—a fact readily confirmed on any standard chest X-ray but commonly overlooked during examination of the patient.

Subdivisions of the lung

The lungs are divided into **lobes**—three on the right and two on the left—which are separated by slit-like invaginations of the pleural space. Each lobe has its own lobar bronchus. Each lobe is further subdivided by incomplete fibrous septa which extend inwards from the pleural surface into **bronchopulmonary segments**. Each bronchopulmonary segment is supplied by its own segmental bronchus and the usual arrangement of the segmental bronchi is shown in Fig. 1.2. Some pathological processes may be limited to particular segments which may be identified radiologically. Smaller incomplete fibrous septa are present within each segment which outline individual **lobules**. Lobules are about 1 cm in diameter and of variable shape but generally they are pyramidal with the apex towards the bronchiole which supplies them. The anatomy of the lobule is illustrated in Fig. 1.3. Each lobule contains three to five **acini**, each supplied by a terminal bronchiole. Acini are sometimes visualized on the chest X-ray when they are filled with secretions or bronchographic contrast medium producing a blotchy appearance sometimes referred to as acinar pattern.

1

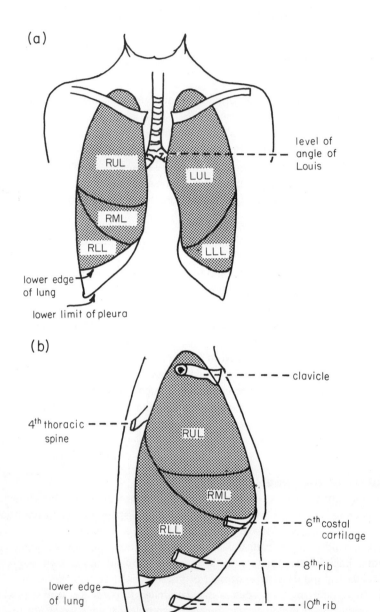

Fig. 1.1. Surface anatomy. (a) Anterior view of the lungs. (b) Lateral view of right side of chest at resting end-expiratory position. RUL, right upper lobe; RML, right middle lobe; RLL, right lower lobe; LUL, left upper lobe; LLL, left lower lobe.

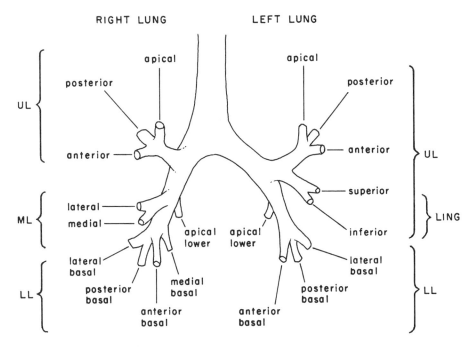

Fig. 1.2. Diagram of bronchopulmonary segments. UL, upper lobe; ML; middle lobe; LL, lower lobe; LING, lingula.

Branching of the airways

The trachea divides into two main bronchi. The left main bronchus is longer than the right and comes off at a more abrupt angle. The right main bronchus is more directly in line with the trachea so that inhaled material tends to enter the right lung more readily than the left. The main bronchi divide into lobar and then segmental bronchi as shown in Fig. 1.2. Further divisions occur in an uneven dichotomous fashion; that is, the branches at a division are not necessarily of the same size.

Bronchi and bronchioles

Bronchi are airways with cartilage in their walls. There are about 10 divisions of bronchi beyond the tracheal bifurcation. Smaller airways without cartilage in their walls are referred to as **bronchioles**. The term **respiratory bronchiole** refers to the peripheral bronchioles with alveoli in their walls. The bronchiole immediately proximal to the appearance of alveoli is known as the **terminal bronchiole**. The number of divisions between the bifurcation of the trachea and the terminal bronchiole varies between about 9 and 32. In general there are fewer branches to acini near the hilum and more branches to the peripherally-situated acini.

The total cross-sectional area of the airways increases at each subdivision so that it is enormously greater at, say, 14 divisions from the trachea than it is in the trachea itself (Fig. 1.4). This means that rate of airflow also diminishes strikingly as air penetrates more deeply into the lungs. This distribution of

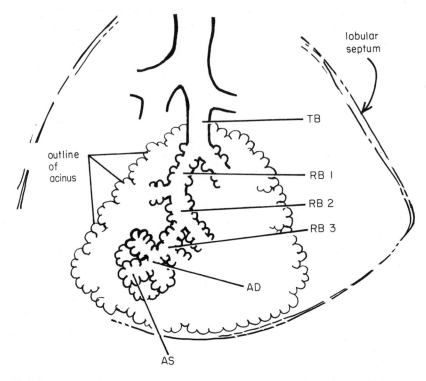

Fig. 1.3. Diagram of the anatomy of the lobule. The lobule lies within incomplete fibrous septa and contains several acini. The borders of individual acini are not normally discernible. Each acinus is supplied by a terminal bronchiole (TB). There are about three orders of respiratory bronchioles with alveoli in their walls (RB 1, RB 2, RB 3) which lead to alveolar ducts (AD) which are formed from the mouths of alveoli and alveolar sacs (AS).

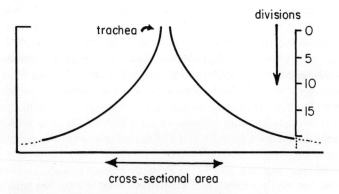

Fig. 1.4. Diagrammatic representation of the increase in total cross-sectional area of the airways at successive divisions.

cross-sectional area and hence rate of airflow has important implications when considering the site of resistance to airflow in health and disease and also when considering mechanisms of deposition of inhaled particulate matter.

Collateral ventilation

Holes in the alveolar walls known as pores of Kohn allow communication between parts of the lobule supplied by different respiratory bronchioles. There is a variable degree of communication at alveolar level between neighbouring lobules. Collateral ventilation through these communications is of importance in panacinar emphysema. In this condition they are increased in size and number as part of the parenchymal destructive process.

Pulmonary vasculature

Pulmonary artery

The pulmonary artery divides into left and right pulmonary arteries which provide branches accompanying the branches of the bronchial tree. The arteries accompanying bronchi are elastic but only have their muscular coats. The arteries accompanying bronchioles have well-developed medial muscular coats which become thinner peripherally. The **arterioles** accompanying terminal and respiratory bronchioles are thin walled and contain little smooth muscle.

Capillary network

The capillary network in the alveolar walls is very dense and provides a very large surface area.

Pulmonary venules

The pulmonary venules do not accompany the arterioles but drain laterally to the periphery of lobules and then pass centrally in the interlobular and inter-segmental septa, ultimately joining to form the four main pulmonary veins which empty into the left atrium.

The bronchial circulation (Fig. 1.5)

Small bronchial arteries usually arise from the descending aorta and travel in the outer layers of the bronchi and bronchioles supplying the tissues of the airways down to the level of the respiratory bronchiole. Most of the blood drains into radicles of the pulmonary vein contributing a small amount of desaturated blood which accounts for part of the 'physiological shunt' observed in normal individuals. The bronchial arteries may be much enlarged in some diseases (e.g. severe bronchiectasis, pulmonary fibrosis).

Structure of the airways

Trachea

The trachea has cartilaginous horseshoe-shaped 'rings' supporting anterior and lateral walls. The posterior wall is flaccid and during coughing, when intratho-racic pressure is raised and the glottis opens, this soft posterior segment billows

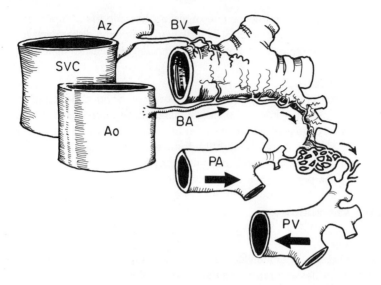

Fig. 1.5. The bronchial circulation. Three or more bronchial arteries (BA) arise from the aorta (Ao) and supply the bronchi down to the level of the terminal bronchiole. They also supply the vessel walls of pulmonary arteries (PA) and veins (PV). The bronchial supply to the large bronchi drains to the right atrium via bronchial veins (BV), the azygos or hemiazygos veins (Az) and the superior vena cava (SVC). Most of the bronchial arterial blood, however, drains to the left atrium via the pulmonary veins; these are plexuses linking the two circulations in the lung periphery.

forwards reducing the lumen of the trachea to a U-shaped slit. This results in a high linear velocity of airflow which produces a shearing effect, hastening the clearance of any excess of secretions. The trachea is lined with ciliated epithelium which contains goblet cells.

Bronchi

The bronchi have irregular plates of cartilage in their walls. Smooth muscle is arranged in spiral fashion internal to the cartilaginous plates and attached to them. The muscle coat becomes more complete distally as the cartilaginous plates become more fragmentary.

The epithelial lining is ciliated and includes goblet cells which become less numerous peripherally. Larger bronchi also have acinar mucus-secreting glands in the submucosa. Hypertrophy of these glands is one of the more striking features of chronic bronchitis.

Bronchioles

The bronchioles have no cartilage in their walls. The muscular layer becomes progressively thinner peripherally but some strands of smooth muscle persist to the level of respiratory bronchioles and possibly beyond. Bronchial smooth muscle and bronchial innervation is considered. The epithelium is made up of a single layer of ciliated cells with only very occasional goblet cells. A granulated cell known as the Clara cell appears in the wall of distal bronchioles and this cell

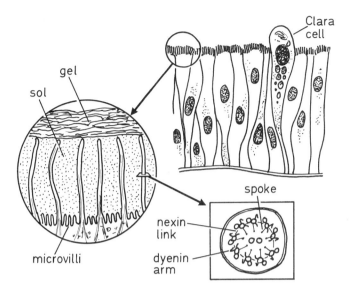

Fig. 1.6. Ciliated epithelium in a bronchiole. The cilia beat in the thin (sol) layer beneath the raft of sticky mucus (gel layer). The sol layer is about 5 μm thick and its water and electrolyte content is regulated by the brush border (microvilli) present on many cells. The main features of a cross-section of a cilium are shown in the rectangle. Cells are about 0.2 μm in diameter.

is suspected of possessing secretory properties. It may contribute mucus to alveolar fluid making up the foundation of the mucous blanket which is propelled upwards by ciliary action.

Other cells are present in distal bronchioles which have a brush border. These are suspected of having a role connected with salt and water regulation of the fluid secretions passed upwards from the alveoli.

Ciliated epithelium

Ciliated epithelial cells possess about 200 cilia each 3–6 μm in length. Cilia beat with a whip-like action very rapidly (the beat frequency is about 20 per second), organized waves of contraction passing regularly from cell to cell. The structure of each cilium is complex (Fig. 1.6). Normal cilia contain longitudinal tubules which are arranged as nine pairs of tubules in an outer circle with a pair of central tubules. The peripheral tubules are connected to each other by structures referred to as nexin links and to the central tubules by radial 'spokes'. One of each pair of outer tubules carries two additional links referred to as dyenin arms. These appear to be responsible for the contractile properties of the cilium. They are absent in some forms of the immotile cilia syndrome where there is gross deficiency of pulmonary mucociliary clearance.

Mucociliary clearance is discussed in Chapter 4.

Alveolar structure

Alveoli are about 0.1–0.2 mm in diameter and take up a variety of shapes depending on the arrangement of adjacent alveoli. The structure of the alveolar

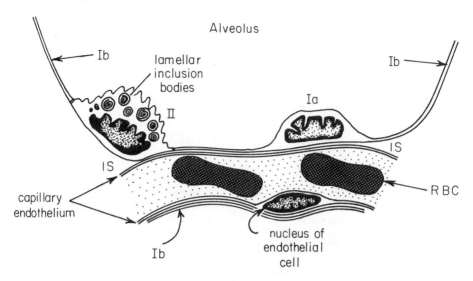

Fig. 1.7. Structure of the alveolar wall as revealed by electron microscopy. Ia, Type I pneumocyte; Ib, Flattened extension of Type I pneumocyte covering most of the internal surface of the alveolus; II, Type II pneumocyte with lamellar inclusion bodies which are probably the site of surfactant formation. IS, interstitial space; RBC, red blood corpuscle. Pneumocytes and endothelial cells rest upon thin continuous basement membranes which are not shown.

wall is represented diagrammatically in Fig. 1.7. The capillaries are completely lined by flattened endothelial cells resting on a complete basement membrane. The alveoli are completely lined by a layer of alveolar cells which are of two types.

Type I pneumocyte

These cells have extensive flattened processes which extend to cover most of the internal surface of the alveoli. Only the nuclei of these cells are evident on light microscopy.

Type II pneumocyte

These cells are less numerous and more globular than the Type I pneumocytes. Electron microscopy reveals that these cells contain bodies with a concentric lamellated structure. It is now generally agreed that these bodies are concerned with the manufacture or storage of surfactant and that the Type II pneumocyte is the principal source of surfactant (p. 28).

Alveoli contain phagocytic macrophages and other cells.

Interstitial space

There is a potential space between the alveolar cells and the capillary basement membrane which is only apparent in disease states when it may contain fluid, fibrous tissue or a cellular infiltrate. It is continuous with the interstitial space surrounding bronchi and blood vessels (see Chapter 25 and Fig. 25.2).

Lymphatic vessels

Lymphatic channels are present in the interstitial space. They accompany the bronchial tree at least as far as the level of the respiratory bronchioles and supply the walls of the airway as well as the pulmonary interstitium. Lymphatics are also found in the interlobular septa and are abundant beneath the pleural surface. Drainage of lymph is towards the intrapulmonary lymph nodes adjacent to the proximal bronchi (hilar lymph nodes) and thereafter to the mediastinal lymph nodes.

Clusters of lymphoid tissue also occur alongside medium and large sized airways in the lung and are termed bronchial associated lymphoid tissue (BALT).

Nerve supply

The lungs receive nerves from the vagus nerves and the sympathetic chain, which entwine to form plexuses which surround both arteries and airways in the lung. The airways seem to receive: (1) a sympathetic supply to the airways which seems to stop short of impinging on bronchial muscle whose receptors are stimulated instead by circulating amines; (2) vagal afferent (sensory) nerves which relay centrally the effects of physical stimulation of the airway, for example by stimulation of irritant receptors as part of the cough reflex and also the output of J receptors and related stretch receptors; (3) vagal efferent nerves which are cholinergic and bronchoconstrictor in effect; and (4) non-adrenergic–non-cholinergic (NANC) nerves. The actions of the latter nerves are not understood, but may include release of vasoactive intestinal peptide, exerting an inhibitory effect on bronchoconstrictor muscle.

The lung appears to have no receptors for pain but vagal efferent stimulation may cause referred pain appreciated diffusely over the chest or up the side of the neck. The parietal pleura appears to be completely insensitive but it receives normal somatic innervation from the relevant intercostal nerves.

Chapter 2
Review of Respiratory Physiology

MECHANICAL CONSIDERATIONS

Breathing

Inspiration is brought about by descent of the diaphragm, by movement of the lower ribs upwards and outwards and by movement of the upper ribs and sternum upwards and forwards. Although the principal effect of diaphragmatic contraction is to cause it to descend, thereby increasing the vertical dimension of the pleural cavity, it also has a variable action on the lower ribs causing them to be elevated. This effect is probably controlled by the degree of contraction of the abdominal musculature (Fig. 2.1). If descent of the diaphragm is opposed by significant abdominal muscle contraction during inspiration then shortening of the elevated diaphragm causes elevation of the lower ribs. Forward and outward movement also takes place as the downward sloping ribs adopt a more

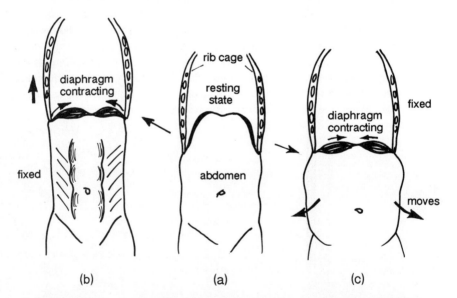

(b) (a) (c)

Fig. 2.1. Effects of diaphragmatic contraction. Diagram of the rib cage, abdominal cavity and diaphragm showing the position at the end of resting expiration (a). If, when the diaphragm contracts, the abdominal wall is lax and atonic, the diaphragm will descend on inspiration (c) and the abdominal wall will move outwards. If, however, the abdominal muscles are in a state of active contraction during inspiration, the diaphragm is unable to descend so that shortening of the diaphragm causes the ribs to be elevated (b), braced by the tense abdominal contents. The extent to which the diaphragm distends the abdomen or encourages elevation of the ribs is modulated by the degree of abdominal muscle contraction.

horizontal orientation (the bucket handle effect). The effect of the diaghragm in raising the lower ribs is most marked at low lung volumes when the peripheral part of the diaphragm is in a vertically dependent position and there is a large area of apposition of the diaphragmatic and costal pleural surfaces (Fig. 2.1). When the diaphragm descends the abdomen moves outwards. There is a close relationship between the anteroposterior movement of the thorax and that of the abdomen. Changes in breathing pattern which increase one component can have an almost equal diminishing effect on the other, and vice versa.

Elevation of the upper ribs and sternum is achieved by contraction of the scalene muscles. These muscles were for a long time regarded as 'accessory muscles' of respiration but electromyographic studies suggest that they are active even in ordinary quiet breathing.

The intercostal muscles play an important part in ensuring that the influences on upper and lower ribs are conducted to all of the ribs. The parasternal intercostal muscles in particular act in concert with the scalene muscles in bringing about elevation of the chest. The intercostal muscles also exert a bracing effect on the chest, countering distortion by external pressure and resisting undue collapse or bulging of the intercostal spaces when significant negative or positive intrathoracic pressures are generated. It was at one time thought that the internal and external intercostal muscles had specific and different effects on expiration and inspiration, but this view is now less widely held.

Inspiration is thus achieved by active muscular contraction. Expiration by comparison is a relatively passive procedure. Inspiratory muscles continue, however, to act during expiration—gradually lessening their force of contraction. The action of the inspiratory muscles during breathing has been likened to a seaman hauling on a rope (inspiration) and then gradually 'paying off' (expiration), rather than merely letting go of the rope.

The abdominal musculature, apart from determining the precise effect of diaphragmatic contraction, has important actions in inspiration and expiration during fast breathing and is the principal driving force in coughing and in achieving extreme expiration (residual volume).

Lung compliance

The inherent elastic property of the lungs causes them to tend to retract from the chest wall producing a negative intrapleural pressure. The strength of the retractive force is related to the degree of stretching of the lung tissue—that is to lung volume. At high lung volumes the intrapleural pressure is more negative than at low lung volumes. The term lung compliance refers to the relationship between this retractive force and lung volume. Lung compliance is expressed as **the change in lung volume brought about by unit change in transpulmonary (intrapleural) pressure** and the units employed are litres per kilopascal or litres per centimetre of water. Figure 2.2 shows intrapleural pressure at varying lung volumes. The slope of the line represents lung compliance. It will be seen that compliance becomes less at high lung volumes (i.e. smaller volume changes follow changes in pressure at high lung volume).

The retractive forces of the lung are balanced by the semi-rigid elastic structure of the thoracic cage and the action of the respiratory muscles. At the

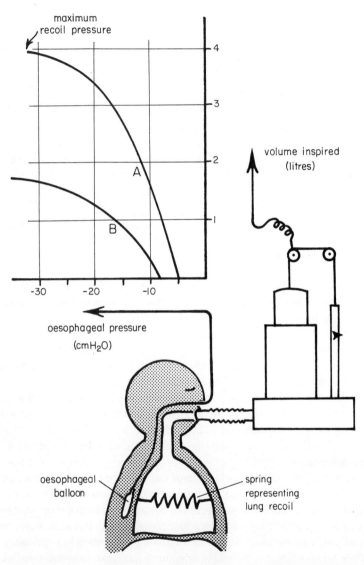

Fig. 2.2. Lung compliance. Oesophageal pressure is noted at a number of different volumes (each held momentarily with glottis open). The relationship between transpulmonary pressure and volume of air inspired is plotted for two individuals, A and B. Lung compliance is an expression of the change in lung volume which accompanied unit change in transpulmonary pressure (lung recoil). In the case of A, lung compliance is normal (= approx. 0.25 litre cmH_2O^{-1} or 2.5 litre kPa^{-1}). In the case of B, a smaller change in volume accompanies each unit change in pressure and compliance is low (= approx. 0.1 litre cmH_2O^{-1} or 1.0 litre kPa^{-1}). Note that lung compliance becomes progressively less as lung volume increases.

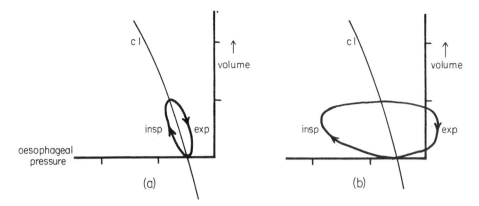

Fig. 2.3. Change in intrapleural (oesophageal) pressure during quiet breathing. (a) In a normal individual. During inspiration the pressure is more negative and during expiration more positive than would be expected from consideration of lung compliance: cl, compliance line. The excessive pressure change is that required to overcome the resistance of the airways. (b) An individual with airways obstruction. Here the pressure changes are even more marked. During expiration, oesophageal pressure is actually above atmospheric pressure, indicating compression of the lungs by expiratory musculature.

end of a quiet expiration, the retractive force exerted by the lungs is nicely balanced by the tendency of the chest wall to spring outwards and the respiratory muscles are at rest.

Airways resistance

During breathing, bigger changes in intrapleural pressure are observed than would be explained by lung retractive forces alone and this is because of the resistance to airflow offered by the respiratory passages (Fig. 2.3). The additional pressure change depends upon the calibre of the airways and also upon the rate of airflow. The greater part of the total airways resistance is situated in the large airway—main bronchi, trachea and larynx—as this is where linear velocity of airflow is highest. When breathing through the nose, about one-third of the total resistance to flow may be imposed by the nasal passages themselves. Although the large airways and upper airway are the site of most resistance, increased resistance occurring in disease generally originates in more peripheral airways. The effects of such increased distal resistance may, however, be complex, and may cause collapse of the larger airways in expiration.

The airways behave differently during inspiration and expiration. During inspiration, pulmonary elastic recoil causes the airways to open. During expiration the pull on the walls of the airways diminishes, so that there is an increasing tendency towards closure of the airways.

The flow-limiting mechanism

Consider the model of the lung described in Fig. 2.4. During expiration the resistance of the distal airway (Res) will cause a drop in pressure between A and B so that the floppy segment will tend to collapse. It will be protected from

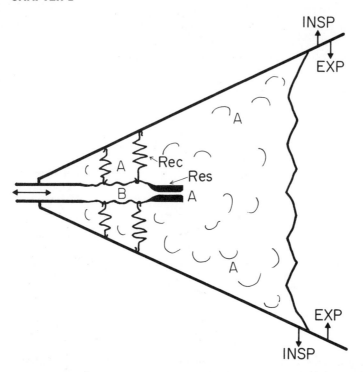

Fig. 2.4. Model of the lung to demonstrate the flow-limiting mechanism (see text). The chest is represented as a bellows. The airways of the lungs are represented collectively as having a distal resistive segment (Res) and a more proximal collapsible or 'floppy' segment. The walls of the floppy segment are kept apart by the retractive force of lung recoil (Rec). EXP, expiration; INSP, inspiration.

collapse by the retractive force of the surrounding lung parenchyma (Rec). The extent of the pressure drop from A to B is proportional to the rate of airflow. There will be a critical rate of airflow which results in B being so much lower than A that the retractive force of the lung is overcome and the floppy segment closes. The closure limits the airflow, leading to a less dramatic pressure drop from A to B, which permits some re-opening of the floppy segment. It will be apparent that the system will control the maximum rate of airflow to a level determined by lung recoil (assuming that the resistance of the upstream segment (Res) remains constant). Lung recoil depends upon how stretched the lungs are and it should now be clear why high expiratory flow rates are obtainable at high lung volumes, but as lung volume decreases during expiration the maximum flow rate progressively diminishes. For each lung volume there is a particular maximum flow rate which cannot be exceeded, no matter how great the expiratory effort.

The shape of the forced expiratory spirogram (Fig. 7.6) is thus determined by inherent mechanical properties of the lung and is to a large extent independent of effort above a certain level. This explains its very remarkable reproducibility.

When airways resistance is increased in disease, a much greater pressure drop occurs between A and B (Fig. 2.4) so that the supporting effect of recoil pressure (Rec) tends to be overcome at more modest rates of expiratory airflow than in the normal. In this situation there is obvious advantage in breathing at a high lung volume which results in a greater lung recoil (Rec).

Forced expiration is discussed further in Chapter 7 in the context of spirometry and the flow–volume loop.

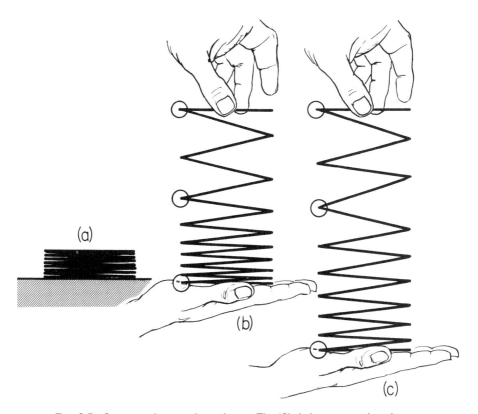

Fig. 2.5. Gravity and regional ventilation. The 'Slinky' spring used to demonstrate greater ventilation of the bases in the normal upright lung. (a) The 'Slinky' spring in its resting condition. (b) The spring extended upwards to represent the normal lung suspended within the pleural cavity in a stretched condition by the effect of atmospheric pressure. The circles mark the top, middle and bottom of the spring (lung) under these conditions. (c) The bottom hand has been lowered to represent inspiration. Most of the increase in length has been contributed by the lower part of the spring; the upper part was already at almost full stretch before 'inspiration'. In the lung the upper zones are relatively more stretched than the lower zones and their compliance is thus less. During inspiration under such conditions more air goes to the bases. This is appropriate since the bases are relatively better perfused than the upper zones.

The 'Slinky' spring also permits exploration of the effects of gravity in abnormal lungs. When lung volume is progressively reduced it is evident that collapse is much more likely to occur in the lower zones. Lung recoil is evidently lower in the lower zones so that the smaller airways are not held open so forcibly. In the presence of diffuse airways obstruction the obstruction tends to be more severe in the lower zones. Many airways in the lower zones close on expiration and ventilation is directed more to the upper zones.

Where does the air go?

During an inspiration the distribution of air within the lungs is uneven because the compliance of different parts of the lungs is not uniform and the resistance of the airways is uneven. One most obvious cause of the uneven distribution of lung compliance is the effect of gravity. The weight of the lungs causes the upper parts to be kept under a greater stretch than the more dependent zones; the upper parts are thus less compliant. During inspiration more air tends to pass into the lower zones. The uppermost parts of the lungs may be regarded as already almost fully stretched and thus less 'receptive'. The analogy of a suspended spring may make the effect of gravity clearer (Fig. 2.5). The greater ventilation of the lower zones during quiet breathing is appropriate as gravity also directs pulmonary blood flow preferentially to the lower zones.

Unevenness of ventilation is also present within the lungs on a more miniature scale—adjacent lobules and even adjacent alveoli may have different compliances and, in response to a change of intrapleural pressure, may accept more or less air than expected. Local differences of airways resistance will also cause some unevenness in the distribution of inspired air. The effect of an increase in airways resistance is to reduce the rate of airflow produced by a given change in intrapleural pressure; this is, to delay filling of the lung or part of the lung. During extremely slow breathing the effect of increased airways resistance will be very small and air will pass into the most receptive (most compliant) parts of the lungs. But when breathing is more rapid, local increase in airways resistance will hamper the acceptance of air by the part of the lung in question because there may be insufficient time for proper filling of the region.

The local differences referred to are probably small in the healthy lung as the network of the lung parenchyma distributes forces fairly evenly, but local differences become important in disease of the lung parenchyma which tend to be patchy in distribution.

Where does the blood go?
(haemodynamics of the pulmonary circulation)

The pulmonary circulation normally offers a much lower resistance to perfusion than the systemic circulation and it operates at a lower perfusion pressure. The difference between the mean pulmonary artery pressure and left atrial pressure in the resting individual is only of the order of 15 mmHg—or less than one-sixth of the effective perfusion pressure of the systemic circulation.

At rest in the erect position gravity exerts a major effect upon the distribution of blood within the lungs. Blood passes predominantly to the bases and there is barely any perfusion of the apices—the pulmonary circulation is not 'full' (Fig. 2.6). If pulmonary artery pressure rises, either through an increase in pulmonary vascular resistance or an increase in cardiac output, then more of the pulmonary circulation in the upper zones is brought into play.

An increase in left atrial pressure secondary to left-sided cardiac disease will dam back blood in the lungs, raising pulmonary venous pressure so that veins further up the lungs become filled. Pulmonary artery pressure must increase if the circulation is to be maintained so that in these circumstances more of the circulation in the upper zones is opened up.

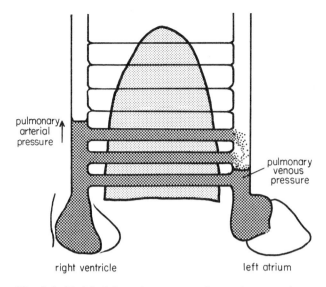

pulmonary
arterial
pressure

pulmonary
venous
pressure

right ventricle   left atrium

Fig. 2.6. Model of the pulmonary circulation. At rest in the erect position, the bulk of the cardiac output passes through the bases and the apices are virtually unperfused because pulmonary artery pressure is not sufficiently high. If pulmonary artery pressure rises because of increased cardiac output, increased pulmonary vascular resistance or increased pulmonary venous pressure, then more of the pulmonary circulation will be filled.

In addition to the major regional effect of gravity, there are other factors which affect the distribution of blood within the lungs and these may be quite localized.

Hypoxia

Hypoxia is a potent pulmonary vasoconstrictor, which seems to be a direct response of arterial smooth muscle to low oxygen tension in the lung surrounding it. By this means blood tends to be diverted away from underventilated areas of the lungs—a process which may be looked upon as a form of autoregulation of pulmonary blood distribution.

Alveolar pressure

The pulmonary capillaries are capable of being compressed as they pass through the alveolar walls if alveolar pressure rises above capillary pressure. Under certain circumstances local increases in alveolar pressure may develop and have an effect upon the distribution of blood flow.

GAS EXCHANGE AND VENTILATION/PERFUSION RELATIONSHIPS

Overall gas exchange

During steady-state conditions the relationship between the amount of CO_2 produced by the body and the amount of oxygen absorbed depends upon the metabolic activity of the body as a whole and is referred to as the respiratory quotient (RQ or R).

$$RQ = \frac{CO_2 \text{ produced}}{O_2 \text{ absorbed}}$$

The actual value is dependent upon the principal metabolic substrate of the body at the time. RQ varies from about 0.7 during pure fat metabolism to 1.0 during pure carbohydrate metabolism and is usually found to be about 0.8 at rest during the day. Overall RQ is important, but consideration of gas exchange in the lung is made much easier if its value is assumed to be 1.0. Oxygen and CO_2 are exchanged in equal amounts in this situation.

Alveolar ventilation

It is obvious that not all of the air drawn into the lungs reaches the alveoli. The volume of air filling the airways down to the level of the terminal bronchiole at the end of an inspiration is termed the anatomical deadspace. It is less obvious that even in the normal lung not all of the inspired air which actually reaches the alveoli participates evenly in gas exchange. Some alveoli are relatively overventilated and some are underventilated relative to the blood flow they receive. To overcome the difficulties of analysing such a complicated state of affairs the expired air can be regarded as being derived from two hypothetical sources: (1) ideal alveoli all of which contain alveolar air with the same partial pressure of CO_2 (Pco_2) as arterial blood; and (2) other areas of lung which do not participate in gas exchange at all. These two components of the total ventilation are termed alveolar ventilation and deadspace ventilation. Alveolar ventilation is effective ventilation. Deadspace ventilation is ineffective ventilation. Deadspace ventilation is normally less than a quarter of the total but the proportion varies with breathing frequency, exercise and other influences.

Effect of changing alveolar ventilation

For the moment discussion will be limited to the situation which exists in an idealized normal lung in which all of the units have well-matched ventilation and perfusion, and all behave identically.

Carbon dioxide

If CO_2 is being produced by the tissues of the body at a constant rate the Pco_2 of alveolar air depends only upon the amount of outside air that the CO_2 is mixed with in the alveoli; that is, the Pco_2 depends only upon alveolar ventilation. If alveolar ventilation is high, the Pco_2 will be low; if alveolar ventilation falls the Pco_2 will rise. Alveolar Pco_2 is inversely proportional to alveolar ventilation.

Oxygen

The level of alveolar Po_2 also varies with alveolar ventilation. If alveolar ventilation is greatly increased the steady uptake of oxygen by the body will only slightly reduce the alveolar Po_2 below the level in the outside air. On the other hand, if alveolar ventilation is very low then the alveolar Po_2 will fall to a low level. Alveolar (or arterial) Po_2 varies directly with alveolar ventilation.

Measurement of arterial Po_2 is less reliable than measurement of Pco_2 as an index of alveolar ventilation because it is profoundly affected by regional changes in ventilation/perfusion ratio as will be shown below.

Measurement of alveolar or arterial Pco_2 is the only reliable guide to the adequacy of alveolar ventilation.

The changes in alveolar ventilation just described are examples of changes in the ventilation/perfusion ratio (V/Q) of the lungs as a whole.

Effect of overall increase in V/Q

If alveolar ventilation increases in relation to perfusion then alveolar Pco_2 will fall and alveolar Po_2 will rise.

Effect of overall fall in V/Q

If alveolar ventilation falls in relation to perfusion, alveolar Pco_2 will rise and alveolar Po_2 will fall.

In the model under discussion, all of the alveoli behave identically and the arterial blood therefore shows the same changes in Pco_2 and Po_2 as the alveolar air.

Relationship between Pco₂ and Po₂

The possible combination of Pco_2 and Po_2 can be explored with the help of the diagram shown in Fig. 2.7. Moist atmospheric air at 37°C has a Po_2 of about 20 kPa (150 mmHg). In our model, O_2 could be exchanged with CO_2 in the alveoli to produce any combination of Po_2 and Pco_2 described by the oblique line which joins Po_2 20 kPa (150 mmHg) and Pco_2 20 kPa (150 mmHg). The position of the cross on this line represents the composition of a hypothetical sample of alveolar air. A fall in alveolar ventilation would result in an upwards movement of this point along the line and conversely an increase in alveolar ventilation would result in a downward movement of the point.

In practice the RQ is rarely 1.0 and it is nearer the truth to say

Alveolar Po_2 + (alveolar Pco_2/RQ) = 20 kPa (150 mmHg).

The interrupted oblique line represents the combinations of Pco_2 and Po_2 encountered when the RQ is 0.8. Point (a) represents the Pco_2 and Po_2 of arterial blood (it lies a little to the left of the RQ 0.8 line because of the small normal alveolar–arterial oxygen tension difference). Point (b) represents the arterial gas tension after a period of underventilation.

This relationship between Pco_2 and Po_2 is very useful clinically. For example, if the arterial Pco_2 and Po_2 were those represented by point (c) it would be clear that the fall in Po_2 was more than could be accounted for on the grounds of reduced alveolar ventilation. An appreciation of the relationship between Pco_2 and Po_2 provides some safeguard against certain errors in blood gas measurement. Even when the RQ is 1.0 the sum of Pco_2 and Po_2 should not exceed 20 kPa (150 mmHg) when breathing air.

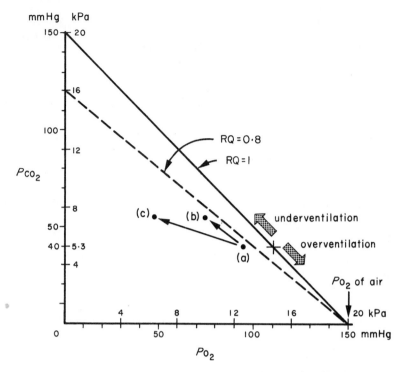

Fig. 2.7. Oxygen–carbon dioxide diagram. The continuous and interrupted lines describe the possible combinations of P_{CO_2} and P_{O_2} in alveolar air when the RQ is 1.0 and 0.8 respectively. (a) A hypothetical sample of arterial blood. (b) Progressive underventilation. (c) P_{O_2} lower than can be accounted for by underventilation alone.

Review of the carriage of CO_2 and O_2 by blood

The quantity of a gas which blood will carry when exposed to different partial pressures of the gas is described by the dissociation curve. The dissociation curves of O_2 and CO_2 are shown together on the same scale in Fig. 2.8. The most important points to be noted are:

1 The amount of CO_2 carried by blood is roughly proportional to the P_{CO_2} prevailing (over the range normally encountered).

2 The quantity of O_2 carried is roughly proportional to the P_{O_2} only over a very limited range—from about 2.7 to 6.7 kPa (20–50 mmHg).

3 Above this level there is less additional O_2 carried with each increase in P_{O_2} and above 13.3 kPa (100 mmHg) the haemoglobin is fully saturated and hardly any additional O_2 is carried.

Effect of local differences in V/Q

In the normal lung the vast majority of alveoli receive ventilation and perfusion in about the right proportion ((a) in Fig. 2.9). In diffuse disease of the lung, however, it is usual for ventilation and perfusion to be irregularly distributed so that a greater scatter of V/Q ratios is encountered (b in Fig. 2.9). Even if the *overall* V/Q remains normal there is a wide local variation in V/Q. Looking at Fig. 2.9 it is tempting to suppose that the effects of the alveoli with low V/Q

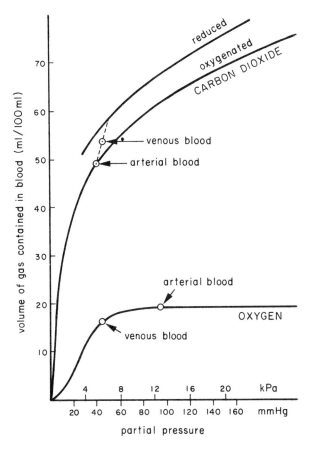

Fig. 2.8. The oxygen and carbon dioxide dissociation curves of blood drawn to the same scale.

might be nicely balanced by the alveoli with high V/Q. In fact this is not the case: the increased range of V/Q within the lung affects the transport of CO_2 and O_2 differently.

In Fig. 2.10, (b) and (c) are regions of low and high V/Q respectively and the result of mixing blood from these two regions is shown at (d) where arterial CO_2 and O_2 contents are represented.

Effect upon arterial CO_2 content

Blood with a high CO_2 content returning from low V/Q areas mixes with blood with a low CO_2 content returning from high V/Q areas and the net CO_2 content of arterial blood may be nearly normal, as the two balance out.

Effect upon arterial O_2 content

Here the situation is different. Blood returning from low V/Q areas has a low Po_2 and a low O_2 content but there is a limit to which this deficit can be made good by mixture with blood returning from high V/Q areas which, although it has a

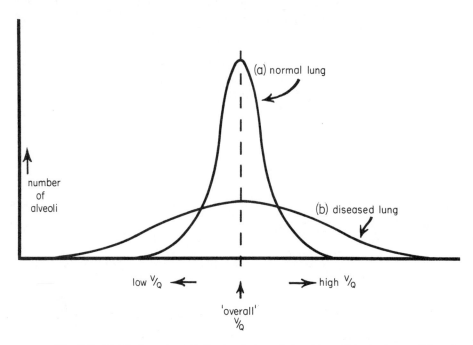

number
of
alveoli

low V/Q ◄——   ——► high V/Q

'overall'
V/Q

Fig. 2.9. Distribution of ventilation/perfusion relationships within the lungs. Although the overall ventilation/perfusion (V/Q) ratio is the same in the two examples shown, the increased spread of V/Q ratios within the diseased lung (b) will result in a lower arterial oxygen tension and content than in the normal lung (a). Arterial $P\text{CO}_2$ will be similar in the two situations shown.

high $P\text{O}_2$, cannot carry more than the 'normal' quantity of oxygen as its O_2 content is limited by saturation of the haemoglobin.

1   Areas of low V/Q result in a rise in arterial CO_2 content and a fall in arterial O_2 content.

2   Increased ventilation of areas of high V/Q may balance the effect upon CO_2 content but will only partly correct the reduction in O_2 content of arterial blood; a degree of hypoxaemia is inevitable.

3   It follows that where arterial oxygen levels are lower than would be expected from consideration of the $P\text{CO}_2$ there are probably local areas of low V/Q present in the lungs.

CONTROL OF BREATHING

The main elements involved in the control of breathing are outlined in Fig. 2.11. The respiratory centre is an anatomically ill-defined group of interconnected neurones, responsible for generating phasic motor discharges which ultimately pass by phrenic and intercostal nerves to the respiratory musculature. The medullary discharge is integrated at spinal level and the final output is matched to the mechanical loading of the lungs and chest through the operation of muscle spindles.

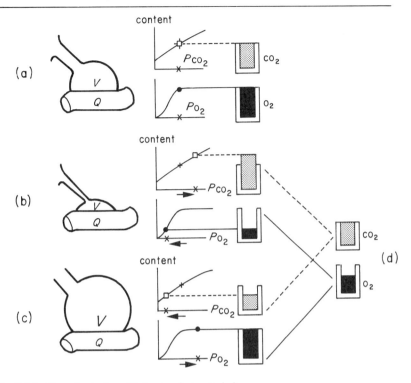

Fig. 2.10. The effect of ventilation/perfusion imbalance.

(a) *Appropriate* V/Q. The ventilation (V)/perfusion (Q) ratio is shown diagrammatically on the left. When ventilation is appropriately matched to perfusion in an alveolus or in the lung as a whole, the P_{CO_2} is about 5.3 kPa (40 mmHg) and the P_{O_2} is about 12.6 kPa (95 mmHg). The dissociation curves shown in the centre of the diagram describe the relationship between the blood gas tension and the amount of gas carried by the blood. The normal blood gas contents are represented very diagrammatically on the right.

(b) *Low* V/Q. Reduced ventilation relative to blood flow results in a rise in P_{CO_2} and a fall in P_{O_2}. Reference to the dissociation curves shows that this produces a rise in arterial CO_2 content and a fall in O_2 content.

(c) *High* V/Q. Increased ventilation relative to blood flow results in a fall in P_{CO_2} and a rise in P_{O_2}. Reference to the dissociation curves shows that this results in a fall in CO_2 content below the normal level but in the case of O_2 there is no increase in content above the normal level.

In health, the vast majority of alveoli have an appropriate balance of ventilation and perfusion and the arterial blood has a normal CO_2 and O_2 content as shown in (a). In many disease states the V/Q ratio varies widely between areas. Such variation always results in disturbance of blood gas content. The effects of areas of low V/Q are not corrected by areas of high V/Q . The result of mixing blood from areas of low and high V/Q is shown diagrammatically on the extreme right of the diagram (d). It will be seen that with respect to CO_2 content, the high content of blood from underventilated areas is balanced by the low content of blood from overventilated areas. However in the case of O_2, the low content of blood from underventilated areas cannot be compensated for by an equivalent increase in the O_2 content of blood from overventilated areas. *Arterial hypoxaemia is inevitable if there are areas of low V/Q* (relative underventilation or overperfusion).

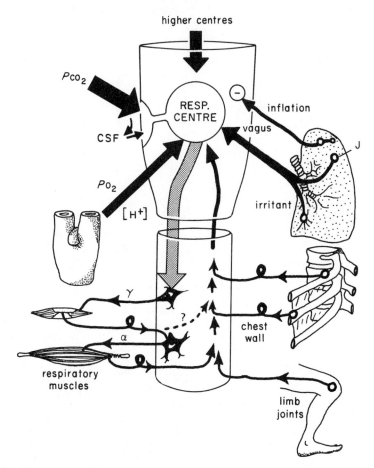

Fig. 2.11. Control of ventilation. Diagram showing some of the more important factors involved (see text).

Chemical factors in the control of ventilation

Carbon dioxide

The P_{CO_2} of arterial blood is the most important factor in the regulation of ventilation. Normal individuals maintain an arterial P_{CO_2} very close to 5.3 kPa (40 mmHg) and an increase above this level provokes hyperventilation. Arterial P_{CO_2} exerts its effect upon the respiratory centre by stimulating sensitive areas on the surface of the medulla which are bathed by CSF. CO_2 may act on these sensitive areas directly and also by diffusing into the CSF which has less efficient buffering properties than blood. Change in CSF P_{CO_2} produces a greater change in $[H^+]$ than that which occurs in blood. The CSF-mediated effect is probably more potent than the direct effect and this may account for certain anomalies encountered in clinical practice. When longstanding disorders of acid–base balance are corrected the ventilatory control may lag behind despite improvement in the acid–base status of the arterial blood.

Hydrogen ion concentration $[H^+]$

Increase in $[H^+]$ (fall in pH) stimulates ventilation. $P\text{co}_2$ and $[H^+]$ are able to stimulate ventilation independently. $[H^+]$ probably exerts its influence by stimulation of the carotid and aortic bodies.

Oxygen

A fall in arterial tension stimulates ventilation. The effect of O_2 tension is very small above a $P\text{o}_2$ of about 8 kPa (60 mmHg). Hypoxia sensitizes the respiratory centre to CO_2 and the effects of a fall in $P\text{o}_2$ and an increase in $P\text{co}_2$ are more than merely additive. Hypoxia exerts its effects by stimulating the carotid and aortic bodies. These receptors are sensitive to reduced delivery arising from circulatory failure as well as that due to reduced arterial tension.

Neurogenic factors

Higher centres

Sleep and coma of whatever cause reduce the response to the normal ventilatory stimuli. Alarm and excitement tend to stimulate ventilation. Part of the ventilatory response to exercise may be initiated by higher centres as hyperventilation commonly precedes the actual start of exercise. Voluntary control can of course override the normal automatic control of breathing.

Brain stem

Breathing is interrupted during coughing, swallowing, phonation and other semi-automatic activities. Damage to the brain stem may cause hyperventilation, hypoventilation or other disturbances of control.

Vagus

The vagus carries afferent stimuli from the respiratory tract which may influence breathing.

Inflation reflex (Hering–Breuer)

In animals, stretching of the lungs causes reflex inhibition of subsequent inspiration. This effect is difficult to demonstrate in man and probably unimportant.

J receptors

These are situated deep in the parenchyma of the lung and excitation stimulates ventilation. Pulmonary embolism and pulmonary oedema are among the conditions thought to excite the receptors.

Irritant receptors

These receptors are probably situated in the distal bronchioles. Irritation and local distortion are thought to stimulate them and this results in increased ventilation. It is possible that these receptors may play a part in the production of the hyperventilation which accompanies asthma, inhalation of irritant vapours and gases, pulmonary embolism, pneumonia, etc. Bronchoconstriction appears to be a part of the reflex response.

Cough receptors

The larger bronchi and the trachea possess vagally innervated receptors which are sensitive to contact and irritants. Stimulation provokes the cough reflex and a variable degree of bronchoconstriction.

Spinal cord

Stretch receptors in muscle tendons and joint position receptors are stimulated by chest movement and may be particularly sensitive to chest deformation caused by increased respiratory effort. The central effect of this sensory information is uncertain. Stimulation of joint receptors in the limbs enhances ventilation and this may be a contributory cause of the hyperpnoea of exercise.

Exercise

Ventilation increases in direct proportion to work during exercise. P_{CO_2}, P_{O_2} and [H^+] generally remain normal and cannot explain the ventilatory response. Psychic factors and the limb joint reflex already mentioned are similarly inadequate explanations. A number of hypotheses have been suggested which explain the observed facts but no comprehensive analysis of the control of ventilation has attained general acceptance.

Respiratory sensations

An awareness of the behaviour of the lungs and of the act of breathing may be compiled from several sources. These include vision, hearing, the sensation of movement and temperature change in the upper respiratory tract, sensations originating in vagal irritant and cough receptors, and sensations of chest wall movement.

Appreciation of breath size and resistance to breathing is probably mainly derived from muscle tendon and joint receptors in the thorax, although the skin receptors may contribute some information. Muscle spindles may provide further sensory signals. Afferent discharge from the spindles enhances the main spinal motor discharge to the muscle when there is a mismatch between the length set by the spindle and that achieved by the muscle. It is not known whether this afferent traffic from the spindle is accessible to higher centres as an index of muscular achievement.

Dyspnoea

This is one of the most important symptoms of respiratory disease and its mode of production is probably complex. It may be defined as an awareness of increased respiratory effort which is unpleasant and recognized as inappropriate. Dyspnoea is *not*:

Hyperventilation

This term is reserved for breathing which is in excess of the body's needs and which therefore results in a lowering of alveolar and arterial P_{CO_2}.

Hyperpnoea

This merely indicates an increased level of ventilation, such as occurs during exercise: it is appropriate to the situation and is not unpleasant.

Tachypnoea

This refers to increased rate of breathing.

Experimental work using such techniques as curarization and local anaesthesia of the vagi and chest wall suggest that vagal input, muscular action, chest wall movement and other sensations are probably all important in the genesis of dyspnoea. There is little to suggest a single source or pathway.

Appreciation of dyspnoea involves recognition of an unsatisfactory ventilatory movement relative to the drive to breathe, or an excessive drive to breathe relative to the prevailing circumstances, or both. Breathing movements, drive and circumstance are in some way compared with the integrated past experience of each.

Chapter 3
Surface Tension and Alveolar Stability

Surface tension and small bubbles

Surface tension acting at the curved internal surface of a bubble tends to cause it to decrease in size. The smaller the bubble, the greater this contracting force; small bubbles tend to empty into bigger ones (Fig. 3.1a). Very small bubbles are very unstable and tend to collapse completely. Alveoli are essentially small bubbles and surface tension would make the lungs impossibly difficult to distend if it were not for the presence of surfactant.

Surfactant

Source and nature of surfactant

Surfactant is almost certainly derived from the Type II pneumocyte. It is composed of lipoprotein, largely dipalmitoyl lecithin, which is insoluble and forms a thin (probably monomolecular) layer at the air–fluid interface. The molecules probably change their orientation relative to the surface, with change in the surface area of the film.

Action of surfactant

Surfactant modifies the surface tension of the alveolar fluid film. Whereas the tendency of a bubble to collapse increases as the bubble becomes smaller, surfactant has the effect of causing surface tension to fall off markedly as the size of the surface is reduced, so that a small bubble remains quite stable. Small bubbles no longer empty into bigger ones, but there is instead a tendency for bubbles to adjust to the same size (Fig. 3.1c). Fluid surfaces with surfactant activity exhibit hysteresis—the surface tension lowering effect of surfactant is improved by a transient increase in size of the surface. During quiet breathing there may be a tendency for occasional alveoli to be underventilated and gradually decrease in size. A deep breath re-expands such alveoli and restores the performance of the surfactant layer. Occasional deep breaths or sighs are a feature of normal breathing and there is some evidence that minute areas of collapse may develop if sighing is prevented. In normal individuals, restriction of movement of the chest wall with strapping results in the development of patchy radiological collapse and an increase in intrapulmonary shunting over the course of some hours. These effects are reversed by one or two deep breaths.

Significance of surfactant in pulmonary disease

It is difficult to measure surfactant activity quantitatively. Surfactant activity is undoubtedly defective in a number of parenchymal lung disorders, but in most of these the defect is probably a consequence of lung damage rather than the cause.

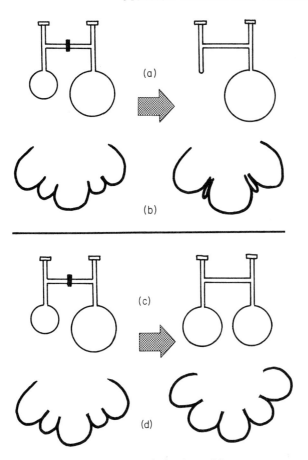

Fig. 3.1. Surface tension and alveolar stability.
(a) No surfactant. Small bubbles exert greater retractive force than larger bubbles. In a closed system such as that illustrated, small bubbles tend to empty into larger ones.
(b) Diagram of the equivalent situation at alveolar level. Although alveoli are not interconnected by a closed system they exert retractive forces on each other by virtue of their side-by-side and back-to-back arrangement in the lung.
(c) Surfactant present. Surfactant reduces surface tension as the surface area is reduced. Small bubbles then exert only a small retractive force. Larger bubbles tend to empty into them until the bubbles are of similar size.
(d) Equivalent situation at alveolar level. Small alveoli are now stable and there is a tendency for alveoli to adopt a uniform size.

Defective surfactant activity plays a central role in respiratory distress syndrome of the newborn and may play some part in the evolution of, and recovery from, pulmonary oedema, lung collapse, pneumonia, etc.

Patients with painful abdominal wounds, factured ribs or thoracic cage deformity and patients on long-term artificial ventilation may have shallow tidal breathing and be prevented from taking adequate sighs. All are prone to patchy lung collapse, particularly at the lung bases. It seems possible that failure to maintain surfactant activity may have some part to play in the evolution of the collapse.

Production of surfactant is impaired if pulmonary perfusion is severely reduced, and this may explain the collapse associated with pulmonary embolism. A number of other factors, including the presence of blood in the alveoli, appear to impair surfactant activity or production.

Surfactant and the neonate

The first breath

At birth the lungs are filled with amniotic fluid. The first breaths draw the fluid–air interface into the lungs. For the infant to be able to inflate the lungs the fluid surface must have a low surface tension when the surface area is small (small bubbles must be stable). Otherwise the lungs will tend to collapse completely at every expiration. The fluid within the lungs is absorbed via the pulmonary lymphatics in the first hours of life. This is also dependent on the surface tension of the fluid being low.

Respiratory distress syndrome of the newborn (RDN, hyaline membrane disease)

Pathogenesis of RDN

The syndrome is due to deficient surfactant activity, usually because of prematurity. Surfactant activity is normally developed at around 32–35 weeks of gestation. In affected infants, the alveoli have no stability and the lungs tend to collapse almost completely at the end of each expiration. Lung compliance is extremely low and the infant is unable to maintain adequate ventilation. Severe hypoxia results from underventilation, shunting of blood through airless parts of the lungs and from the re-opening of foetal right to left shunts as a consequence of hypoxic pulmonary vasoconstriction.

Autopsy specimens of lung are largely airless. Some alveolar ducts may be aerated and contain a layer of proteinaceous material—hyaline membrane—probably derived from plasma proteins which have leaked from damaged alveolar capillaries. Hyaline membranes of this sort are not specific for RDN and are seen in other forms of peripheral lung damage, at all ages.

Clinical features

1 *Features of prematurity.*
2 *Respiratory distress.* Tachypnoea, sternal recession, grunting, cyanosis and tachycardia may be evident from the first few minutes but may not develop until after an hour or two.
3 *Chest X-ray.* This will show general haziness, sometimes of a ground-glass appearance, against which air-filled bronchi are visible. The chest X-ray helps to differentiate the condition from other possible causes of early respiratory distress, such as diaphragmatic hernia, congenital heart disease, pulmonary malformations and aspiration.
4 *Test for surfactant.* A test using polarized microscopy of the airway fluid has recently been developed and promises to be useful.

Management

This requires specialist skills and includes the following elements:

1 *Oxygen administration.* This is usually given in an incubator maintaining an arterial or capillary Po_2 of about 8 kPa (60 mmHg). Oxygen levels must be monitored, as high Po_2 (above 20 kPa (150 mmHg)), may cause blindness from retrolental fibroplasia.

2 *Ventilation (intermittent positive pressure ventilation—IPPV)* . Ventilation by cuffed endotracheal tube is needed in more severe cases. A slight positive pressure throughout the breathing cycle is usually employed (positive end-expiratory pressure—PEEP).

3 *Surfactant administration.* This is still a novel treatment but is likely to become standard when existing bovine or human extracted surfactant is replaced by genetically engineered synthetic material.

Outcome

Complications include pneumothorax and interstitial emphysema (air in the connective tissue planes of the body). Once recovery has occurred the condition does not recur. Deaths usually occur in the first 2 days and are related to degree of prematurity. Most surviving infants go on to complete recovery with no obvious consequences for future pulmonary health.

Chapter 4
Defence Mechanisms Protecting the Lung

The lungs bring the whole of the cardiac output into intimate relationship with the outside world, and therefore offer the opportunity for immediate, potentially devastating access by noxious agents of all sorts: particles, toxic vapours, micro-organisms, etc. A variety of mechanisms oppose such invasion and these merit separate consideration, not least since the breakdown of any of them may be associated with pulmonary disease. Defence mechanisms are summarized in Fig. 4.1.

Particle penetrance and deposition

Particle size

Penetration of airborne particles into the respiratory tract is largely dependent upon their size. In practice aerodynamic shape also plays a part, and the relevant index is referred to as mass median diameter (MMD). In a mixture of the inhaled particles, ranked according to particle diameter, this is the diameter of the particles at the point where half of the mass of the mixture comprises particles which are smaller and half particles which are larger.

Deposition

The geometry of the airway plays an important part in preventing ingress of inhaled particles. Particles more than about 3 µm are largely removed by the nose; those of 5–10 µm penetrate the tracheobronchial tree; and particles smaller than about 3 µm may reach alveoli. Some particles actually change size as they enter the respiratory tract through hygroscopic attraction.

Particles become deposited on the airway surfaces mainly by impaction and sedimentation. Heavier particles tend to be flung outwards where there is a change in direction of airflow. A high proportion thus make contact with the wall in the turbulent upper airways (impaction) and others reaching lower down become impacted where bronchi divide. In particles of intermediate size which reach the bronchi, deposition may to a large extent be determined by slow gravitational settling (sedimentation). Even though the airstream is moving more or less continuously, particles tend to move downwards in the airstream and a proportion make contact with the wall. Very small particles forming a perfect aerosol may impact by chance brownian movement, though this is not thought to be very important; particles of this size are largely exhaled without deposition. Figure 4.2 shows the relationship between size of particle and deposition in the upper respiratory tract, tracheobronchial tree and alveoli.

Implications

Patterns of deposition have most immediate relevance in the context of occupational lung disease: some impressively dusty occupations may not be

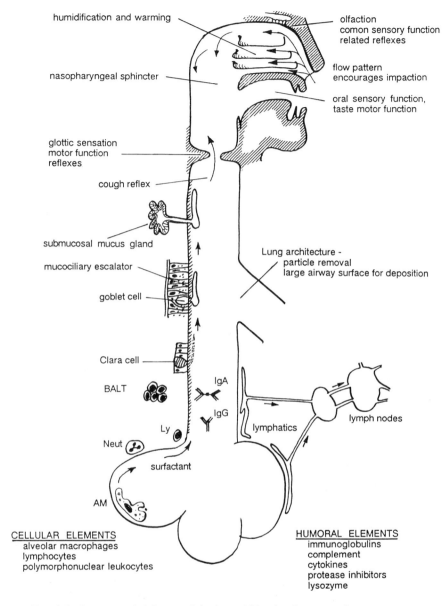

Fig. 4.1. Summary of defences of the lung. AM = alveolar macrophage; BALT = bronchial associated lymphoid tissue; Ly = lymphocyte; Neut = neutrophil.

threatening if particles are relatively large and not harmful to clearance mechanisms; other occupations with less impressive dust which penetrates deeply and impedes clearance may result in serious disease. Virus particles, when excreted in droplet form, dry to a very small desiccated nucleus of less than 0.5 μm. On being inhaled by the host they may behave as very small particles, but they may rehydrate very rapidly during inhalation and impact like larger

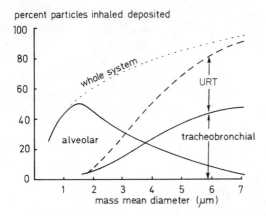

Fig. 4.2. Deposition of inhaled particles. Graph showing percentage of particles inhaled which is deposited in the airways—divided into tracheobronchial section and upper respiratory tract (URT)—and the percentage deposited at alveolar level. Particles with a diameter of less than about 3 μm are more likely to be retained at alveolar level than to be removed at a higher level. (After Hatch, 1966).

particles. Consideration of particle size and deposition is obviously of importance in the administration of therapeutic aerosols.

The upper airway

Nose

The nose plays an important part. Both smell and non-olfactory detection of irritants in the air can lead to the avoidance of harmful inhalation. Nose breathing removes an important proportion of inhaled particles of all sizes (virtually all particles above 20 μm, and some smaller). The nose and pharynx 'condition' the inspired air; thus over a very wide range of combinations of external temperature and humidity, the air in the trachea is fully saturated and at normal body temperature. This prevents drying of the airways which would otherwise lead to crusting of mucus and failure of the mucociliary escalator.

Larynx

Proper sensory and motor function of the larynx is crucial to the protection of the airway from inhalation by food and secretions. The aryepiglottic folds and the false and true vocal cords offer a three-layered defence. Apart from its action in swallowing, the larynx may close the airways instantly in a reflex response to olfactory and other stimuli and it also plays a part in the cough reflex.

Cough

The cough comprises the following actions: (1) sometimes a preliminary inspiration; (2) closure of the glottis (vocal cords); (3) contraction of the abdominal musculature and bracing by intercostal musculature; (4) sudden release of the glottis.

The reflex is provoked by physical or chemical stimulation of irritant receptors in the larynx, trachea or bronchial tree (particularly near bifurcations), or by inflammation in these sites.

The result is a forceful expiratory blast, which may remove inadvertently inhaled solid or fluid material. The force of expiration in a vigorous cough is accompanied by a large pressure drop from the alveoli to the trachea and major bronchi, which causes compression with invagination of the posterior non-cartilaginous part of the wall. This narrows the airway down to a U-shaped slit resulting in very high flow rates, very close to the surface of the mucous membrane, which imparts a shearing force promoting upward movement or actual expulsion of inhaled material or collections of abundant mucus.

Mucociliary escalator

Cilia

Cilial action
Ciliated cells are present from the terminal bronchiole to the larynx. They are very sparse peripherally and become the predominant cell proximally. The upward movement of a 'raft' of mucus (the gel layer) on the surface of thinner fluid (the sol layer) propelled by the forward movement of the tips of cilia, beating in organized waves, is a wonderful clearance mechanism which is crucial to pulmonary health (Fig. 1.6).

Cilial performance
Cilial structure is considered in Chapter 1. The function of cilia can be assessed by observing ciliary beat frequency in epithelial cells from the nasal mucosa, using a specially adapted microscope linked to a photocell. Normal cilia beat at about 14 beats s^{-1}. Cilial function disorders are considered in Chapter 12.

Assessment of mucociliary clearance
The effectiveness of mucociliary clearance can be assessed experimentally by using a gamma camera to observe the rate of clearance of an inhaled radiolabelled aerosol, which has deposited on the airways. Other methods involve observing the movement of tiny discs, introduced into the central airways, either radiographically or using photography or bronchoscopy. The rate of movement of the mucus blanket seems to be faster peripherally than centrally, where it is about 1 mm min^{-1}. Material deposited in the airways is normally completely cleared within 24 hours.

Agents affecting cilia
Cilial performance is adversely affected by smoke, acidosis and toxins. The products of certain bacteria are harmful; viral infection can result in the widespread shedding of ciliated respiratory cells. Cilial beat performance is enhanced by β-agonist drugs. Mucus clearance is also enhanced by methylxanthines. Cholinergic drugs enhance clearance and atropine-like agents cause slowing. Ipratropium seems to have no effect.

Airway mucus

Regulation of the composition of the airway secretion is probably complex. Alveolar fluid, containing lipid surfactant together with material contributed by Clara cells, forms the layer peripherally. The quantity and composition of the sol layer seems to be regulated by the brush border of ciliated cells (overall considerable reabsorption of fluid is needed as branching airways come together). Goblet cells (throughout the larger airways) and mucus glands (bronchi and trachea) provide mucus itself.

Mucus glycoprotein, the main component, is responsible for the visco-elastic properties of sputum and is composed of a central polypeptide core, from which come long chains of sugars. Bonds between these chains give mucus its stability. Viscosity and elasticity of the mucus layer are probably important to ciliary effectiveness; both are complex and difficult to study. A certain elasticity (or recoverable stretching) of mucus by each cilial beat is essential if the mucus is to move forward whilst the cilia recover for the next beat. A degree of viscosity, to retard the recovery of the deformed mucus sheet, is also important for movement. Excessive viscosity, however, impedes the movement of the cilia.

Mucus secretion by goblet cells appears to be increased by local inflammation; mucus gland secretion is under vagal control. Increased mucus production has a protective function, limiting penetration of noxious soluble substances and increasing the likelihood of impaction of particulate matter, but excessive quantities of mucus produced, for example in chronic bronchitis, lead to less effective clearance.

Most agents designed to modify mucus are ineffective. Inhalation of an aerosol of hypertonic saline (7.1%) produces a marked increase in secretion and this effect is harnessed in attempts to diagnose suspected infection by pneumocystis (see Chapter 11). Inhaled water, by vapour or aerosol, has no effect.

Humoral mechanisms

Apart from mucus glycoprotein, respiratory secretions contain proteins derived from plasma, some of which are represented in proportions determined by their intravascular concentration and molecular size, others being concentrated or manufactured locally. Immunoglobulins and antiproteases are the most important defensive proteins.

Immunoglobulins

All classes of immunoglobulins are present in lung secretions, but the proportions are different from those found in plasma. The principal immunoglobulin in lung secretions is IgA whereas in plasma it is IgG. It is now thought that most of the immunoglobulin present in normal secretions is manufactured locally, in the lungs, by lymphoid cells such as plasma cells in the interstitium and walls of the airways, or by bronchial associated lymphoid tissue (BALT, see p. 9). Most of the IgA in secretions is in the form of twin molecules (dimers), linked by a special protein (secretory component) which is derived from the respiratory epithelium during the process of secretion. The linkage may improve transfer into the lumen, or act to protect part of the molecule against destruction by products of micro-organisms. Resistance to infection in populations has been shown to be related to IgA concentrations; IgA production is defective in malnutrition and reduced in smokers. IgG present in lung secretions is probably also largely produced locally. The amounts are small and IgG is probably of minor importance in initial resistance to respiratory infection. Small amounts of IgD and IgE have been identified in respiratory secretions. IgM is present in negligible amounts, being confined to the intravascular compartment by its large size.

Complement

Components of the complement system are present in small quantities, derived either from macrophages or from plasma. Complement components are recruited in the course of the inflammatory process, but the role of complement in protection of the lungs against infection is not well understood.

Cytokines

These are peptides, released by cells, which have an activating effect on other cells. Cytokines include interferons, the interleukins, chemotactic factors and tumour necrosis factor. Chemotactic factors include those derived from macrophages, damaged lung tissue, complement components and factors produced by micro-organisms.

Protease inhibitors

Lung secretions contain antiproteases derived from plasma α-1 protease inhibitor—formerly known as α-1 antitrypsin), or produced locally (e.g. anti-leukoprotease). They protect the tissues against digestion by proteolytic enzymes, released from neutrophils, macrophages and micro-organisms in the course of the response to infection. Antiprotease deficiency is discussed in Chapter 18.

Lysozyme

Lung secretions contain lysozyme, an ill-understood bactericidal enzyme present in tears and other body secretions.

Cellular mechanisms

Alveolar macrophages

Macrophages are normally present within alveoli and within the interstitium of the lung parenchyma. They are ultimately of bone marrow origin, although they appear able to reproduce locally. Recruitment to the lung is increased by inflammation and products of tissue necrosis. Macrophages are actively phagocytic and largely responsible for disposing of particulate matter that reaches alveolar level. Some macrophages are drawn up on the mucociliary escalator; some appear able to pass through cell junctions peripherally, with their burden of ingested matter, eventually reaching the lymphatics. Prior opsonization of micro-organisms may be required before the macrophage is able to ingest them. Phagocytic function of macrophages may be impaired by factors such as air pollutants (for example, smoke and ozone), viral infection, alcohol ingestion and malnutrition. In addition to their phagocytic role, macrophages are able to secrete enzymes, internally and externally. They can kill ingested micro-organisms by intracellular production of superoxides in an intense phase of metabolic activity which follows phagocytosis—the 'respiratory burst'. They produce proteases (and antiproteases), complement components, neutrophil chemotactic factor (NCF) and other chemoattractants, interferons, interleukins and a large number of other active substances. Macrophages also appear to act as antigen presenting cells, in the course of a specific immune response in the lungs.

Neutrophils

There are normally very few neutrophils present in the airway. They appear as part of the inflammatory response, probably in response to the release of cytokines like NCF by macrophages and lymphocytes, and the presence of other chemoattractants. Neutrophils contain lysozomal enzyme and also proteases (especially elastase) which may damage lung tissue. Eosinophils and mast cells are normally present in negligible numbers, but play a part in hypersensitivity inflammatory responses (see Chapter 15).

Lymphocytes

Small numbers of intraluminal lymphocytes are normally present and have an uncertain defensive role. Scattered lymphocytes, found throughout the interstitium and lymphoid accumulations (BALT), have been referred to above and are almost cetainly the site of immunoglobulin manufacture. Some are presumably members of T-cell subsets—helper, suppressor and killer cells. The latter may protect against the development of neoplasia. The full range of cellular and humoral, immunological, inflammatory and some healing reactions is available within the lung tissue itself, constituting a further set of defences which will not be reviewed here. Fully developed inflammatory tissue, especially that associated with suppurative lung disease, derives its principal blood supply from the bronchial circulation.

Pulmonary lymphatics

Increased lymphatic drainage is a highly effective means of controlling the increased transudation from capillaries which accompanies physical or toxic insult to the airway or lung parenchyma. Lymphatics also remove particulate matter, micro-organisms and the by-products of inflammation and necrosis. Intrapulmonary, hilar and mediastinal lymph nodes constitute further defences against generalized infection.

Chapter 5
The History—Symptoms of Respiratory Disease

Assessment of the patient with respiratory disease hinges on thorough, unhurried history-taking and not upon tests of pulmonary function or the chest X-ray. The aim, as in all history-taking, is to obtain a clear impression of particular symptoms and combinations of symptoms and most importantly to build up a clear picture of their progress or variation with time. The following notes are not intended to be exhaustive but they may be helpful in suggesting ways in which enquiry may be extended.

Dyspnoea

Character
What words does the patient use? 'Tightness' may indicate airways obstruction or angina; 'gasping' and 'panting' suggest hyperpnoea—excessive but not necessarily laboured or obstructed breathing. The patient may liken the dyspnoea to the sensation which normally follows running. Is there accompanying noise? A wheezing sound is suggestive of airways narrowing (which may accompany disease not primarily affecting the airways, such as pulmonary embolism or incipient pulmonary oedema). A frothy bubbling may accompany frank pulmonary oedema. It is often helpful when in doubt, to mimic the sounds in question (wheezing can be reproduced by first breathing quietly right out, almost to residual volume, and then giving a further sharp forced expiration).

Circumstances
Is it related to time of day, exercise, meals, posture, etc? Patients with long-standing overinflation dislike bending intensely; asthma has a characteristic diurnal variation; and so on.

How severe is it?
The effect upon a patient's activities is the best guide to severity. Exercise tolerance may be crudely but usefully graded as follows:

	Grade
Short of breath at rest	4
Short of breath walking about the house and undertaking light activity such as washing	3
Has to stop even when walking at own reduced pace on the level	2
Asks friends of own age to slow down but keeps going at own reduced pace on level	1
Able to walk with friends at normal pace on level but unable to keep going on hills or when hurrying	0

Inexperienced clinicians are peculiarly prone to preoccupation with the detailed assessment of the nature and severity of current disability and may fail to make a penetrating assessment of its duration and rate of progress—both of which may contain information of critical diagnostic importance. Useful insight may sometimes be gained into the rate and progress of disability, by noting change in a patient's *range*. When was he or she last shopping in a distant centre, when last shopping locally or visiting park or pub? When was the patient last beyond the street in which he or she lives, the garden gate, the front door, one floor of the house, one room, chair or bed?

Cough and sputum

The duration and annual or daily pattern of cough and sputum production should be clearly established. Nocturnal cough is particularly likely to be associated with asthma or left heart failure. The approximate volume, texture and colour of sputum should be recorded. Black particles usually only reflect local atmospheric pollution, yellow sputum usually indicates a high cellular content due to bacterial infection, but in asthma, eosinophil clumps can produce similar appearances. Regular production of green sputum may indicate bronchiectasis, as may longstanding daylong production of large volumes of sputum. Enquiry should be made regarding previous *haemoptysis*, its quantity and possible association with epitaxis, fever, chest pain or other respiratory symptoms.

Chest pain

The association of chest pain with respiratory movement, coughing or turning over will suggest a pleural origin. It is sometimes helpful to mimic the wince and grunt which an inspiration evokes in the presence of pleural pain—this is generally recognized immediately by patients who have experienced the symptom. Normal individuals may experience occasional pleural pain, which is transient and relieved by gradually taking a deep breath in small steps; this phenomenon is referred to as the 'Catch syndrome'. Sometimes localized anterior chest pain of this sort is accompanied by tenderness of one costochondral junction and this is referred to as Tietze's syndrome or costochondritis: a benign condition. Obese individuals are sometimes troubled by brief costal margin pain interrupting a breath, related to a rib (usually the ninth) rolling over the rib above (clicking rib). Shoulder-tip pain suggests irritation of diaphragmatic pleura; radiation of precordial pain to the neck and arms suggests a myocardial origin. Precordial pain may also accompany mediastinal enlargement, pericarditis and oesophagitis, all of which may have special additional features. Pain in the epigastrium and around the costal margin is common in severe airways obstruction and may be related to peptic ulceration, oesophagitis and extreme muscular effort.

Previous respiratory illness

If a patient reports previous episodes of 'bronchitis', 'influenza', 'pneumonia', etc. it is important to obtain a clear account of the nature of the illness and not merely to accept the offered diagnosis at face value. Careful enquiry may reveal that a reported episode of 'bronchitis' had features very suggestive of asthma or that 'pneumonia' might in fact have been pulmonary embolism. The extent of previous investigations and the response to treatment may provide valuable clues. Enquiry should always be made regarding previous X-ray examinations; a surprising proportion of the adult population in the UK has had a chest X-ray at some time or other and, if previous films can be located, they may sometimes provide invaluable information.

Associated allergies

Asthma is so common that enquiry should always be made about previous skin disorders (eczema, 'dermatitis'), hay fever, recurrent or persistent colds, nasal obstruction, nasal operations etc., all of which have an association with asthma.

Family history

A similar enquiry should be made regarding allergic disorders in the family and this should be extended to include 'bronchitis', wheezing and excessive cough and breathlessness, as well as tuberculosis. It is worthwhile pausing whilst the patient reviews each generation in turn; if enquiry is hurried it is very likely to be negative.

Occupational history

A clear sequential account of a patient's previous occupations including descriptions of the actual tasks and names of materials encountered may be vital (see especially sections on asthma, extrinsic allergic alveolitis, asbestos related disease and pneumoconiosis).

Smoking history

It is important to obtain a clear account of total smoking exposure and not to be misled by patients who may have recently reduced their consumption or stopped smoking.

Chapter 6
Examination of the Chest

Some important clues relating to the respiratory system may be evident from the moment the patient is first seen, and these signs should be noted carefully, lest they be overlooked during formal examination of the chest. They include the character of the breathing and its relationship to activity and speech, the shape of the shoulders (Fig. 6.1) and spine and the character of the cough. The presence of partial nasal obstruction, or of stridor, may be apparent when the patient first speaks, but overlooked later.

Inspection

Cyanosis

Cyanosis is generally apparent when about $5 \text{ g } 100 \text{ ml}^{-1}$ of haemoglobin is present in the reduced state within the blood vessels of the skin.

Peripheral cyanosis

This is commonly due to local circulatory slowing resulting in more complete extraction of oxygen from the blood. The regions in question are commonly cool.

Central cyanosis

This is said to exist when the bluish colouration involves areas not normally prone to local circulatory changes. The best site to examine is the tip of the tongue. The lips may sometimes appear blue due to local pigmentation or local circulatory change, but the tip of the tongue always has adequate blood supply. Central cyanosis indicates that there is desaturation of arterial blood. When using tissue

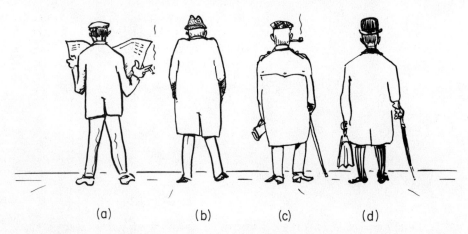

(a)   (b)   (c)   (d)

Fig. 6.1. Which man has airways obstruction? (Answer at foot of p. 53.)

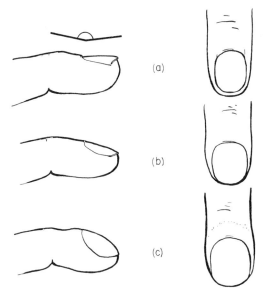

Fig. 6.2. Clubbing. (a) Normal, showing the 'angle'. (b) Early clubbing; the angle is absent. (c) Advanced clubbing. The nail shows increased curvature in all directions, the angle is absent, the base of the nail is raised up by spongy tissue and the end of the digit is expanded.

colour to assess arterial oxygenation, note should obviously be taken of the pinkest area visible. Arterial oxygenation cannot be worse than the level suggested by this area. When there is frank central cyanosis, arterial Po_2 will almost always be below 6 kPa (45 mmHg) depending on haemoglobin content and arterial pH.

Clubbing

Clubbing is easier to recognize than to define rigidly. There is increased curvature of the nail and the nail-bed is raised so that the normal angle between the proximal part of the nail and the skin over the dorsum of the terminal phalanx is lost (Fig. 6.2). The base of the nail may be palpable through the skin and an abnormal sponginess may be apparent when pressure is applied over it. Clubbing is associated with:

1   Bronchial carcinoma.
2   Bronchiectasis and other forms of chronic suppurative lung disease.
3   Pulmonary fibrosis.
4   Pleural and mediastinal tumours.
5   Subacute bacterial endocarditis.
6   Cyanotic congenital heart disease.
7   Cirrhosis and coeliac disease.

Breathing pattern

From the beginning of the encounter with the patient there will be the opportunity to observe whether he appears to be breathless or distressed, grunting or in pain, wheezing or panting, etc. and these important features should be carefully noted. If it is suspected that the **respiratory rate** may be increased, it should be counted over a whole minute as the error inherent in counting for a shorter period, such as 15 seconds, is large and reduces the value of the observation, particularly if the rate is being counted serially.

The character of the cough

The sound produced by a cough is a most valuable (and widely ignored) physical sign. The patient should be requested to give several sharp coughs (not merely clearing the throat). A rattling sound may give clear indication of the presence of abundant bronchial secretions. A 'bovine cough' lacking the usual explosive onset may suggest vocal cord paralysis. Most importantly, a muffled wheezy cough may provide a very vivid indication of the presence of otherwise quite unsuspected airways obstruction.

Stridor

This (often sinister) sign is likely to be noticed early in the interview as the patient draws breath whilst talking rather than during formal examination of the chest. It can be imitated by breathing in and out with the vocal cords held in the position of the whispered word 'air'. It indicates localized obstruction of the larynx, trachea or large bronchi.

Jugular veins

Examination of the jugular veins should never be omitted. The patient should be examined in a semi-reclining position with the trunk between 30 and 45 degrees from the horizontal. It is very important that the head should be in line with the trunk and fully supported so that the sternomastoid muscles are relaxed and soft (if not in use as accessory muscles of respiration). The jugular veins reflect intrathoracic pressure changes; assessment of the level and character of the jugular venous pulse can be difficult when breathing is laboured, but useful information can still be obtained if the patient is asked to take one or two extremely slow, shallow breaths. If he or she is requested to stop breathing briefly, then the glottis is generally closed and the venous pressure is spuriously raised.

Inspection of the chest

Inspection of the chest should begin with an overall view of the shape of the chest and thoracic spine to note any obvious kyphosis, asymmetry, scars, prominent veins, etc. It is then helpful for the patient to adopt the semi-reclining position described above. Flattening, overinflation or other asymmetry may then be assessed by viewing from the front.

Respiratory movements

Regional asymmetry. Despite its semi-rigid nature, the chest reflects filling of the underlying lung remarkably well in its movements. The diseased side always moves least. Movement of the upper part of the chest may be more easily appreciated by placing the hands exactly symmetrically on either side of the upper sternum. Contraction of pectoralis major sometimes complicates this observation.

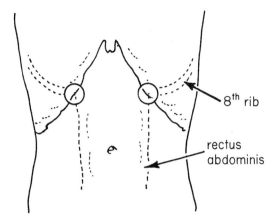

Fig. 6.3. Movement of the costal margin. The position for observing costal margin movement with the fingertips is indicated by the circles.

Expansion of the lower zones may be appreciated by spreading the hands with the fingers directed backwards and the thumbs close to the mid-line. The relative movement of the two hands and the separation of the thumbs is then observed closely.

Movement of the costal margin. Observation of the movement of the costal margin may reveal a lateralized abnormality; it may also provide a very valuable clue to the presence of airways obstruction. The observation is made in the semi-recumbent position described and movement is best appreciated by placing the fingertips on the costal margin just lateral to the outer edge of rectus abdominis in the position of the circles shown in Fig. 6.3. As the patient breathes, the fingertips should follow the costal margin and the distance separating the fingertips of the two hands is closely observed (Fig. 6.4).

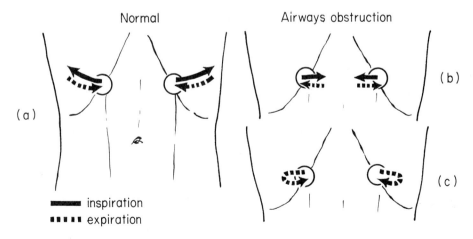

Fig. 6.4. Movement of the costal margin. The arrows indicate the direction of movement in normal individuals and in those with severe airways obstruction (see text p. 46).

1   In normal quiet breathing the hands move apart on inspiration and towards each other on expiration.

2   In severe airways obstruction the hands may move towards each other on inspiration and apart again on expiration.

3   Sometimes in severe airways obstruction the main abnormality is in expiration, when there is an outward and then an inward movement.

Patterns (2) and (3) are referred to here as costal margin paradox. The sign is associated with a high inspiratory impedence at a high lung volume. Clinical observation supports the following conclusions:

1   When costal margin paradox is observed there is substantial airways obstruction present.

2   Where severe airways obstruction is already known to be present (by use of a spirometer) but costal margin movement is in the *normal* direction, this is unusual and there is almost always either:

(a) some factor limiting the volume of the lungs (diffuse fibrosis, infiltration, kyphosis, etc.) or

(b) severe emphysema present.

Costal margin paradox is most commonly seen in association with severe chronic obstructive lung disease. It is also seen in infants with bronchiolitis and in subjects of all ages with severe asthma. A change from paradoxical costal margin movement to normal outward movement is a reassuring sign of improvement in an asthmatic crisis, which is particularly useful in those unable to perform simple ventilatory tests. The sign is not present in other causes of dyspnoea such as pulmonary fibrosis or heart failure—with the occasional exception of those cases of pulmonary oedema in which wheezing and airways obstruction are prominent.

Movement of the sternum. In patients with laboured breathing, the movement of the sternum should be observed carefully either by viewing from the side or by placing the fingertips of one hand lightly over the lower third of the sternum. Attention is paid to the *anteroposterior* movement of this point. Normally the whole sternum moves forwards during inspiration and backwards during expiration. If the reverse is observed (i.e. indrawing of the lower sternum during inspiration) it generally indicates a high inspiratory impedence at a low lung volume. The sign is referred to here as lower sternal paradox and it is seen in very severe pulmonary fibrosis, in which the lungs are contracted and stiff, and in localized upper airways obstruction (for example, tracheal narrowing or a blocked endotracheal tube). The sign may help in distinguishing between severe upper airways obstruction causing stridor and severe diffuse airways obstruction.

Summary: costal margin paradox = high volume impeded breathing;

lower sternal paradox without costal margin paradox

= low volume impeded breathing.

Palpation

Cervical and axillary lymph nodes

These nodes should always be carefully sought by palpation.

Position of the mediastinum

This is assessed by localization of the trachea above and the cardiac apex below.

Ribs

Particularly where there is chest pain the ribs should be palpated carefully, seeking localized tenderness, suggesting fracture, or swelling, suggesting bony metastasis. It may help to compress the chest gently but firmly, laterally and anteroposteriorly; localized pain suggests rib fracture.

Percussion

All areas should be percussed, paying particular attention to comparison of the note obtained with the finger placed exactly symmetrically on the two sides. The presence or absence of hepatic and cardiac dullnesses should be noted—they disappear when the lungs are overinflated (for example, during a deep breath). The position of tympanitic gastric resonance on the left may provide a clue to the position of the diaphragm. When percussing the back it may be helpful to ask patients to place one elbow on top of the other in front of them—this has the effect of bringing the scapulae forwards out of the way.

Auscultation

The effect of lung tissue on the transmission of sound gives important information to the clinician (Fig. 6.5).

Source of sound

With the exception of abnormal added sounds (crackles, wheezes, etc. dealt with later), the sources of audible sound in the lungs are: (1) turbulent air flow in the larynx and central airways; and (2) the voice. Both have high- and low-pitched components; these are transmitted differently by normal and abnormal lung.

Normal breath sounds

These amount to a faint, low-pitched rushing sound with a gentle beginning and end during inspiration and again rather briefly during expiration. The source of the sound is the larynx and upper airway; normal lung attenuates the higher frequencies, leaving the small amount of medium- and low-pitched sound typical of normal breathing. There is some variation in the intensity and character of normal breath sounds consequent upon the thickness of the chest wall, breathing pattern, body size, etc. Breath sounds are normally harsher anteriorly in the upper zones particularly on the right. Two further terms are still occasionally used to describe breath sounds. 'Vesicular breathing' is synonymous with 'normal breath sounds' and derives from an age when it was believed that the entry of air into alveoli generated the sound. 'Air entry' is a loose term used to indicate that breath sounds have been heard with greater or lesser ease. Both of these terms are redundant.

Bronchial breathing

This can be heard over consolidated areas of lung. These areas conduct the high-frequency 'hiss' component from the larger airways quite well. Bronchial

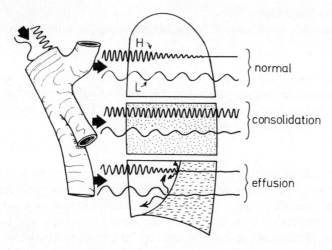

Fig. 6.5. Summary of sound transmission in the lung. Sound is generated either by turbulence in the larynx and large airways, or by the voice. Both sources are a mixture of high (H) and low (L) pitched components. *Normal aerated lung* filters off the high-pitched component but transmits the low-pitched component quite well. This results in soft low-pitched breath sounds, well-conducted vocal resonance and easily palpable very low-pitched sound (vocal fremitus). *Consolidated lung* transmits high-pitched sound well and filters off some of the lower pitched sound. This results in loud high-pitched breath sounds (bronchial breathing), high-pitched bleating vocal resonance (aegophony) and easy transmission of the high-pitched consonants of speech (whispering pectoriloquy). *Pleural effusion* causes reduction in the transmission of all sound—probably because of reflection of sound waves at the air–fluid interface. Breath sounds are absent, vocal resonance much reduced and vocal fremitus is absent.

breathing is characteristically rather similar in inspiration and expiration and there is a momentary silent pause between the two. The sound can be imitated by listening with a stethoscope over the larynx whilst the subject breathes in and out with the vocal cords held in the position of a whispered 'ee'.

Vocal resonance

The character of vocal resonance—observed by auscultation over the chest during speech—provides further evidence of the lung's ability to transmit or filter different sound frequencies. Normal aerated lung transmits the booming low-pitched components of speech and attenuates the high frequencies. Consolidated lung on the other hand filters off the low frequencies and transmits the higher frequencies, so that speech takes on a telephonic or bleating quality (aegophony). The facilitated transmission of high frequencies can be demonstrated by the clear transmission of whispering over consolidated lung (whispering pectoriloquy). Pleural fluid reduces the intensity of all frequencies, most especially low frequencies.

Vocal fremitus

(Included here because it concerns sound transmission.) Normal aerated lung transmits *low* frequencies well and a sonorous voice produces easily palpable fremitus (a buzzing vibration) over the chest wall. Consolidated lung transmits fremitus less well and pleural fluid very severely dampens it and may obliterate the vibrations altogether.

Added sounds (adventitiae)

Semantic difficulties arise here. The term *râle* is taken by some to mean any added sound and by others as synonymous with crackle; for this reason it is perhaps best avoided.

Wheezing (rhonchi)

Wheezes or rhonchi are sustained musical sounds of varying length and pitch. They may be heard during inspiration or expiration (more commonly the latter) and they are then produced by a flow-limiting mechanism (see p. 13). They tend to be heard in the presence of airways obstruction but they are not inevitably present in this situation and are generally a poor indication of the severity of the obstruction.

Crackles (formerly called crepitations)

A series of very brief clicking sounds which may be loud and coarse or fine and high-pitched. Fine high-pitched crackles can be imitated by rolling a few hairs together close to the ear. The sounds are probably produced by the opening of previously closed bronchioles. The timing of crackles is of some significance.

Early inspiratory crackles

These are associated with diffuse airways obstruction. A series of clicks are commonly heard very close together at the beginning of inspiration with relative silence afterwards. These sounds do *not* indicate pulmonary oedema, left ventricular failure, etc.

Pan-inspiratory or late inspiratory crackles

These are associated with diffuse fibrosis, pulmonary oedema (actual or incipient), bronchiectasis and partial consolidation (Fig. 6.6).

Probable explanation. During inspiration, areas of lung open up in sequence according to their compliance (distensibility). Compliant areas open up first, and

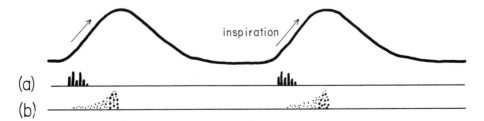

Fig. 6.6. Timing of crackles. Diagrammatic representation of: (a) early inspiratory crackles—commonly associated with airways obstruction; (b) pan-inspiratory or late inspiratory crackles—commonly associated with early pulmonary oedema, lung fibrosis, etc.

then as the retractive forces in the lung increase, increasingly stiff areas participate in receiving inspired air.

In the case of airways obstruction there may be widespread terminal airways closure during expiration, particularly in relatively compliant (floppy) parts of the lung. During inspiration these areas accept air most readily and the clicks are probably produced by the opening of their airways early in inspiration.

The disorders associated with late inspiratory crackles cause reduced lung compliance (increased stiffness) which is to some extent patchily distributed. During inspiration air passes first to the more compliant parts—that is to the more normal parts—and only begins to enter the stiffer abnormal areas later in inspiration as lung recoil forces build up in the stretching lung.

Pleural rub

Pleural rubs are commonly creaking or groaning sounds and sometimes take the form of an interrupted dry scuffing sound. They are often quite localized and indicate roughening of the normally slippery pleural surfaces.

The sputum

The sputum should *always* be inspected. Truly clear sputum is unusual in city dwellers and if it is thin, slimy and bubbly the specimen is probably saliva. Greyish mottled fragments are usually present in the true mucoid sputum. In asthma, mucoid sputum may be so tenacious that it is impossible to tip it out of a container and it frequently has a glary refractile appearance. If the sputum is creamy or yellow it is referred to as purulent; this appearance commonly reflects active bronchial bacterial infection. Green or khaki coloured sputum indicates delay in production of sputum and suggests bronchiectasis or chronic lung abscess. Brown sputum may be produced by intra-alveolar haemorrhage or a resolving haemoptysis. Solid chunks of sputum are seen in asthma and small bronchial casts may sometimes be seen hanging like fronds below the surface, if sputum is suspended in water. A transparent container is an advantage when inspecting sputum, particularly if there is a large amount of saliva, and an ordinary universal container is useful in this context.

SIGNS OF LOCAL LUNG DISEASE

Warning

Certain distinctive combinations of physical signs have for generations been recognized as allowing some crude but useful assessment of the type of gross pathological change within the chest. The correlation between the signs and the underlying changes is, however, much looser than is the case in cardiological examination and it is as well to be aware of the limitations of physical examination. In developed countries it is realistic to regard the chest X-ray as a normal extension of physical examination where there is good reason to suspect localized lung disease. The appearance of the chest X-ray frequently modifies the interpretation of the physical signs.

Signs of consolidation (airless but not collapsed lung)

Movement of the affected side may be less.

Percussion note is dull—not usually profoundly so.

Vocal fremitus may be somewhat reduced.
Bronchial breathing may be heard.
Crackles may be heard (pan-inspiratory or late inspiratory).
Vocal resonance may have a bleating quality (aegophony).
Whispering pectoriloquy may be heard.

Summary

Moderate dullness, often crepitations and characteristically well-conducted high-pitched sound.

Signs of collapse

Reduction in lung volume may be apparent from movement of the *trachea* towards the collapsed side. The chest wall may appear flattened on the affected side. The apex may be displaced towards the collapse. Movement of the affected side may be reduced. The gastric resonance may be exceptionally high in left-sided collapse.

Breath sounds are usually diminished over the collapsed lobe. In addition to these signs there may be signs of consolidation as outlined above—collapse and consolidation commonly occur together.

Note. These signs may be present in massive collapse but sometimes negligible signs accompany collapse, particularly of a lower lobe.

Summary

Perhaps evidence of localized loss of lung volume, with reduction in movement, breath sounds and moderate dullness on percussion.

Signs of pleural effusion

Trachea and apex may be displaced away from the effusion if it is massive.
Movement of the affected side may be reduced.
Dullness on percussion. This is the most important sign of pleural fluid and is maximal at the base and in the axilla. At least 500 ml of fluid seems to be necessary before dullness becomes detectable.
Vocal fremitus is reduced or absent over pleural fluid.
Breath sounds are reduced or absent. Towards the upper part of an effusion there may be signs of consolidation.

Summary

Striking dullness on percussion with reduction of breath sounds and vocal fremitus.

Signs of pneumothorax

Without tension

In a small pneumothorax there may be *no* signs at all.
Percussion is usually unremarkable ('hyperresonance' is usually unconvincing).
Breath sounds are absent or much reduced and this may be the only sign. A clicking sound in time with the heart is sometimes heard in small left-sided

pneumothoraces due to intermittent contact of the two pleural surfaces over the heart. Other signs are generally lacking.

Tension pneumothorax
Trachea and apex are displaced away from the affected side (important).
Movement of the side may be reduced and the chest may appear fuller on that side.
Percussion may yield a hyperresonant note.
Breath sounds are absent over the pneumothorax.
Vocal resonance and fremitus are somewhat reduced. Tachypnoea and respiratory distress are usual and there may be hypotension, sweating and congestion of neck veins.

Summary
Absent or reduced breath sounds without dullness or signs of consolidation. In tension pneumothorax: displacement of the mediastinum, reduced movement, overdistension and signs of circulatory embarrassment.

Signs of pleural thickening
This is difficult to diagnose with certainty from signs alone.
Movement of the side may be reduced if thickening is extensive.
Dullness on percussion is usual but may not be striking.
Breath sounds are reduced.
Vocal resonance and fremitus are impaired.
Other signs: a pleural rub may be audible but other signs are generally lacking.

Summary
Signs suggestive of a small pleural effusion with sometimes reduced movement of the side in question.

Signs of local pulmonary fibrosis
This is difficult to distinguish from collapse. Upper lobe fibrosis (usually related to old tuberculosis) may produce deviation of the trachea towards the affected side with flattening and reduced movement of the upper chest. Slight dullness, bronchial breathing and crepitations may be evident over the upper lobe.

SIGNS OF DIFFUSE LUNG DISEASE

Diffuse pulmonary fibrosis (p. 185)

Pulmonary oedema (p. 259)

Bronchiectasis (p. 128)

Signs of diffuse airways obstruction
Note. The only really important signs of airways obstruction are provided by a spirometer or a peak flow meter (see p. 58 and p. 56). There are a number of

signs which are regularly associated with airways obstruction (described below and see p. 45) but they are not particularly reliable as indicators of its presence or severity, and it is quite easy for experienced observers to overlook severe airways obstruction. The assessment of airways obstruction does not hinge upon the amount of wheezing audible on auscultation.

The character of the cough is wheezy or muffled—a convenient and very valuable sign.

Signs of overinflation. These can be mimicked by taking in a full breath when it will be found that:

1   The shoulders are high (Fig. 6.1).
2   The antero-posterior diameter of the chest is increased.
3   Accessory muscles of respiration are in operation.
4   Further expansion is limited and accompanied by *inward* movement of the costal margin (Fig. 6.4) and sometimes by descent of the larynx.
5   Percussion reveals absent hepatic and cardiac dullness.

Movement of the costal margin. Inward movement of the costal margin on inspiration is an important sign of severe airways obstruction. An outward movement of the costal margin early in expiration has similar significance. Absence of these signs does not exclude severe airways obstruction (see Figs 6.3 and 6.4 and accompanying text).

Breathing pattern. In severe airways obstruction the patient appears to snatch at inspiration and to have a (relatively) prolonged expiration. In less severe obstruction, prolonged expiration is not very obvious. Pursed lip breathing may be noted.

Wheezes (rhonchi). These may be of high or low pitch and tend to be more marked towards the end of expiration. Very severe airways obstruction can exist without rhonchi. The loudness of rhonchi is related to breathing pattern and is a very poor indicator of severity of obstruction. Prominent inspiratory rhonchi are suggestive of asthma.

Crackles. Early inspiratory crackles and clicks may be heard (p. 48, Fig. 6.5).

Prolonged forced expiratory time. A maximum forced expiration from a position of full inspiration can normally be completed within about 5 seconds. Prolongation beyond this time generally indicates airways obstruction. The end of expiration can be determined by auscultation over the trachea.

From Fig. 6.1: (b) has airways obstruction. Note the high position of the shoulders.

Chapter 7
Pulmonary Function Tests and Blood Gases

Despite the bewildering profusion of sophisticated investigations now employed in testing pulmonary function, it (happily) remains possible to obtain most of the information relevant to clinical practice with the aid of a few fairly simple tests. In this section the emphasis will be on simplicity and practicality.

SIMPLE TESTS OF VENTILATORY FUNCTION
Ventilation refers to the process of moving air into and out of the lungs.

Normal values
Ventilatory performance varies widely with body size, age and sex (Fig. 7.1). Tables and nomograms are available which take these variables into account and display 'predicted normal values' for individuals of particular age and height. These 'predicted' values are the *mean* values derived from study of a normal population and it should be understood that there is considerable variation about this mean (Fig. 7.2). For example, the standard deviation of the mean predicted

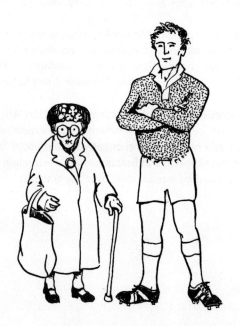

FEV$_1$	1.12	4.32	(litres)
FVC	1.60	5.80	(litres)

Fig. 7.1. Normal values.

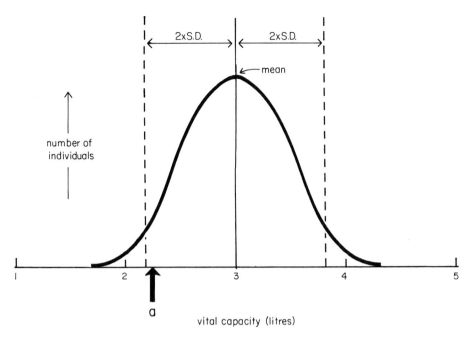

Fig. 7.2. Distribution of vital capacity in normal individuals of one particular age, height and sex (see text).

value for vital capacity is about 500 ml. In effect this means that if a medium-sized adult has a vital capacity which is 1 litre below the predicted normal value (a in Fig. 7.2), the low result *may* by the result of respiratory disease but, on the other hand, the value is only about 2 standard deviations from the mean and perhaps 5% of normal individuals of the same age and size will be found to have a lower vital capacity than this. The practice of expressing results as a 'percentage of predicted normal' is thus potentially misleading: the finding of a vital capacity of 75% of the predicted value does not indicate a 25% disability and is still compatible with normality.

Vital capacity

The vital capacity (VC) is the volume of air expelled by a maximal expiration from a position of full inspiration; this can be measured with any spirometer (Fig. 7.3).

Vital capacity is reduced in the following circumstances:

1 Reduced lung compliance (lung fibrosis, infiltration, loss of lung volume, pulmonary oedema, etc.).

2 Deformity of the chest (kyphoscoliosis, ankylosing spondylitis, etc.).

3 Muscular weakness (myopathy, myasthenia gravis, etc.).

4 Airways obstruction. (Although the main defect is a limitation in rate of airflow, reduction in vital capacity is almost inevitable.)

Strictly, VC should be measured by a slow exhalation from full inspiration. In busy clinical practice, however, the measurement is often derived from a

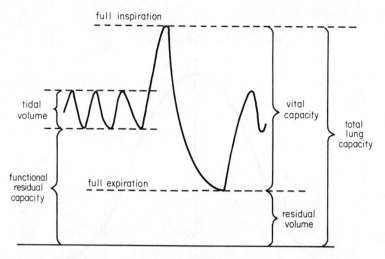

Fig. 7.3. The more commonly used subdivisions of total lung capacity.

forced expiratory spirogram, in which case it is correct to refer to it as forced vital capacity (FVC, see below). In normal individuals, VC and FVC are very similar, but in patients with airways obstruction air-trapping occurs during forced expiration, so that the FVC may be significantly smaller than the slow VC.

Peak expiratory flow (PEF)

This is measured with a peak flow meter (Fig. 7.4). It is the maximum *rate* of airflow which can be achieved during a sudden forced expiration from a position

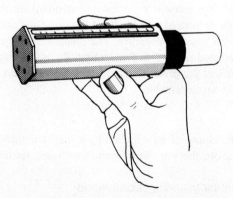

Fig. 7.4. Measurement of peak expiratory flow (PEF). The Wright Mini Peak Flow Meter. The subject takes a *full inspiration*, applies the lips to the mouthpiece and makes a sudden maximal expiratory blast. A piston is pushed down the inside of the cylinder, exposing more and more of a slot in the top, until a position of rest is reached. The position of the piston is indicated by a marker and PEF read from a scale. It is customary to take the best of three properly performed attempts as the PEF.

Two models (high and low reading) are available. The original Wright Peak Flow Meter was a more expensive piece of precision engineering which is now rarely used outside the research field.

of full inspiration. The best of three attempts is usually accepted as the PEF. The value achieved is a little dependent on effort, but is mainly determined by the calibre of the airways. The forced expiration must be performed from the full inspiratory position. The results must be related to body size. PEF is particularly impaired in the presence of diffuse airways obstruction, but it is also somewhat impaired in conditions which reduce lung volume.

The importance of measurement of peak flow rate stems from its reproducibility, speed, simplicity and convenience. It is particularly important in asthma, in which airways obstruction varies considerably (Chapter 17). Occasional measurements of pulmonary function made in the laboratory or clinic are of limited relevance in this condition and much more information about severity, provoking factors and response to treatment (and even about the diagnosis of asthma itself) can be obtained from frequently repeated measurements, made by the patient in his or her own home or work environment. This illustrates the fact that sophisticated sensitive tests of pulmonary function do not necessarily yield more discriminatory or relevant information.

The forced expiratory volume in one second (FEV_1) and the forced vital capacity (FVC)

The FEV_1 is the volume of air expelled in the first second of a maximal forced expiration from a position of full inspiration. The forced vital capacity is obtained by continuing the forced expiration until no further air can be expelled.

The FEV_1 is reduced in any condition which reduces vital capacity but it is particularly reduced when there is diffuse airways obstruction. The relationship between FEV_1 and FVC is clinically very useful as it is to a large extent independent of body size and age.

In a forced expiration about 75% of the air is expelled in the first second ($FEV_1/FVC = 0.75$; this is sometimes referred to as the forced expiratory ratio). In the presence of diffuse airways obstruction a smaller proportion of the air is expelled in the first second (the forced expiratory ratio is reduced).

'Restrictive' and 'obstructive' patterns of ventilatory impairment

When lung volume is restricted by pulmonary fibrosis or infiltration or by rigidity of the chest wall, the VC is reduced and the FEV_1 is also reduced in proportion so that the forced expiratory ratio is normal, or even higher than normal. This pattern of ventilatory impairment is described as a **restrictive defect**.

In the presence of airways obstruction, VC and FEV_1 are again reduced but the FEV_1 is proportionately greater affected than the VC. The forced expiratory ratio is reduced and this pattern is referred to as an **obstructive defect**.

The division of ventilatory defects into obstructive and restrictive patterns is clinically useful, but it should be noted that, although diffuse pulmonary fibrosis and parenchymal infiltrations generally produce a restrictive defect, sometimes an obstructive pattern is seen. Pulmonary function tests always require to be interpreted in the light of all additional available information concerning the individual patient.

The forced expiratory spirogram

Any spirometer equipped with a fast-moving recording chart may be used to record the forced expiratory spirogram, from which the FEV_1 and FVC may be read. It is important that a true maximum forced expiration is achieved. This can be checked by observing the striking reproducibility of the true forced expiratory spirogram. The FEV_1 and FVC are generally taken as the best of three closely reproducible attempts. Comparison of successive attempts and other useful features of the spirogram can be observed most readily with spirometers, which are equipped to start the expired tracing at the same point at each attempt. A widely available self-triggering bellows type spirometer (Vitalograph) possesses this important facility, as well as a number of other features of practical importance (Fig. 7.5). Some commonly encountered patterns of forced expiratory spirogram are shown in Fig. 7.6.

In addition to FEV_1 and FVC, a number of other indices may be calculated from a forced expiratory spirogram. Probably the most useful additional measurement is the maximal mid-expiratory flow rate measured over the middle half of the forced expiration ($FEF_{25-75\%}$); this measurement is dependent upon age and height, normal values lying between 1.5 and 3.5 litre s^{-1} in women and 1.5 and 5.5 litre s^{-1} in men.

A further useful feature is the forced expiratory time. Normally this is less than 4 seconds and the expiratory curve should be virtually flat at this time. If a substantial proportion of forced expiration is exhaled after 4 seconds then airways obstruction can be assumed to be present. Although the chart of the Vitalograph spirometer moves only for the first 6 seconds (later models 12 seconds), this is sufficient to observe whether the curve is flat or continuing (Fig. 7.6 c,d,e).

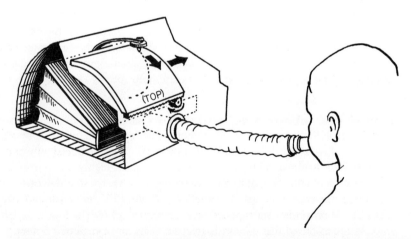

Fig. 7.5. Schematic view of Vitalograph dry spirometer. The main components are a bellows and a moving record chart. An arm attached to the bellows carries a writing point which moves forwards across the chart as air enters the bellows. As soon as the bellows moves a microswitch is triggered and a motor causes the record chart to move steadily from left to right. The combination of lateral movement of the chart and forward movement of the writing point causes an oblique line to be inscribed upon the chart (see Fig. 7.6).

FEF$_{25-75\%}$ and observation of forced expiratory time are helpful in borderline cases of airways obstruction and where there appears to be a mixed ventilatory defect. Amongst elderly women in particular, airways obstruction (sometimes due to asthma) may be reflected by reduction in VC with the FEV$_1$ being reduced more or less in proportion, so that the forced expiratory ratio is close to 0.75. Inspection of FEF$_{25-75\%}$ and forced expiratory time reveals the true nature of the defect.

The flow–volume loop

In recent years there has been greater interest in another method of displaying maximum (or forced) ventilatory manoeuvres—the flow–volume loop. This is at first a little harder to interpret than the familiar spirometer trace (which represents a plot of volume against time), but it is helpful to bear in mind that the flow–volume loop is merely another way of looking at the same information. There are a number of ways of obtaining an instantaneous record of airflow. One way is to use a pneumotachograph, which is a transducer comprising a small resistance to airflow through which the subject breathes. Pressure drop across this specially designed laminar flow resistance is directly proportional to airflow. The pressure is converted to an electrical signal and displayed on an oscilloscope or plotter. The **volume** of air moved can be derived from electrical integration of the flow signal, or it can be obtained independently using a spirometer. The flow–volume relationship is usually displayed as in Fig. 7.7, with lung volume on the horizontal axis and flow on the vertical axis. Conventionally, full inspiration is to the left and expiration to the right. The horizontal line (Z–Z in Fig. 7.7) itself represents no flow. Expiratory flow is represented above the line and inspiratory flow below. The combined expiratory and inspiratory limbs form a loop—the **flow–volume loop**. The shape of the normal loop is as shown and it is quite distinctive. Peak expiratory flow is reached early in expiration from total lung capacity (TLC) and it is somewhat faster than peak inspiratory flow. There is a steady fall in the maximum expiratory flow that can be achieved as expiration progresses. The expiratory limb is highly reproducible: the subject finds it impossible to break out of the boundary of the loop (Fig. 7.8a). The line describes the maximum flow that can be achieved at each particular lung volume. Inspiration is rather less reproducible; maximum inspiratory flow is achieved in mid-inspiration.

The flow–volume curve may be used to derive indices of maximum flow towards the middle or end of expiration (for example, the maximum flow after 50% or 75% of the vital capacity has been expired (FEF$_{50\%}$ or $\dot{V}_{max50}$; FEF$_{75\%}$ or $\dot{V}_{max75}$). These indices may be more sensitive to increased resistance in the small airways (in contrast to PEF and FEV$_1$ which are predominantly influenced by diffuse changes affecting medium sized and larger airways) and they have found some applications in research. A further application of the flow–volume loop is in the elucidation of localized narrowing of the large airways (Fig. 7.8). In practice there is quite often difficulty in diagnosing obstruction of the large airways: usually because the possibility is not considered in the first place. It is

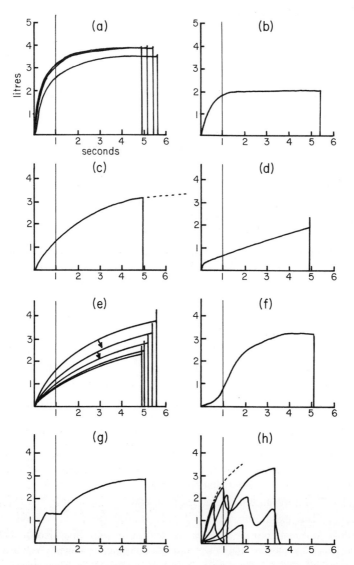

Fig. 7.6. Forced expiratory spirogram tracing obtained with a Vitalograph spirometer.
(a) *Normal.* Four expirations have been made. Three of these were true maximal
forced expirations as indicated by their *reproducibility.* The FEV$_1$ is 3.2 litres and the
FVC is 3.8 litres. The forced expiratory ratio (FEV$_1$/FVC) is 84%.
(b) *Restrictive ventilatory defect.* Patient with pulmonary fibrosis. The FVC in this case
was 2 litres less than the predicted value for the subject. The FEV$_1$ is also reduced
below the predicted value but it represents a large part of the FVC. The forced
expiratory ratio is greater than 90%.
(c) *Obstructive ventilatory defect.* The FEV$_1$ is much reduced. The rate of airflow is
severely reduced as indicated by the reduced slope of the curve. Note that the forced
expiratory time is increased—the patient is still blowing out at 5 seconds. The vital
capacity has not been adequately recorded in this case because the patient did not
continue the expiration after the chart stopped moving; he or she could have expired
further (this is a common technical error).

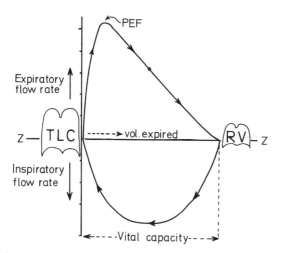

Fig. 7.7. The flow–volume loop. Air flow is represented on the vertical axis and lung volume on the horizontal axis. The line Z–Z represents zero flow. Expiratory flow appears above the line; inspiratory flow below. PEF, peak expiratory flow; TLC, total lung capacity; RV, residual volume.

Fig. 7.6. (continued)

(d) *Severe airways obstruction.* The FEV_1 is about 0.5 litres. FVC is also reduced but not so strikingly as FEV_1. Forced expiratory ratio 23%. Very low expiratory flow rate. This pattern of a very brief initial rapid phase followed by a straight line indicating little change in maximal flow rate with change in lung volume is sometimes associated with severe emphysema.

(e) *Airways obstruction and bronchial hyperreactivity.* Five expirations have been made, FEV_1 and FVC become lower with each expiration. Patient with asthma. This feature suggests poor control of asthma and liability to severe attacks.

(f) *A non-maximal expiration.* Compare with (a). In a true forced expiration the steepest part of the curve always occurs at the beginning of expiration which is not the case in (f). A falsely low FEV_1 and forced expiratory ratio are obtained. Usually the patient has not understood what is required or is unable to co-ordinate his actions. Some patients wish to appear worse than they really are. This pattern is unlikely to be mistaken for a true forced expiration because of its shape and because it cannot be reproduced repeatedly.

(g) *Escape of air* from the nose or lips during expiration.

(h) *Inability to perform the manoeuvre.* Five attempts have been made. In some the patient has breathed in and out. Other attempts are either not maximal forced expirations or are unfinished. Bizarre patterns such as this are often seen in patients with psychogenic breathlessness and in the elderly and demented. Even with poor co-operation it is often possible to obtain useful information. In the example shown (h) significant airways obstruction can be excluded because of the steep slope of at least two of the expirations which follow an identical course and show appropriate curvature (dotted line) and the FVC can be estimated as not less than 3.2 litres. The pattern seen in large airways obstruction is shown in Fig. 7.9.

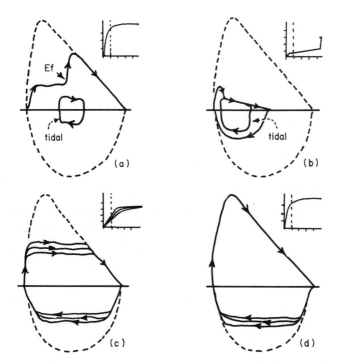

Fig. 7.8. Further flow–volume loops. The dotted outline represents a typical normal loop. The small graphs show the appearances of a forced expiration on a Vitalograph spirometer (as in Fig. 7.6).

(a) *Demonstration of maximum flow.* A normal individual makes an unhurried expiration from full inspiration and then about halfway through the vital capacity, a maximal expiratory effort (Ef) is made. The flow–volume tracing rejoins the maximum flow–volume curve which describes the highest flow which can be achieved at that lung volume. Also shown in (a) is the flow–volume loop of typical tidal breathing. At the resting lung volume there is an abundant reserve of both inspiratory and expiratory flow available.

(b) *Very severe airways obstruction* in an individual with emphysema. Maximum expiratory flow is very severely reduced. There is a brief peak (probably caused by airways collapse) after which flow falls very slowly. Also shown in (b) is a loop representing quiet tidal breathing. It is clear that every expiration is limited by maximum flow. Expiratory wheezing or purse lip breathing would be expected. There is some inspiratory reserve of flow but hardly any expiratory reserve. Ventilation could be increased slightly by adopting an even higher lung volume and be speeding up inspiration.

(c) *Fixed intrathoracic large airways obstruction:* for example, tracheal compression by a mediastinal tumour. Here the peak inspiratory and expiratory flows have been truncated in a characteristic pattern.

(d) *Variable extrathoracic obstruction.* Severe extrathoracic obstruction results in inspiratory collapse of the airway below the obstruction (but still outside the thorax). In this example expiration is normal, and this suggests a variable check-valve mechanism such as might be caused by bilateral vocal cord paralysis.

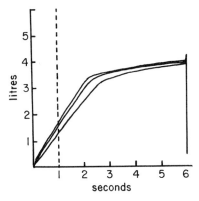

Fig. 7.9. Large (central) airways obstruction. Typical tracing obtained with a Vitalograph spirometer. The subject has made three maximal forced expirations. Each shows a striking straight section which then changes relatively abruptly, at about the same volume to follow the expected curve of the forced expiratory spirogram. The straight section is not as reproducible as a normal spirogram. A 'family' of similar tracings is thus obtained, each with straight and curved sections. *Explanation:* Over the straight section flow is limited by the fixed intrathoracic localized obstruction. This is little influenced by lung recoil so the critical flow is similar during expiration and the spirogram appears straight. A lung volume is eventually reached where maximum flow is even lower than that permitted by the central obstruction. The ordinary forced expiratory spirogram is described after this point. In the example shown there must be an element of diffuse airways obstruction, as forced expiratory time is somewhat prolonged (see also Fig. 7.8c).

therefore of some importance to be able to recognize the pattern produced by fixed intrathoracic large airway obstruction using an ordinary spirometer (Fig. 7.9).

BLOOD GAS MEASUREMENT

Alveolar ventilation

Measurement of P_{CO_2}

The only satisfactory means of assessing the adequacy of ventilation is measurement of alveolar or arterial P_{CO_2} (see p. 19).

Measurement of P_{CO_2} by rebreathing technique

Changes in arterial P_{CO_2} are mirrored by changes in mixed venous P_{CO_2} (provided CO_2 production and cardiac output are not grossly disturbed). The rebreathing technique first described by Campbell and Howell permits mixed venous P_{CO_2} to be measured quickly and conveniently at the bedside or in the consulting room by non-invasive means (Fig. 7.10). The apparatus is cheap and easily maintained—features of relevance in developing countries.

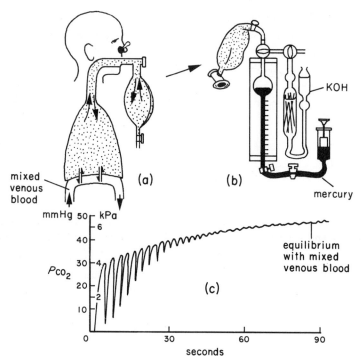

Fig. 7.10. Rebreathe P_{CO_2}. The subject rebreathes from a small bag filled with oxygen until equilibrium between the bag, lungs and venous blood is achieved (a). The CO_2 concentration of the contents of the bag is then measured with modified Haldane gas analysis apparatus (b). (c) shows the result of rapid CO_2 analysis of the bag contents during the procedure. Equilibrium is achieved after about 90 seconds. After this there is a very slow rise in CO_2 concentration of the bag (and the subject's arterial blood). The value for P_{CO_2} obtained at 90 seconds approximates to that of mixed venous blood.

Procedure (abbreviated version of the method)
1   A rubber bag is filled with about 2 litres of O_2.
2   The patient breathes quietly in and out of the bag for 90 seconds.
3   The CO_2 concentration of the mixture in the bag is measured using a modified Haldane apparatus.
During the period of rebreathing the concentration of CO_2 in the bag rises sharply to start with but only very slowly towards the end of 90 seconds (Fig. 7.10). By this time there is equilibrium (with respect to CO_2) between the blood in the pulmonary capillaries (mixed venous blood) and the air going back and forth between bag and lungs. Mixed venous P_{CO_2} is then the same as the P_{CO_2} of the contents of the bag. The latter is obtained by multiplying the percentage concentration of CO_2 in the bag by the available barometric pressure (barometric pressure less water vapour pressure at 37°C).

The mixed venous P_{CO_2} measured by this means is about 1.2 kPa (9 mmHg) higher than the arterial P_{CO_2}. For most clinical purposes it is justifiable and convenient to subtract this amount and to quote the result as an 'arterial' P_{CO_2} (rebreathe method).

Arterial P_{CO_2} is normally between 4.8 and 6.1 kPa (36 and 46 mmHg).

Measurement of arterial P_{CO_2} by electrode

Arterial P_{CO_2} is almost always measured with an electrode of the Severinghaus type. It is now common for this to be miniaturized and incorporated within an automated system, together with electrodes measuring pH and P_{CO_2} enabling small samples to be handled in a standardized manner. The CO_2 electrode comprises a pH electrode with a thin film of bicarbonate kept in position over its tip by a polypropylene membrane and fitted into a small sample chamber. When blood comes into contact with the membrane, CO_2 diffuses rapidly across into the bicarbonate solution and the pH in the solution stabilizes at a value related to the sample P_{CO_2}. The meter is calibrated to read P_{CO_2} directly and the electrode is calibrated using gases of solutions of known P_{CO_2}.

Measurement of P_{CO_2} by calculation from pH and bicarbonate level

It is now quite common for pH, P_{CO_2} and plasma bicarbonate all to be measured directly in the laboratory. If any two of these are known the third may be calculated or read from a graphical representation of the Henderson–Hasselbalch equation such as that shown in Fig. 7.15.

Measurement of P_{O_2}

See p. 73.

ACID–BASE BALANCE

Background

Relationship between $[H^+]$ and P_{CO_2}

If a solution of bicarbonate is brought into equilibrium with several gas mixtures in turn, each with a different P_{CO_2}, and if hydrogen ion concentration, $[H^+]$, is measured after each equilibration it will be found that there is a direct relationship between P_{CO_2} and $[H^+]$ (Fig. 7.11). This relationship between P_{CO_2} and $[H^+]$ is a representation in graphic terms of the Henderson-Hasselbalch equation.

Dissolved CO_2 forms carbonic acid which dissociates into H_2O and CO_2 in a constant relationship:

$$K = \frac{[H^+][HCO_3^-]}{[H_2CO_3]}$$

The $[H^+]$ can be expressed thus:

$$[H^+] \propto \frac{[H_2CO_3]}{HCO_3^-}$$

The concentration of H_2CO_3 is directly related to the prevailing partial pressure of CO_2 so the formula can be written:

$$[H^+] \propto \frac{P_{CO_2}}{[HCO_3^-]}$$

In other words there is a direct linear relationship between P_{CO_2} and $[H^+]$ of the sort shown in Fig. 7.11.

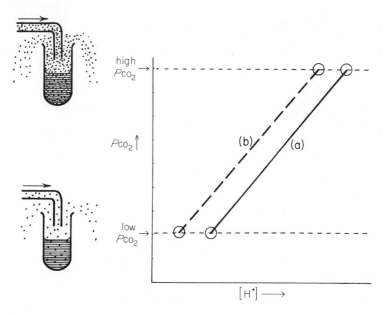

Fig. 7.11. Relationship between P_{CO_2} and hydrogen ion concentration in a bicarbonate solution. A solution of bircarbonate is equilibrated with two gases of known P_{CO_2}. H^+ is measured. (a) shows the relationship between P_{CO_2} and H^+ for that solution (the buffer line). (b) shows the relationship for a solution with a higher bicarbonate concentration.

If in this model some bicarbonate is added to the solution and the same procedure repeated, it will again be found that there is a direct relationship between P_{CO_2} and $[H^+]$ but at each level of P_{CO_2} the $[H^+]$ will be lower than previously ((b) in Fig. 7.11).

$[H^+]$ is generally expressed as pH, which is the negative logarithm of $[H^+]$, but this does not prevent a convenient linear plot of pH against P_{CO_2} if the latter is given a logarithmic scale (Fig. 7.12). For any particular bicarbonate solution a line may be plotted which describes the relationship between pH and P_{CO_2} in that solution. Interpretation of acid–base status requires knowledge of pH, P_{CO_2} and bicarbonate concentration.

Bicarbonate concentration

Bicarbonate concentration can be calculated if P_{CO_2} and pH are known (see Fig. 7.15) and it can also be measured directly: the *actual bicarbonate* concentration. *Standard bicarbonate* is a calculated value indicating what the bicarbonate concentration would be at a standard P_{CO_2} (of 5.3 kPa or 40 mmHg). Two other expressions can also be obtained by calculation if haemoglobin is known; they are *base excess* and *buffer base*. These expressions recognize the fact that there are other buffers apart from bicarbonate in the blood. There is little to choose between these parameters of the buffering capacity of blood—actual or standard bicarbonate, buffer base and base excess—it is a matter of individual preference which is employed. They all behave in a similar fashion in disturbances of acid–base homeostasis.

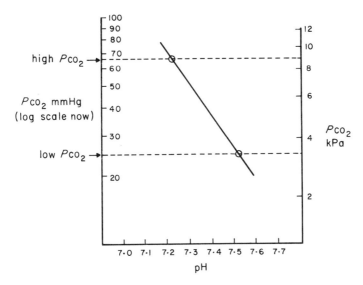

Fig. 7.12. Plot of P_{CO_2} and pH. This figure shows the same relationship as in Fig. 6.8. The $[H^+]$ scale has been converted into the more widely used pH. pH is the negative logarithm of $[H^+]$. High $[H^+]$ is now on the left and low $[H^+]$ on the right and the buffer line now slopes the other way. Because pH is a logarithmic term, P_{CO_2} has been given a logarithmic scale so that the straight line relationship between the two is retained.

Review of patterns of disturbance of acid–base balance

Although there are other buffering systems in the body, the CO_2 bicarbonate system is the most accessible and the most responsive: for clinical purposes, disturbances of acid–base balance are usually discussed in terms of the changes observed in it. pH is determined by the ratio of P_{CO_2} to bicarbonate concentration. Changes in pH which are caused primarily by an alteration in P_{CO_2} are termed **respiratory**; P_{CO_2} is determined by alveolar ventilation. Changes in pH which are brought about by changes in bicarbonate concentration are termed 'non-respiratory' or, by convention, **metabolic**. The renal tubule modulates bicarbonate concentration in response to the prevailing P_{CO_2} but this is very slow. (The kidney has other important functions in acid–base regulations which will not be reviewed here.)

Acid–base diagrams

It is usual to employ a diagram to assist discussion of this topic. The three variables: pH, P_{CO_2} and bicarbonate, can be displayed by several graphical means, all based upon the Henderson–Hasselbalch equation and all having about equal merit. The format already described, with axes comprising log P_{CO_2} and pH, is a convenient base from which to start. In the following section, outlining the principal types of disturbance, the reader should refer frequently firstly to Fig. 7.13 which allows the three components to be related to each other and secondly to Fig. 7.16 which shows the direction in which disturbances from the normal are observed to occur in well-defined experimental or clinical

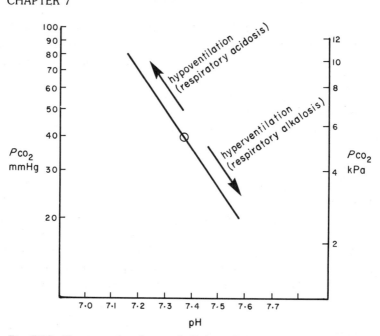

Fig. 7.13. 'Respiratory' acidosis and alkalosis. If the bicarbonate concentration remains unaltered then changes in pH of the blood must be due to changes in P_{CO_2}. P_{CO_2} is determined by alveolar ventilation. Hyperventilation causes a fall in P_{CO_2} and a rise in pH and movement of the arterial point downwards along the buffer line as shown above. Hypoventilation causes an increase in P_{CO_2} and an upward movement of the arterial point.

situations, where there is an uncomplicated 'pure' disturbance of either ventilation (respiratory) or bicarbonate (metabolic) compounds.

Respiratory acidosis (acute)

Reduction in alveolar ventilation causes an increase in arterial P_{CO_2}. In the short term there is insufficient time for renal compensation by reabsorption of bicarbonate so that the bicarbonate concentration remains almost unchanged. The change in pH is entirely due to change in P_{CO_2} and the arterial blood point is plotted in the direction indicated in Fig. 7.16.

Note: In practice the changes *in vivo* are slightly different from the expected changes because of the operation of other buffering systems apart from bicarbonate (see Fig. 7.16).

There is *some* increase in the bicarbonate level because increase in P_{CO_2} leads to increase in dissolved CO_2. Dissolved CO_2 is a small part of the total and the change in bicarbonate in pure respiratory disturbances is small (Fig. 7.15).

Causes. An acute underventilation–obstruction of the airway, opiate overdosage, massive neurological damage, paralysis, etc.

Pattern. pH reduced, P_{CO_2} raised, bicarbonate normal.

Respiratory alkalosis

Alveolar hyperventilation causes a fall in P_{CO_2} and the arterial point is plotted in the direction indicated (Fig. 7.16). Bicarbonate concentration is virtually unchanged and the change in pH is due principally to the change in P_{CO_2}. In long-sustained respiratory alkalosis there is some renal adaption with reduction in plasma bicarbonate (restoring pH towards normal) but this compensation is slow and partial.

   Causes. Any form of acute hyperventilation—pulmonary embolism, acute asthma, salicylate poisoning, anxiety and hysteria, etc.

   Pattern. pH raised, P_{CO_2} reduced, bicarbonate normal.

Metabolic acidosis

The primary disturbance is generally an increase in acid. This has an effect on the equilibrium $H^+ + HCO_3^- \rightleftharpoons H_2O + CO_2$ pushing it to the right. The CO_2 produced is removed by increased ventilation and the net result is a lowering of plasma bicarbonate. An acute fall in bicarbonate results in an acute shift of the 'buffer line' to the left (Fig. 7.14). In practice the resulting fall in pH causes further respiratory stimulation so that the P_{CO_2} is reduced promptly and the arterial point moves in the direction indicated in Fig. 7.16—the lowering of P_{CO_2} ensures that

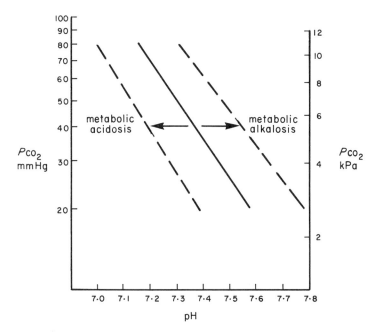

Fig. 7.14. 'Metabolic' acidosis and alkalosis. The position of the buffer line has already been noted to be dependent upon the bicarbonate concentration of the solution. Changes in the level of plasma bicarbonate are the result of non-respiratory metabolic changes. pH change, which is largely the result of altered bicarbonate buffering, is loosely referred to as 'metabolic'. The buffer line moves to the left with fall in bicarbonate (metabolic acidosis) and to the right with increase in bicarbonate (metabolic alkalosis). In the Siggard–Anderson plot of P_{CO_2} and pH various indices which reflect bicarbonate content and buffering capacity of the blood can be read directly from the intersection of the line with special nomograms.

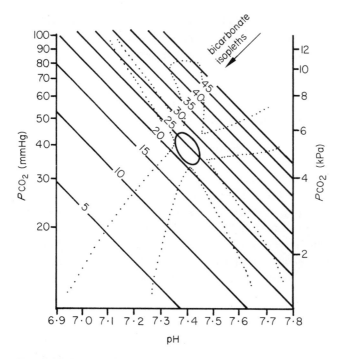

Fig. 7.15. Relationship between P_{CO_2}, pH and actual bicarbonate ion concentration (compare with Figs 7.13 and 7.14). If two of the indices are known the third may be estimated from the diagram. The oval indicates normal values. The dotted areas indicate the direction of the main patterns of acid–base disturbance; these are shown in Fig. 7.16.

the change in pH is much less dramatic than would otherwise have been the case. This respiratory compensation is an inevitable accompaniment in metabolic acidosis—acute and chronic—unless there is some other factor limiting ventilatory function or responsiveness.

Causes. Diabetic ketoacidosis, acute circulatory failure and other forms of lactic acidosis, renal tubular acidosis, etc.

Pattern. pH reduced, P_{CO_2} reduced, bicarbonate reduced.

Metabolic alkalosis

Increase in bicarbonate concentration has the effect of moving the 'buffer line' to the right (Fig. 7.14). In practice the P_{CO_2} usually increases a little, so that the change in pH is a little less than would otherwise have occurred. This compensatory fall in alveolar ventilation is usually slight and the correction partial.

Causes. Administration of excessive alkali, loss of acid through vomiting, reabsorption of bicarbonate, e.g. in hypokalaemia.

Pattern. pH raised, P_{CO_2} normal or slightly raised, bicarbonate raised.

Chronic respiratory acidosis

(Sometimes called chronic compensated respiratory acidosis.) If underventilation from whatever cause is sustained for some days, renal tubular reabsorption

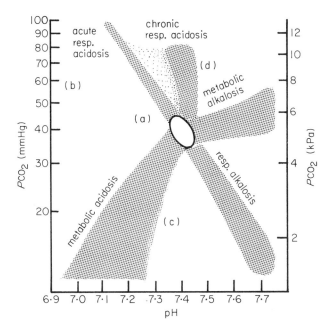

Fig. 7.16. Acid–base disturbances. The oval indicates the normal position. The shaded areas indicate the direction of observed 'pure' or uncomplicated disturbances of acid–base balance. Bicarbonate levels are omitted for clarity but are shown in Fig. 7.15. Letters (a)–(d) are referred to in the text (see Interpretation of mixed disturbances).

of bicarbonate will achieve significant elevation of plasma bicarbonate level, and this has the effect of correcting the acidosis. The arterial point moves on the diagram toward the right (Fig. 7.16). The correction is usually not complete, so that the pH remains a little low.

Causes. Any cause of sustained hypoventilation—most commonly chronic obstructive pulmonary disease.

Pattern. pH normal or slightly reduced, P_{CO_2} elevated, bicarbonate elevated.

Mixed disturbances

These are quite common. Mixed disturbances are represented in Fig. 7.16 by the spaces between the limbs of the shaded area; the nature of the mixed disturbance is indicated by the adjacent limbs. For example, point (a) in Fig. 7.16 (low pH, normal P_{CO_2}, low bicarbonate) indicates a mixed metabolic and respiratory acidosis. Note that an element of respiratory acidosis can be deduced, even though the P_{CO_2} is not significantly raised. This is because the P_{CO_2} is higher than would have been expected in an individual with a 'pure' metabolic disturbance.

Interpretation of mixed disturbances

In mixed disturbances there are usually a number of possible interpretations. For example point (a) (Fig. 7.16) is equally compatible with the following totally different clinical situations:

1   A patient with acute pulmonary oedema who is severely hypoxic and also in low-output cardiac failure. The metabolic acidosis reflects probable lactic acidosis from critically low peripheral oxygen delivery (Chapter 26) and the P_{CO_2} suggests that, despite the ventilatory stimuli stemming from the acidosis, hypoxia and the pulmonary oedema, the patient's ability to hyperventilate is compromised.

2   A patient in renal failure with accompanying acidosis who has been given a narcotic agent which has suppressed the ventilatory response to the acidosis.

Unless the clinical situation is known beforehand, it is generally not possible to interpret the acid–base data beyond describing the components of the mixed disturbance.

Further examples of mixed disturbances (Fig. 7.16)

Point (b). This could represent the situation soon after a cardiac arrest where a severe lactic acidosis exists and the emergency artificial ventilation or the patient's spontaneous ventilation has been insufficient.

Point (c). This could represent the situation in severe aspirin poisoning where aspirin-induced hyerventilation has been complicated by aspirin-induced metabolic acidosis.

Point (d). This could represent the situation of an individual with chronic ventilatory failure due to chronic obstructive lung disease (e.g. previously with P_{CO_2} 75 mmHg, 10 kPa and pH 7.4) who is stimulated to increase ventilation shortly before the sample was taken by physiotherapy, pulmonary embolism, IPPV, etc.

Scope and limitations

Acid–base data in the acute situation:

1   Has limited diagnostic potential considered on its own.

2   May help by indicating that a disturbance is mixed rather than simple.

3   May provide a useful indication of the severity of a disturbance.

4   May provide useful information concerning the trend of a disturance.

5   Only rarely requires direct treatment. Almost always the disturbance is managed by taking measures to reverse the primary process giving rise to the abnormality, rather than by giving acid or alkali.

ARTERIAL OXYGENATION

Oxygen saturation

Oxygenation can now be measured non-invasively and continuously, using a pulse oximeter. This is a relatively expensive instrument which measures saturation by transillumination of either a finger or an earlobe, and measures the transmitted light at particular wavelengths by use of filters in the probe. Reduced and oxygenated blood have different absorption patterns (responsible for the change in colour in cyanosis).

The instrument gives a continuous digital display of saturation and a pulse signal is also produced. Alarms can be set to signal high or low saturation or pulse rate. Some instruments have recording facilities which can be used overnight to assess sleep apnoea.

Oximeters are very valuable in the assessment of ill patients and in adjusting oxygen requirements. Blood gas estimations (below) are, by contrast, invasive, labour intensive and sometimes take a long time where staff and laboratories are not readily to hand.

Saturation is sometimes measured on blood specimens—especially during cardiac catheterization in the investigation of shunts.

Arterial oxygen tension (Pao_2)

A note on arterial blood sampling

Sampling from the radial artery at the wrist has advantages over other sites such as the femoral or brachial arteries:

1   The artery is readily palpable.
2   There is no big vein accompanying it.
3   It is easily compressed against the radius after puncture.
4   If a haematoma does develop, it is soon detected and not hidden beneath clothes.
5   In the unlikely event of the artery becoming damaged there is an excellent collateral circulation via the palmar arch.

There is no need to transfix the artery by a vertical stab; it may easily be entered by an angled approach along the line of the vessel (Fig. 7.17). For clinical purposes it is perfectly acceptable to use a small plastic syringe and a fine needle, provided only light suction is applied and the specimen is analysed promptly. Use of a fine needle followed by good compression causes minimal trauma to the artery and repeated sampling from the same site is possible.

Capillary blood sampled from a warmed earlobe or finger yields blood gas values very close to those of arterial blood and this may be useful in small children.

Measurement

Arterial blood oxygen tension (arterial Po_2 or Pao_2) is measured using a Clark-type platinum polarigraphic electrode, which comprises a platinum cathode and a silver anode in a tiny electrolytic cell, biased by a small voltage and separated from the blood sample by a thin membrane. The current output of the cell is proportional to the availability of oxygen molecules at the platinum surface and hence to Po_2. Transcutaneous oxygen electrodes are now available but they require expert handling and have limited clinical uses.

Interpretation

The normal range in healthy young adults is from about 10.5–14 kPa (80–105 mmHg). In older or immobile individuals, lower values would be expected even in the absence of notable lung disease. Cyanosis in individuals with normal haemoglobin concentration and pH begins to be evident at an arterial Po_2 below about 6.4 kPa (48 mmHg), at which level saturation is about 80%. It is very obvious below 5.3 kPa (40 mmHg) when saturation is below 75%.

Arterial oxygen Po_2 falls reciprocally with the increase in Pco_2 when there is overall (alveolar) underventilation (see Fig. 2.7). Hypoxaemia is also caused by

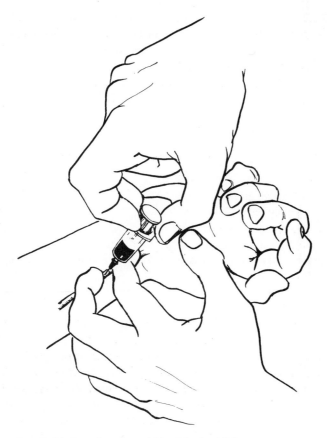

Fig. 7.17. Sampling arterial blood from radial artery.

regional underventilation. One form of this is represented by a widened spread of ventilation/perfusion ratios—a common disturbance in lung disease (see Fig. 2.10). Sometimes hypoxaemia during exercise reveals impairment of pulmonary function. Faster transit of blood through the alveolar capillaries and greater desaturation of the venous blood returned to the lungs exaggerates the effects of impaired gas transfer and of ventilation/perfusion disturbance respectively. For a discussion of hypoxia see Chapter 31.

Saturation or tension?

There is little to choose between the two forms of oxygen measurement up to a Po_2 of about 9.3 kPa (70 mmHg) and one may be obtained from the other if the pH of the blood is known. Oxygen tension is more widely used, perhaps because it is also useful in the higher range above a Po_2 of 70 mmHg, where saturation hardly changes at all.

SI units—pressure

The unit of pressure employed is the kilopascal (kPa) which is equivalent to 7.5 mmHg. To convert kPa to mmHg multiply by 7.5. To convert mmHg to kPa multiply by 0.13 (add one-third and divide by 10).

TRANSFER FACTOR

Transfer factor (T_{LCO}) is also known as diffusing capacity (D_{LCO}). It expresses the overall ability of the lungs to transfer carbon monoxide from the alveoli to the blood. Another term, K_{CO} (transfer coefficient), is an expression of this ability corrected for the volume of lung (see below).

Background

The important influence of ventilation/perfusion relationships upon gas exchange has already been noted. At one time the ability of gases to diffuse across the alveolar–capillary membrane was thought to be the principal factor limiting gas exchange in disease. This led to the concept of 'diffusing capacity'—a measurement of the rate at which gas passes from the alveoli to the bloodstream.

Diffusing capacity = quantity of gas transported across in each minute for every unit of pressure gradient.

The measurement was found to be clinically useful. Later when it was realized that many factors apart from diffusion affected gas transfer in the lungs, the expression was renamed 'transfer factor'.

Oxygen transport is obviously of most interest to clinicians, but special difficulties are encountered in studying this gas because transport stops when haemoglobin becomes saturated. The difficulties can be partly overcome by using very low concentrations of oxygen, which do not permit saturation of the blood, but other problems are then encountered. Carbon monoxide is usually employed in the measurement of transfer factor. Very low concentrations are used so that the blood remains avid for the gas during its passage through the pulmonary capillary.

Outline of measurement

Two pieces of information are required:
1 The quantity of CO transferred per minute.
2 The pressure gradient across the alveolar membrane (this is in effect the alveolar partial pressure of CO as blood CO tension can be ignored).

Steady–state method

The patient breathes air containing a known low concentration of CO from a Douglas bag and expired air is collected in another Douglas bag over a timed period of some minutes. The rate of CO transfer (a) can be calculated from the difference between inspired and expired concentrations. The alveolar CO level (b) is more difficult to establish because it varies during each breath, as CO is lost into the blood. A mean alveolar level can be calculated by estimating deadspace ventilation for CO_2 and assuming that this same volume was filled with unchanged inspired CO mixture. The shortfall in expired CO must then be entirely due to a lower concentration in the alveolar fraction, which can be calculated.

Single-breath method

This is more widely used. The patient takes a measured breath containing small amounts of both helium (He) and CO, holds the breath for 10 seconds and then breathes out. A sample of expired air is obtained (after the initial deadspace air has escaped) and the concentration of CO is measured.

The expired concentration of He is lower than the inspired because it has been diluted by mixture with air already in the lungs at the beginning of the breath (but, being insoluble, no actual absorption has occurred). The volume of air in the lungs during the breath-hold can be calculated. The expired concentration of CO is also lower than the inspired level but the fall is proportionately greater than in the case of He because some CO has been absorbed into the bloodstream.

The calculation of the rate of CO transfer (a) and alveolar CO tension (b) is based on the assumption that the CO is instantly diluted in the same proportion as He at the beginning of the breath-hold and that the alveolar CO concentration then falls exponentially towards the expired level (Fig. 7.18). Integration yields an expression of the relationship between rate of fall of concentration of CO and alveolar concentration of CO. When account is taken of the volume of air involved, the rate of CO transfer in millilitres per minute per mmHg partial pressure of CO can readily be calculated.

Normal values and units

Transfer factor is normally of the order of 20 ml min^{-1} mmHg^{-1}, but varies with age, sex and body size. Transfer factor in SI units is expressed as mmol

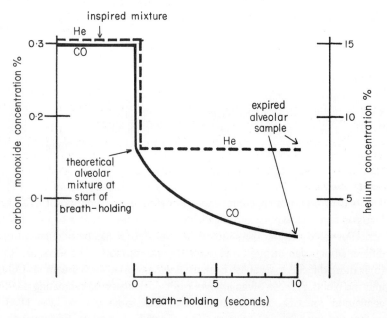

Fig. 7.18. Measurement of transfer factor by the single-breath method. Schematic representation of the helium and carbon monoxide concentrations in the inspired mixture and in alveolar air during breath-holding.

min^{-1} kPa^{-1} and is normally of the order of 6.7 mmol min^{-1}kPa^{-1} (to convert from SI units to 'old' units, multiply by 3).

Factors influencing transfer factor

Transfer factor is influenced by many considerations which include:

1   Ventilation/perfusion imbalance—in disease much of the inspired gas may not reach perfused alveoli.
2   The thickness of the alveolar–capillary membrane.
3   The area of the membrane.
4   The pulmonary capillary blood volume.
5   The haemoglobin concentration.
6   The rate of reaction of CO with haemoglobin.

Impairment of transfer factor does not necessarily mean impairment of diffusion. Despite the number of factors which perturb it, transfer factor remains an extremely useful measurement (the same could be said of the ESR).

Transfer coefficient (Kco)

This is obtained by dividing transfer factor by the alveolar volume (the volume in which the He became diluted is usually used for this purpose). It is an expression of gas transferring ability per unit volume of lung. It assists interpretation when a reduced transfer factor is encountered. For example, an individual who has had one lung removed will have a reduced transfer factor but a normal Kco; diseases which cause lung shrinkage produce the same effect. Where, however, the lung parenchyma becomes damaged by disease (for example in fibrosing alveolitis or in emphysema), lowered transfer factor is accompanied by lowering of the Kco. Normal values for Kco depend on age and sex. Fit young adults have values around 1.5 (SI units are mmol min^{-1} kPa^{-1} litre^{-1}); the very elderly may have normal values as low as 1.0.

Interpretation

In the presence of normal ventilatory function, the finding of a significantly reduced transfer factor is a strong indication of the presence of a parenchymal lung disorder involving the alveoli or their blood supply.

In the presence of a restrictive ventilatory defect, an impairment of transfer factor suggests fibrosis, oedema or infiltration if the reduction is more severe than would be expected from simple reduction in lung volume—that is to say, if Kco is also reduced to about the same extent. In diffuse parenchymal disease, measurement of transfer factor may provide a crude index of severity and progress.

The significance of impairment of transfer factor in the presence of an obstructive ventilatory defect is more difficult to assess and depends to some extent on the relative severity of the two defects and upon clinical circumstances. Persistent impairment of transfer factor and Kco provides support for a diagnosis of emphysema.

EXERCISE TESTS

Exercise tests may provide valuable insight into the performance of the cardiorespiratory apparatus as a whole. Often very useful information may be obtained by merely walking with a patient on the level or up stairs. More precise information is obtained if pulse, minute ventilation and oxygen uptake are measured during graded exercise, using an ergometer. Measurement of maximum exercise tolerance is useful but not without hazard in the elderly and those with cardiac disease. It is sometimes helpful to measure arterial blood gas tensions or steady-state transfer factor during exercise, particularly when the cause of dyspnoea is obscure.

SUMMARY OF THE BASIC TESTS OF PULMONARY FUNCTION

PEF	Peak flow meter	Allows detection of major degrees of airways obstruction. Its major role is in recording patterns of *change* in severity of obstruction by means of frequent recordings in the home and at work. This helps both diagnosis and assessment of treatment.
FVC FEV$_1$	Spirometer, e.g. Vitalograph	Permits recognition of defects of ventilation and provides information about their nature, e.g. obstructive or restrictive.
P_{CO_2}	Arterial blood/ CO_2 electrode	Allows assessment of alveolar ventilation. Together with pH and/or bicarbonate concentration, gives information relating to acid–base status.
Oxygen saturation	Pulse oximeter	Rapid or continuous assessment of oxygenation
P_{O_2}	Arterial blood/ O_2 electrode	Assessment of oxygenation. Allows assessment of ventilation/perfusion mismatch.
Transfer factor and K_{CO}	Steady-state or single-breath methods	Provide useful non-specific information relating to gas transfer function of the lungs which may not be readily gained by other means.
Exercise testing		Assessment of global cardiopulmonary performance.

Chapter 8
Elements of Radiology of the Chest

The interpretation of physical signs, particularly of local disease, is a valuable skill but far from infallible, and the ready availability of chest radiography in developed countries makes it important that the clinician should be familiar with the elements of interpreting chest radiographs, almost as an extension of physical examination.

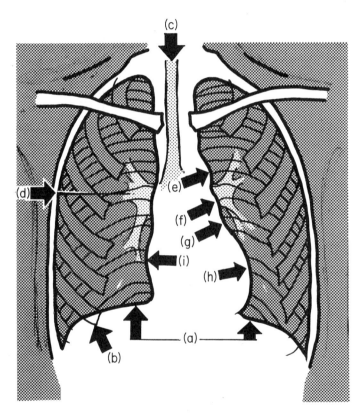

Fig. 8.1. Diagram of chest X-ray (PA view). The right hemidiaphragm is 1–3 cm higher than the left (a) and on full inspiration it is intersected by the shadow of the anterior part of the sixth rib (b). The trachea (c) is vertical and central or very slightly to the right. The horizontal fissure (d) is found in the position shown, or slightly lower and should be truly horizontal. It is a very valuable marker of change in volume of any part of the right lung. The left border of the cardiac shadow comprises: (e) aorta; (f) pulmonary artery; (g) concavity overlying the left atrial appendage; (h) left ventricle. The right border of the cardiac shadow normally overlies the right atrium (i) and above that the superior vena cava.

The normal chest X-ray

Some of the more useful landmarks of the normal chest X-ray are indicated in Fig. 8.1. It is desirable that the film should be examined systematically to avoid missing useful information. The centring and penetration of the film should be quickly noted as these factors have considerable influence on the shape of the heart and mediastinum and upon the character of the vascular markings in the lung fields. The shape and bony structures of the chest wall should be surveyed and the position of the diaphragms and trachea noted. The heart's shape and size and the appearance of the mediastinum and hilar shadows are examined. On the right side the horizontal fissure is a particularly useful landmark and should be carefully identified. The size, shape and disposition of the vascular shadows are next noted and the pattern of the lung markings in different zones carefully

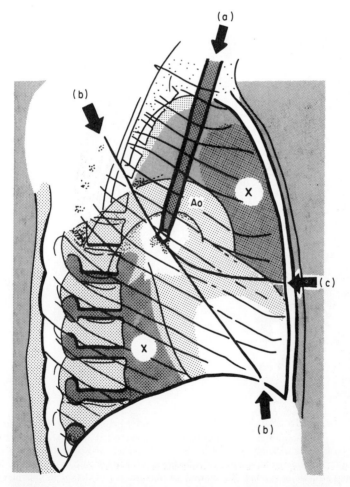

Fig. 8.2. Diagram of chest X-ray (lateral view). (a) Trachea. Ao: aorta. (b) Oblique fissure. (c) Horizontal fissure. It is useful to note that in a normal lateral view the radiodensity of the lung field above and in front of the cardiac shadow is about the same as that below and behind (X).

compared. Whenever a localized abnormality of any sort is evident or suspected, a lateral film becomes essential for accurate localization. The main features of the lateral film are indicated in Fig. 8.2.

Collapse

Collapse of a lobe is usually evident from shift of landmarks (fissures, mediastinum, blood vessels) and the collapsed lobe itself *may* cast a character-istic shadow (Fig. 8.3). However, the changes are often very difficult to see on a postero-anterior (PA) chest film and lateral or even oblique or lordotic views may be required to identify the collapsed lobe. Note that in right middle lobe collapse, there may be little to see on the PA film apart from lack of definition of the right border of the heart. This is a useful sign which helps to distinguish it from lower lobe collapse, where the right border of the heart remains clearly defined. In left lower lobe collapse, there may be a triangular area of increased

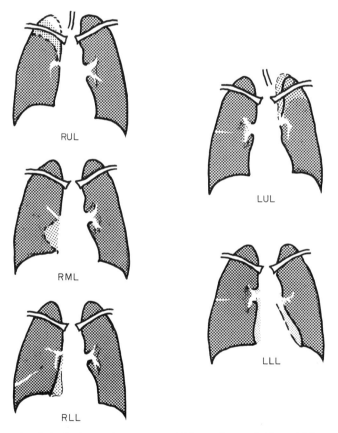

Fig. 8.3. Radiographic patterns of lobar collapse. Collapsed lobes occupy a surprisingly small volume and are commonly overlooked on the chest X-ray. In the above diagram note the position of the diaphragms in each case. Helpful information may be provided by the position of the trachea, the hilar vascular shadows and the horizontal fissure. RUL, right upper lobe; RML, right middle lobe; RLL, right lower lobe; LUL, left upper lobe; LLL, left lower lobe.

density visible behind the heart shadow, but this may not be evident and lateral or oblique views may be required. In complete collapse of the left lower lobe, some small upward curving linear shadows often appear in the left lower zone, just outside the apex of the heart on the PA film.

Consolidation

Consolidated areas of lung appear as uniform areas of opacification which conform to the outline of a lobe or segment; there is often a variable amount of collapse present.

The silhouette sign (Fig. 8.4)

The sharp edge of structures such as heart, mediastinum and diaphragm is due to the contrast between aerated lung and pleural surface. When there is abnormal shadowing overlying such a border in a postero-anterior X-ray, the silhouette sign may enable the observer to decide where exactly the abnormal area is in the chest. If the sharp outline, for example that of the heart border, is lost then the abnormal pulmonary shadowing must be adjacent to the structure rather than merely projected so as to overly it. If the sharp outline, or silhouette, is visible through the pulmonary shadowing then the reverse is true and the shadowing does not abut against the structure at that point.

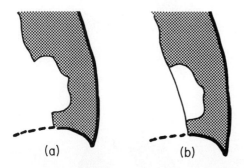

(a)   (b)

Fig. 8.4. The silhouette sign. Diagram showing abnormal lung shadowing in the left lower zone. Where the sharp outline of mediastinal structures or diaphragm is lost because of abnormal lung opacification, it can be concluded that the shadowing is immediately adjacent to the structure (and vice versa). In example (a) the shadowing must be anterior and next to the heart as the sharp outline of the heart is lost. In (b) it must be posterior as the heart outline is preserved.

Pleural effusion

Small pleural effusions (of 300–500 ml) cause no more than blunting of a costophrenic angle; larger effusions cast a characteristic shadow with a curved upper edge rising into the axilla (even though the upper level in fact runs horizontally round the chest wall). Very often, effusions cause uniform opacification of one side of the chest and there may be shift of the mediastinum towards the opposite side.

Fibrosis

Localized fibrosis causes streaky shadows with evidence of traction upon neighbouring structures. Upper lobe fibrosis causes traction upon the trachea and also elevation of the hilar vascular shadows. Generalized interstitial fibrosis produces a hazy shadowing, sometimes with a fine reticular (net-like) or nodular pattern. Advanced interstitial fibrosis results in a honeycomb change which is apparent on the chest X-ray as diffuse opacification containing multiple circular translucencies a few millimetres in diameter.

Rounded shadows

Carcinoma of the lung is by far the commonest cause of rounded shadows of the lung; other causes include:

Metastatic tumour (? multiple).
Tuberculoma (? calcification).
Lung abscess (usually cavitates in time).
Pulmonary infarct (not usually round; tends to disappear).
Rare primary benign tumours (haematoma, adenoma, etc.).
Encysted interlobar effusion.
Hydatid cyst (rare, ? hair-like outline).
Arteriovenous malformation (? adjacent vascular shadow).

Early thoracotomy is indicated in the case of rounded shadows without obvious cause, as they are so often due to surgically curable carcinoma and diagnosis is commonly impossible by other means.

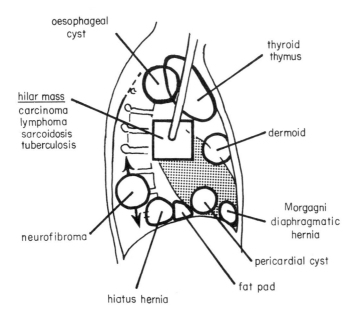

Fig. 8.5. Mediastinal masses. Diagram of lateral view of the chest, indicating the sites favoured by some of the commoner mediastinal masses.

Miliary mottling

This term is used to describe the appearance produced by numerous minute opacities in the lung fields 1–3 mm in diameter (which may resemble millet seeds)—an appearance which may be caused by a very large number of pathological processes, some of the commoner causes being:

Miliary tuberculosis.
Pneumoconiosis.
Sarcoidosis.
Fibrosing alveolitis.
Lymphangitis carcinomatosa.
Pulmonary oedema (usually perihilar, transient and accompanied by larger fluffy shadows).

Mediastinal masses

Metastatic tumour or lymphomatous involvement of the mediastinal lymph nodes is the commonest cause of an abnormal mediastinal shadow, but other masses may cast shadows and the particular site of the mass may give a clue to its cause (Fig. 8.5).

SPECIAL TECHNIQUES

Tomography

In this technique the film and the X-ray tube move in opposite directions along parallel axes pivoting about a point situated at the level of particular interest within the chest. The movement causes blurring of shadows except those situated in the plane of the pivotal point, which remain fairly sharply defined, giving the effect of a cross-section at this level. Adjustment of the apparatus allows several 'cuts' to be made in the region under scrutiny. The technique may yield useful information in the investigation of pulmonary opacities, particularly those situated near the hilum which may be difficult to distinguish from vascular shadows. Tomography may give a clearer outline of a pulmonary shadow, reveal the presence of calcification or cavitation not evident on a plain film and may demonstrate the relationship between a shadow and adjacent bronchi and blood vessels.

Bronchography

A variety of techniques are employed for the introduction of an iodized oily contrast medium into the trachea, generally under local anaesthesia. It is an uncomfortable procedure. Immediately after instillation of about 20 ml (for one side) of the medium the patient is rolled and tipped into lateral, supine, prone and head-down positions to fill the main bronchopulmonary segments. Oblique, postero-anterior and lateral views are taken. Bronchography may be useful where it is important to confirm the presence or extent of bronchiectasis or in the investigation of bronchial obstruction especially where this is beyond the range of the bronchoscope. Bronchography should not be undertaken lightly— particularly in the presence of asthma or severe respiratory disability.

Fluoroscopy ('screening')

This is generally carried out with the aid of image-intensifying equipment. It permits movement of the lungs and diaphragms to be observed which may be important in the investigation of suspected diaphragmatic paralysis. Movement of the paralysed side is defective and if the patient sniffs, the paralysed diaphragm will show paradoxical upward movement. Screening may also permit air-trapping in large localized areas of lung to be observed.

Computerized axial tomography (CAT or CT)

CT has had rather less impact on the diagnosis of pulmonary disease than it has had on disease elsewhere, probably because the air in the lungs has always provided excellent contrast for plain X-ray investigation.

Nevertheless, CT has found a number of uses which include investigation of the following:

1   Suspected mediastinal masses.

2   Staging of lung cancer pre-operatively.

3   Pleural tumours—e.g. distinguishing features of mesothelioma from pleural effusion and thickening.

4   Bronchiectasis—this may be demonstrated without bronchography (effective in severe disease; mild disease cannot be excluded if CT normal).

It has revealed points of interest in interstitial disease, such as the peripheral involvement of the lung in most cases of fibrosing alveolitis. It is able to detect smaller nodular lesions than plain radiography (about 3 mm, whereas a diameter of about 5 mm is usually needed in plain radiography). It is able to identify emphysema more securely than plain radiography but this is not a regular clinical application.

Interpretation of CT images will normally be carried out by an expert radiologist, but some familiarity with the main features is useful to the clinician. Figure 8.6 shows the principal mediastinal structures, with horizontal lines indicating the levels of the CT sections illustrated diagrammatically in Fig. 8.7. The legend to Fig. 8.7 offers help in assessing the level of a CT image.

CT may also allow earlier non-invasive diagnosis of mesothelioma particularly where appearances are obscured by pleural effusion or pleural adhesions following repeated pleural aspiration.

CT has found some application in the staging of lung cancer, but decisions on the question of operability are not usually based on the results of the investigation alone. The technique finds its most important thoracic application in the diagnosis of mediastinal masses and their differentiation from normal structures and in particular in distinguishing deposits of fat from other structures.

Pulmonary angiography

Radio-opaque contrast material is injected into the pulmonary artery through a catheter which has been passed from a peripheral vein through the right side of the heart. The usual indications are: (1) confirmation of pulmonary embolism; and (2) identification of arteriovenous malformations.

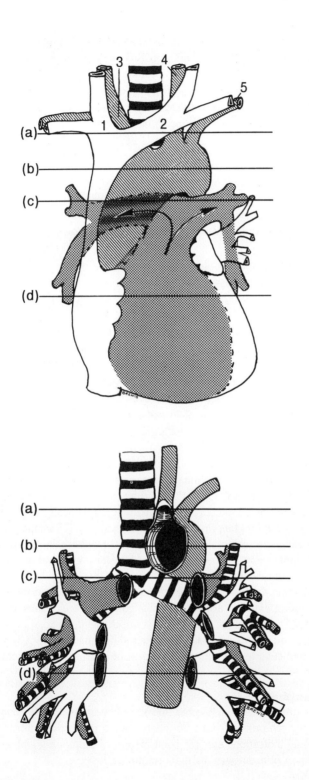

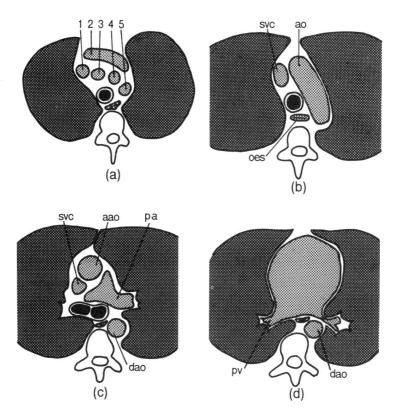

Fig. 8.7. Principal mediastinal structures on computerized tomography (CT). The sections (a) to (d) are at levels (a) to (d) in Fig. 8.6. The sections should be regarded as being **viewed from below** (i.e. the left of the thorax is on the right of the figure). (a) *Section above the aortic arch.* Many large vessels and an anterior sausage shape are seen; the trachea has not bifurcated (black circle). Numerals refer to Fig. 8.6 and its legend. (b) *Section at the level of aortic arch.* A large oblique sausage shape representing the aortic arch is seen (ao); svc = superior vena cava; oes = oesophagus which is visible in all of the sections. (c) *Section below the aortic arch.* Both ascending (aao) and descending (dao) aorta are visible, the trachea is bifurcating and the pulmonary arteries are seen; pa = left pulmonary artery. (d) *Section at the level of pulmonary veins (pv).* Lower lobe intrapulmonary arteries and bronchi are not shown in the diagram.

Fig. 8.6. (*see opposite*) Mediastinal structures. Principal blood vessels and airways. *Above:* Heart and major blood vessels showing the aorta curling over the bifurcation of the pulmonary trunk into left and right pulmonary arteries (arrows). The horizontal lines (a) to (d) indicate the levels of the CT sections illustrated in Fig. 8.7a–d. 1 = right brachiocephalic vein; 2 = left brachiocephalic vein; 3 = innominate or brachiocephalic artery; 4 = left common carotid artery; 5 = left subclavian artery.
Below: Structures with the heart removed. The aorta curls over the left main bronchus which lies behind the left pulmonary artery. Pulmonary arteries are shown stippled, pulmonary veins unstippled and bronchi are shown striped. In general the arteries loop downwards like a handlebar moustache; veins radiate towards a lower common destination—the left atrium. The veins are applied to the front of the arteries and bronchi and take a slightly different path to the respective lung segments. On the right, the order of structures from front to back is vein–artery–bronchus; on the left the pulmonary artery loops over the left upper lobe bronchus and descends behind so that the order is vein–bronchus–artery.

Radio-isotope lung scanning

The major application of isotope scanning is in the diagnosis of pulmonary embolism and this is described in Chapter 24.

Perfusion scanning

Isotope-tagged albumin particles are injected intravenously and lodge in the lungs in proportion to local blood flow. The distribution of the isotope is displayed using a scanning gamma counter or a gamma camera. Dissolved Xenon-133 may be injected as an alternative (this is rapidly evolved into perfused alveoli which can provide additional information but also leads to practical difficulties).

Ventilation scanning

The patient breathes a mixture containing radioactive Xenon-133 in a closed-circuit spirometer. Krypton-81 is easier to use and has a very short half-life enabling several images to be undertaken at one examination.

A gamma camera is used to demonstrate the distribution of the gas. Insight into regional ventilation is gained by observing the rate of 'washing in' and later 'washing out' of the isotope after the patient has begun and ended the period of closed-circuit breathing. The technique may be helpful in providing additional information about lungs involved by bullae, carcinoma or other disease where extensive surgical resection is being considered. It has also proved useful in small children and babies with wheezing dyspnoea where localized bronchial obstruction—for example by a foreign body—may be difficult to distinguish from generalized airways obstruction.

Chapter 9
Acute Respiratory Infection

Most acute respiratory infections are of viral origin. A variety of different viruses are responsible (Table 9.1). Some viruses are regularly associated with a particular clinical pattern, most are capable of producing differing respiratory illnesses depending upon such factors as severity of infection, age of the patient and the presence of pre-existing disease.

Diagnosis in acute respiratory infections goes only so far as identification of the clinical pattern or the level of the respiratory tract which is principally affected. Pursuit of the actual organism is usually only carried out in severe disease, in special centres or in the study of epidemiology. Methods include direct immunofluorescence, isolation in cell culture and detection of a rising titre of serum antibody.

PRINCIPAL PATTERNS OF ILLNESS

Common cold

Rhinorrhoea, nasal obstruction and variable conjunctivitis and epiphora are the main features sometimes associated with a scratchy mild pharyngitis. Nasal secretions become thick and cellular in a few days.

Agents
Causal organisms include: rhinoviruses, coronaviruses, respiratory syncytial virus, parainfluenza virus and influenza virus. The organism is transmitted by droplet spread from an individual in the first 2–4 days of infection.

Treatment
No treatment is usually required. Nasal decongestants based on pseudo-ephedrine may control severe rhinorrhoea but cause mild drowsiness. Aspirin may reduce malaise.

Acute pharyngitis
The common 'sore throat' is more usually associated with fever and a variable degree of malaise. The throat and soft palate are reddened and the tonsils may be inflamed and swollen. After a day or two the tonsillar lymph nodes may be enlarged.

Agents
In young people about 25–33% of sore throats are due to infection by a haemolytic streptococcus; the proportion seems to be falling. Sore throat due to streptococcus is indistinguishable from that due to viral infection.

Table 9.1. Principal respiratory viruses.

Virus	Disease	Notes
Rhinovirus	Common cold, pharyngitis, chronic bronchitic exacerbations	More than 100 serotypes; identification and study difficult
Coronavirus	Common cold	Numerous serotypes; identification difficult
Adenovirus	Pharyngitis, conjunctivitis, severe bronchitis in childhood, rarely severe pneumonia	About 30 serotypes
Respiratory syncytial virus	Bronchiolitis in infants, common cold in adults	One serotype, winter epidemics
Influenza A	Influenza—may be severe	Epidemics, continuous antigenic variation
Influenza B	Influenza	Milder illness, minor epidemics
Parainfluenza	Croup, other URT infections, some bronchiolitis	Serotypes 1–4, a and b
Measles	Measles, severe illness with pneumonia in immunocompromised	Vaccination effective
Cytomegalovirus	Silent infection or minor respiratory illness, pneumonia in immunosuppressed	One serotype
Herpes simplex	Stomatitis, rarely pharyngitis, pneumonia in immunosuppressed	One serotype, severe infection treatable with acyclovir or vidarabine
Herpes zoster	Pneumonia in adult infection	Severe infection treatable with acyclovir, leaves scattered calcific lesions
Coxsackie, enteroviruses and ECHO viruses	Minor part in respiratory infection, Coxsackie A may cause herpangina; B causes 'pleurodynia' and pericarditis/myocarditis	Local epidemics
Epstein–Barr (EB) virus	Pharyngitis, lymphadenitis, infectious mononucleosis	Heterophile antibody test, typical blood picture

Herpes virus and adenovirus may cause vesicular pharyngitis. Some infections are due to *Mycoplasma pneumoniae*. Pharyngitis may be a prominent component of infectious mononucleosis caused by the Epstein–Barr virus.

Treatment
Usually no treatment is necessary. In patients thought to have had acute rheumatic fever or acute glomerulonephritis, penicillin should be given orally if they are not already on regular effective prophylaxis.

Acute laryngitis

This term is used when temporary hoarseness or loss of voice (due to oedema of the vocal cords) accompanies pharyngitis or a common cold. Speech and swallowing may be painful. Causal agents are the same and generally no treatment is necessary.

Acute epiglottitis

This is commonest in children but can occur in adults and may be life-threatening. The patient is usually ill and pyrexial and the symptoms are those of sore throat and laryngitis, sometimes with pronounced painful dysphagia together with worsening upper airways obstruction. The diagnosis of epiglottic swelling may be made by lateral neck X-rays.

Agents
Haemophilus influenzae is the most prominent causal agent followed by *Streptococcus pneumoniae* (pneumococcus).

Treatment
Careful observation of the adequacy of the airway is essential. Hospitalization is necessary in any child with severe pharyngitis who has noisy breathing. Sometimes tracheostomy is necessary. Antibiotic treatment with cefuroxime is preferable to ampicillin in this potentially serious condition, so as to avoid treatment failure due to ampicillin resistant strains of *H. influenzae.*

Acute tracheobronchitis

Cough is the principal symptom. In the early stages it is irresistible, repetitive and unproductive. A barking sound is often produced by flapping vibrations of the posterior wall during coughing. Audible wheezing is sometimes present, but if this is a repeated feature of upper respiratory infections, asthma is a likely diagnosis.

Agents
Respiratory viruses, in particular adenoviruses and *Mycoplasma pneumoniae*, are usually responsible. After the initial infection, *H. influenza* and/or pneumo-coccus may infect the airways—particularly in adults who smoke cigarettes and have chronic bronchitis.

Treatment
Acute tracheobronchitis in an adult who is not otherwise ill requires no treatment. If the sputum is frankly purulent and recovery is delayed, amoxycillin, tetracycline or co-trimoxazole may shorten recovery. Tetracycline should never be given in pregnancy. Uncontrollable cough causing sleeplessness may be helped by codeine linctus.

Croup (acute laryngo-tracheobronchitis)

This term is used to describe the association of stridor, particularly on inspiration, with acute upper and lower respiratory infection in childhood.

Agents
About half of cases are caused by the parainfluenza virus. Influenza virus, RSV and other respiratory viruses can sometimes be implicated.

Treatment
Usually no treatment is required and intubation is rarely necessary. Antihistamines are sometimes found useful, probably because of their mildly sedative effect. If recovery is delayed, ampicillin may be used. Tetracyclines should never be used in children under about 10 years because of effects on teeth and bone.

Influenza

The lay public uses the term influenza or 'flu' to describe almost any pyrexial illness, but in particular acute illness in which the symptoms of malaise and particularly myalgia seem out of proportion to upper respiratory tract symptoms. Any respiratory viruses may underly the symptoms, or there may be a non-respiratory cause.

More specifically, influenza is an acute, highly infectious disease due to influenza A or B viruses causing more or less severe respiratory and generalized symptoms, which usually occur in epidemics—local or world-wide. Minor epidemics occur every winter and pandemics every 4 or 5 years. Some pandemics have been associated with large mortality—generally from complicating bacterial pneumonia, due especially to staphylococcus. Mortality is highest in those with pre-existing lung damage or poor nutrition, but death may also occur in previously healthy individuals. The patient is commonly prostrate, anorexic and pyrexial for 3–4 days and may feel unwell and easily tired for a fortnight or so. A few patients develop continuing lethargy and depression lasting many weeks. The diagnosis can be confirmed by immunofluorescent microscopy of nasal secretions, or by serology.

Treatment
There is no specific treatment, but suspected pneumonia should be treated with agents effective against *Staphylococcus aureus*.

Prophylaxis
Vulnerable individuals (e.g. with advanced cardiac or respiratory disease) may be protected against the currently prevalent strain of influenza A and B by vaccination using killed vaccine. Viral strains vary in antigenic make-up from year to year, which limits the effectiveness of the population's immunity and of immunization. The public's wide faith in the effectiveness of 'flu jabs' in preventing winter coughs and colds in general is not justified.

Acute bronchiolitis

Acute bronchiolitis is an acute disease of the lower airways which affects babies between 1 and 6 months and occurs in winter epidemics. Initial upper respiratory tract symptoms, irritability and difficulty in feeding are followed by cough, wheezing and grunting respiratory distress with inspiratory rib recession accompanied by evidence of overinflation and, in severe cases, signs of respiratory failure. The baby is not usually pyrexial. The illness normally lasts 3–4 days and a rattly cough may last for 2–3 weeks. In severe cases, respiratory distress may persist longer and it may be complicated by respiratory failure and exhaustion, requiring artificial ventilation. Bronchopneumonia is a rare complication.

Agents
Respiratory syncytial virus is almost always the causal organism. Infection is commonest at about 3 months and is unusual before 1 month or later than 6 months, generally occurring in winter epidemics. Maternal IgG antibody does not confer immunity. Resistance to infection requires the development of specific IgA in the respiratory secretions.

Treatment
Antibiotics have no effect. Treatment is directed towards preserving adequate hydration, oxygenation and feeding, until spontaneous improvement occurs. Very occasionally, progressive respiratory failure and exhaustion require the use of artificial ventilation—a specialist procedure not lightly undertaken. In severe deteriorating cases, suspicion of staphylococcal superinfection may lead to administration of flucloxacillin.

Pneumonia
The term pneumonia infers inflammation of the lung parenchyma. Fever, tachypnoea, sometimes with pleural pain, and cyanosis together with clinical and radiological signs of consolidation are the main features. There may be profound systemic upset with delirium and circulatory collapse. (Pneumonia is discussed in more detail in the next two chapters.)

Chapter 10
Pneumonia

Definition

Pneumonia is a general term denoting inflammation of the gas exchange region of the lung. Usually it implies an infective cause. Increasingly the term 'pneumonitis' is used to denote inflammation due to physical, chemical or allergic processes.

The terms bronchopneumònia and lobar pneumonia have little clinical relevance, but are still in widespread use. Bronchopneumonia implies patchy pneumonia and especially that due to peripheral extension of active bronchial infection due to chronic bronchitis or to short-term inadequate clearance of the bases of the lungs. Lobar pneumonia describes consolidation more or less conforming to the radiographic borders of lobes. At one time lobar pneumonia was common and generally due to the *Streptococcus pneumoniae* (pneumococcus); now it is uncommon and not necessarily due to this organism.

Causative agent—relationship to circumstance

Clinical features of pneumonia give little indication of which agent is responsible, although the circumstances of the illness may give some clues (Fig. 10.1). The probabilities are different depending on:

1 the age of the patient;
2 whether pneumonia was acquired in the community or in hospital;
3 whether it developed on a background of previously normal health or established illness;
4 season and geographical locality.

Pneumonia in severely immunosuppressed individuals, and in particular those with AIDS, is dealt with in the next chapter.

Age of the patient

Viral infection is responsible for most community-acquired pneumonia in small children. Respiratory syncytial virus (RSV), adenovirus, influenza and parainfluenza viruses are most common. Measles may cause pneumonia, particularly if there is associated immunosuppression due to leukaemia or lymphoma (histology shows giant cell pneumonia). Bacterial pneumonia in children is less common but usually more severe than viral pneumonia. Infants may develop chlamydial pneumonia from the mother's genital tract. Previously ill children and those in hospital may develop pneumonia due to *Staphylococcus, Pseudomonas, E. coli* and anaerobes; particularly where there is aspiration.

In older children the pneumococcus seems to be the most common cause, then viruses and *H. influenzae*.

Previously well infant
1 RSV
2 Adenovirus and other viruses
3 Bacterial

Previously ill infant
1 *Staphylococcus*
2 *E. coli* and Gram-negative bacteria
3 Viruses and opportunistic organisms

Children
1 Viruses
2 *Pneumococcus*
3 *Mycoplasma*
4 Others

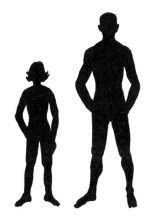

Previously fit adults
1 *Pneumococcus*
2 *Mucoplasma*
3 *H. influenzae*
4 Viruses
5 *Staphylococcus*
6 *Legionella*
7 Others

Previous respiratory illness;
elderly and debilitated
1 *Pneumococcus*
2 *H. influenzae*
3 *Staphylococcus*
4 *Klebsiella* and
   Gram-negative organisms

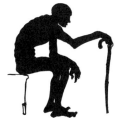

If no response think of:
TB, *Mycoplasma, Legionella,*
carcinoma

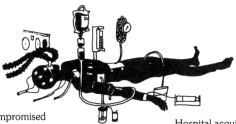

Severely immunocompromised
and AIDS (see Chapter 11):
1 *Pneumocystis,* pneumonia
2 Cytomegalovirus
3 Adenovirus
4 Herpes simplex
5 Bacteria (*Legionella,*
   Staphylococcus, Pneumococcus)
6 Opportunistic mucobacteria;
   tuberculosis

Hospital-acquired pneumonia
1 Gram-negative bacteria
   (*Pseudomonas, Klebsiella,*
   Proteus)
2 *Staphylococcus*
3 *Pneumococcus*
4 Anaerobic bacteria, fungi
5 NB aspiration pneumonia
6 Others

Fig. 10.1. Likely causes of pneumonia in different clinical circumstances. Age and
previous health are important factors.

Community- or hospital-acquired pneumonia

In community-acquired pneumonia in adults, no cause is identified in about 50% of cases investigated. Where a cause is identified, the important organisms and approximate percentage of the total are as follows:

Streptococcus pneumoniae	(50%)
Mycoplasma pneumoniae	(15%)
Haemophilus influenzae	(12%)
Viruses (especially influenza)	(15%)
Staphylococcus aureus	(3%)
Legionella pneumophila	(3%)
Others	(2%)

In hospital-acquired (nosocomial) pneumonia in adults, Gram-negative organisms such as *Klebsiella, Pseudomonas* and *E. coli* are most important:

Gram-negative bacteria	(50%)
Staphylococcus aureus	(20%)
Streptococcus pneumoniae	(15%)
Anaerobes and fungi	(10%)
Others	(5%)

Associated disease

Pneumonia may develop from a breakdown of normal defence mechanisms of the lungs (Chapter 4), for example from failure to clear secretions or frank aspiration due to impaired consciousness, age or weakness. Gram-negative bacteria and anaerobes are usually responsible. Overwhelming bronchial infection associated with chronic bronchitis may lead to *H. influenzae* pneumonia; obstruction due to carcinoma may also lead to pneumonia. Malnutrition, alcoholism, diabetes or immunosupression, due to disease or drugs, predispose to pneumonia. In the presence of important associated disease (and especially that associated with previous administration of antibiotics), the distribution of organisms resembles that of hospital-acquired pneumonia.

Season and geographical locality

In community-acquired pneumonia there is a seasonal effect. Parainfluenza, *Legionella* and, in epidemic years, *Mycoplasma* pneumonias are commonest in the autumn and early winter. RSV infections are most prevalent in December and January. Influenza and bacteraemic pneumonias are more common in late winter.

In developing countries, a proportion of patients presenting with pneumonia may have tuberculosis. In North America, histoplasmosis may need to be considered. Typhoid is an important cause of pneumonia is some tropical countries.

Cases of *Legionella* pneumonia may develop in a cluster around a faulty humidification system or water supply.

Pathology

The common feature of pneumonias is the presence of a cellular exudate in the alveolar spaces. In secondary bacterial pneumonia, suppuration may cause necrosis and damage to the lung architecture, producing abscesses, cysts or damage to the respiratory bronchioles, resulting in centrilobular emphysema. In lobar pneumonia due to pneumococcus and in some viral pneumonias, resolution of the inflammatory intracellular exudates occurs, largely through the action of macrophages, and the lung tissue may return to its former state.

Clinical features

The severity of the illness and precise manner of presentation vary considerably. There is almost always malaise, fever and cough. There is commonly pleural pain and sometimes dyspnoea. Examination may reveal tachypnoea, tachycardia and sometimes cyanosis. There may be signs of consolidation, sometimes associated with a degree of collapse, or evidence of accompanying airways obstruction.

In severe pneumonia there may be severe prostration, delirium, jaundice, oliguria and peripheral circulatory failure.

In the elderly, or in overwhelmingly severe pneumonia, there may be no fever.

Investigation

Chest X-ray

Shadowing, in at least one section of the lung field, is virtually always seen. The X-ray may reveal important evidence of related disease such as carcinoma, tuberculosis, heart disease, or features suggesting pulmonary embolism. It may also show development of complications such as empyema and lung abscess.

Sputum examination

A Gram-stained sputum specimen may give a valuable and rapid clue to the responsible organism in an ill patient. Often, however, results are uncertain. A Ziehl–Neelsen stain should be carried out at some stage.

Sputum culture

This should always be done. The yield is only moderate due to contaminating organisms from mouth and pharynx and to previously administered antibiotics. The organism obtained may not be causative. Where there are virological facilities available, immunofluorescent techniques can make an early diagnosis in some instances (notably influenza and RSV infections). Culture for tuberculosis should always be included in cases of pneumonia.

Blood culture

In severely ill patients, blood culture is important. Pathogenic organisms obtained by blood culture are almost always significant and appropriate treatment is imperative.

Pleural aspiration

This occasionally yields a causative organism or reveals empyema.

Lung aspiration, bronchoscopy

Invasive investigations may be indicated in severe illness—for example patients requiring artificial ventilation or those who may be severely immunosuppressed. Direct needle aspiration of lung may be undertaken. Bronchoscopy is carried out for limited diagnostic lavage of secretions. Secretions are examined by immunofluorescent techniques and cultured.

Antigen detection

Immunological detection of the presence of pneumococcal antigen has increased the positive rate of diagnosis. Antigen can be identified in the sputum, urine, pleural fluid or blood.

Serological tests

Serological tests allow a retrospective diagnosis of pneumonia if a rising titre to one of the commoner viral agents, or to *Legionella,* can be demonstrated. Accurate identification of *Legionella* infection can be important for public health reasons.

Management

General

Mild pneumonia in a robust individual, with a capable family member to provide domestic nursing, can be managed in the home. Where there is cyanosis, hypotension and altered consciousness, hospital admission is desirable. The following measures are frequently necessary:

1   Encouragement of oral fluid intake to avoid dehydration.
2   Aspirin or paracetamol for severe fever, malaise and aching.
3   Stronger analgesics such as codeine or morphine for pleural pain. (Beware patients with previous airways obstruction if opiates are used, as respiratory failure may be precipitated.)

Severe illness

More severely ill patients may require:

Oxygen

If cyanosis is present and respiratory drive is good, oxygen should be given by nasal catheter, or whatever method is best tolerated and in sufficient concentration to relieve cyanosis. Care is again required if there is associated airways obstruction as the patient may have unsuspected chronic respiratory failure.

Intravenous fluids

Severely ill patients with tachycardia, hypotension and a cool periphery may have low plasma volumes, reflected by a low central venous pressure. Large volumes of saline or dextran may be required before central venous pressure rises and adequate circulatory filling is restored.

Corticosteroids

In very severely ill patients, intravenous hydrocortisone is generally felt to be beneficial, although clear evidence in support of this is lacking.

Antibiotic treatment

Community-acquired pneumonia

In most cases of pneumonia, the target organism is the pneumococcus and it is appropriate to give ampicillin or amoxycillin by mouth. This will usually cover *H. influenzae* infection in patients with co-existent chronic bronchitis. In penicillin sensitive persons, erythromycin should be used.

If *Mycoplasma* pneumonia or *Legionella* pneumonia is suspected, erythromycin is appropriate.

In severe pneumonia, it is important to cover possible staphylococcal infection (especially in influenzal epidemics) with flucloxacillin and *Legionella* infection with erythromycin.

Hospital-acquired pneumonia

In the absence of severe illness, ampicillin or amoxycillin may be appropriate. Where there is a severe infection and a high chance of a Gram-negative organism, it may be necessary to give a modern intravenous cephalosporin such as ceftazidime together with an aminoglycoside such as gentamicin or tobramycin. Alternatively an aminoglycoside can be used with a penicillin active against pseudomonas such as azlocillin or ticarcillin. Modern cephalosporins and modified penicillins for intravenous use are very expensive.

Treatment of pneumonia in the severely immunosuppressed and in persons with AIDS is discussed in the next chapter.

Failure to respond

Successful treatment is usually accompanied by signs of improvement in 24–48 hours even though subsequent recovery may be slow. If the patient fails to respond, the clinician should be alert to the possibility of underlying malignant disease or inadequate treatment for Gram-negative infection, tuberculosis, mycoplasmal infection or *Legionella* pneumonia.

Complications

Severe pneumonia may lead to respiratory failure, circulatory failure, renal failure and hepatic failure. Death is virtually inevitable if all are seen. Pneumonia due to staphylococcus may produce cavitation and abscess formation fairly early in the course. *Klebsiella* pneumonia may be very slow to respond and commonly leads to abscess formation and to empyema.

Lobar collapse may complicate any pneumonia and bronchoscopy may be felt necessary if it persists, in order to exclude intraluminal obstruction by carcinoma, foreign body or secretions. Bronchiectasis and localized pulmonary fibrosis may follow severe pneumonia.

Prognosis

The outlook in pneumococcal pneumonia occurring in previously well individuals is good, and the mortality is of the order of 5%. Adverse prognostic factors include: advanced age; altered consciousness; hypoxia; hypotension; multiple lobe involvement; low white cell count (<3000 mm^{-3}) or very high white cell count ($>30\,000$ mm^{-3}).

In severe pneumococcal pneumonia in which more than one lobe is involved and where there is hypotension, hospital series have recorded mortalities of over 20%. Much the same applies to *Legionella* pneumonia. *Klebsiella* pneumonia still carries a mortality of about 45%. Staphylococcal pneumonia is always serious, even in previously well patients, and the mortality is about 20%. Other important factors affecting prognosis relate to host resistance. Factors such as advanced chronic cardiac or pulmonary disease, diabetes, alcoholism, malnutrition and immune incompetence secondary to disease or drugs all weigh heavily against a successful outcome.

NOTES ON SOME INDIVIDUAL FORMS OF PNEUMONIA

Pneumococcal pneumonia

The pneumococcus *Streptococcus pneumoniae* is a paired, capsulated Gram-positive organism. There are numerous serotypes and those causing pneumonia are generally not those found as common upper respiratory commensals. The organism is still the commonest cause of acute pneumonia. The involvement of the lungs is commonly, but not always, lobar in distribution. The affected lobe usually maintains its normal shape and size when it becomes consolidated. Early in untreated pneumonia the alveolar exudate contains abundant red cells and the term 'red hepatization' was used by pathologists to describe the liver-like change in the lung, in those dying soon after the onset. Later the exudate contains abundant white cells and alveolar macrophages, and the term 'grey hepatization' was employed to describe the naked-eye appearance. These labels are of little more than historical significance.

The clinical features are those of an acute pneumonia (see above) and vary greatly in severity. Sometimes recovery is protracted and radiological improvement delayed, but the outcome is usually satisfactory. Pneumococcal meningitis is a rare but serious complication.

Staphylococcal pneumonia

The organism may be identified in Gram stains of sputum as a Gram-positive clustered coccus. Staphylococcal pneumonia has no special early features, but tends to be severe and is a recognized sequel to influenza A infection in epidemics. Even fit young adults may be victims of overwhelming pneumonia. Shock may be present early in the illness and after a few days cavitation, overdistended air-cysts and localized lung abscesses may occur. Remote septic systemic emboli may occur. Hospital organisms and many community-acquired ones are penicillin resistant. Flucloxacillin 500 mg should be given by mouth or intravenously, four times daily, until improvement occurs. Several times this dose may be given, together with large doses of soluble penicillin, in the very ill even if penicillinase-producing organisms are responsible (resistance to penicillin is relative rather than absolute).

Klebsiella pneumonia

This condition is also referred to as Friedlander's pneumonia. The organism responsible, *Klebsiella pneumoniae*, is a Gram-negative capsulated rod-shaped organism. It generally presents as an acute severe pneumonia in patients who either have pre-existing lung disease (e.g. bronchiectasis) or impaired resistance to infection (alcoholism, malnutrition, diabetes and other underlying diseases). It may present with lobar or multilobar involvement of the lung and causes profound illness. Rapid destruction of lung tissue occurs with cavitation. The course is usually stormy and protracted, despite appropriate antibiotic therapy. *Klebsiella pneumoniae* is sensitive to cephalosporins, aminoglycosides and chloramphenicol. Antibiotic treatment appropriate for *Pseudomonas* will be effective against *Klebsiella*.

Haemophilus influenzae pneumonia

Pneumonia attributed to this Gram-negative bacillus usually arises in a severe exacerbation of chronic bronchitis and chronic obstructive lung disease. As well as the features of the pre-existing lung disease there may be fever, pleural pain, a pleural rub, localized crepitations and irregular radiological shadowing, which lead to the diagnosis of pneumonia. A lobar pattern is uncommon. *Haemophilus influenzae* is frequently recovered from the sputum in this situation and presumed to be the cause of the pneumonia. The pneumococcus is commonly recovered at the same time. Treatment with either amoxycillin or cotrimoxazole is appropriate. Resistance to amoxycillin is uncommon but increasing. It is in part a consequence of β-lactamase production by the organism. Augmentin combines amoxycillin with clavulinic acid, which inactivates β-lactamase.

Pseudomonas aeruginosa pneumonia

Infection with this organism almost always arises in debilitated individuals with pre-existing lung disease or recently acquired bronchial obstruction, aspiration pneumonia, etc. It is particularly likely to occur in desperately ill patients who are elderly, who have had antibiotic therapy in hospital, who are undernourished, who are receiving intravenous therapy over a long period, who are being artificially ventilated and who have a tracheostomy (all of these factors individually and together predispose to *Pseudomonas* pneumonia). Diagnosis can be difficult because the organism can very often be cultured from such individuals, whether or not they have pneumonia. Blood culture may be helpful. The condition is always serious. A combination of intravenous azlocillin with gentamicin or tobramycin is often used for treatment. Alternatively, intravenous ceftazidime or cefotaxime may be given.

Legionnaires' disease

This is a severe form of pneumonia caused by a relatively recently discovered bacterium (*Legionella pneumophila*) and it takes its name from an American Legion Convention in 1976, where the first recognized outbreak occurred. The infection is derived from contaminated sources of water. The organism is widely distributed in nature and flourishes at about 24°C. In western temperate societies, it may contaminate humidification plants and water heating circuits and infection is associated with large buildings with such heating and air-conditioning. Affected individuals may live some distance downwind from the source. The incubation period is short; pneumonia may be evident after 3 or 4 days of malaise, myalgia and fever and is accompanied by the usual symptoms and signs. The illness is usually severe, with marked confusion and sometimes acute renal failure. It is not unusual for artificial ventilation to be necessary. The mortality is about 15–20%. The recovery period may be protracted. The diagnosis may be confirmed by a fourfold rise in serum antibody titre; it is difficult to culture or to identify the organism antemortem.

Erythromycin is the drug of choice for treatment and may bring about dramatic sudden improvement. Complete or near-complete resolution of pulmonary changes is usual. Tetracycline may be almost as effective.

Primary atypical pneumonia

This is now a redundant expression. It was formerly used to indicate pneumonia in which there was less severe illness than expected, and no obvious indication of the cause. Some of these cases were due to mycoplasmal infection.

Pneumonia caused by *Mycoplasma pneumoniae*

Mycoplasma pneumoniae (Eaton agent) belongs to a group of the smallest organisms capable of replication outside living cells. It may cause fever, sore throat, myringitis or pneumonia. It tends to attack in winter, occasionally causing local epidemics within families and closed communities. Children and young adults are the usual sufferers.

The pneumonia may be characterized by dramatic radiological shadowing, usually in both lower lobes, which may contrast with rather mild illness. Sometimes fever and symptoms of pneumonia may be very protracted if the cause is not recognized. Permanent damage or serious complications are rare.

The diagnosis is usually suspected on clinical and radiological grounds, supported by a prompt response to tetracycline and confirmed by a rising titre of complement-fixing antibody over 10 days. Cold agglutinins to type O human red cells are usually demonstrable in Mycoplasma pneumonia. The organism is sensitive to tetracyclines and erythromycin.

Psittacosis/ornithosis

These names refer to the illness in man produced by *Chlamydia psittaci* which is a rickettsial type of organism transmitted from infected birds either of the psittacine type (parrots, parakeets, budgerigars) or others (e.g. pigeons).

The illness begins with a high swinging fever and dramatic prostration with headache, photophobia and sometimes delirium. There may be widespread myalgia and severe neck stiffness. This may lead to an initial diagnosis of meningitis. Splenomegaly may sometimes be detected. Attention is often not drawn to the chest until a chest X-ray is carried out although a persistent cough may be present. A few fine crepitations localized to one or more areas of the lungs are usually the only pulmonary signs. Enquiry usually reveals obvious contact with birds and occasionally the recent acquisition of a sick bird.

The chest X-ray reveals some pulmonary shadowing which is usually rather undramatic and may be limited to one segment. Confirmation of the diagnosis is provided by demonstration of a rising titre of complement-fixing antibody.

Aspiration pneumonia

Aspiration of food, drink, saliva and gastric contents can lead to pneumonia. Factors which predispose to aspiration are:

1 *Altered consciousness*—particularly due to anaesthesia, drug overdosage and alcohol.

2 *Muscular weakness or inco-ordination.* Particularly in individuals with bilateral cerebrovascular events and consequent pseudobulbar palsy, brainstem stroke, motor neurone disease, myasthenia, etc.

3 *Laryngopharyngeal anaesthesia*—due, for example, to nerve damage from disease, surgery, radiotherapy or topical anaesthesia.

4 *Oesophageal disease.* Oesophageal obstruction may lead to pooling of food and secretions in the oesophagus which overflows on reclining and during sleep. Causes include carcinoma, achalasia, large hiatus herniae. Rarely a tracheo-oesophageal fistula develops in the course of carcinoma of the bronchus or oesophagus causing aspiration of fluid and saliva, which usually leads to rapidly fatal pneumonia.

5 *Artificial ventilation* by cuffed endotracheal tube, commonly accompanied by a degree of inhalation of secretions despite the protection of the cuff.

If these factors are accompanied by other risk factors for pneumonia such as diabetes, malnutrition, old age, etc. then the chances of aspiration pneumonia are high.

Mendelson's syndrome is a condition of severe pulmonary oedema caused by inhalation of acid gastric contents (see Chapter 25). The clinical features are those of pneumonia and of the circumstances predisposing to aspiration. A test drink with clean water will often reveal incompetent swallowing and a barium swallow will confirm this if there is doubt. The patient generally has abundant purulent sputum, which may be greenish, and a regular, sometimes ineffective cough. The chest X-ray shows lower zone changes, or sometimes right upper lobe changes. The 'axillary subsegments' of the anterior and posterior segments are common sites for pneumonia; recurrent changes in this site are always suspicious of aspiration.

Organisms present include Gram-negative bacteria and anaerobes. It is common to obtain no pathogens on culture of the sputum.

Aspiration can be reduced or prevented, for example by starving patients before anaesthesia for 6 hours, by careful positioning and sometimes gastric suction in those who are unconscious, and by careful observation of vulnerable patients with neuromuscular disease whilst they eat and drink.

Treatment comprises, firstly, arrest of the inhalation by: (1) relief of oesophageal obstruction; (2) semi-solid diet, tracheostomy, nasogastric or parenteral feeding in the case of neurological causes; and (3) careful nursing and gastric aspiration in the case of the unconscious. Antibiotic treatment with penicillin or ampicillin is usually adequate if the patient is not ill, grossly immunosuppressed or artificially ventilated. In the latter case treatment suitable for Gram-negative organisms such as *Pseudomonas* is needed (e.g. intravenous gentamicin and azlocillin or ceftazidime).

Lipoid pneumonia

This is a special form of aspiration pneumonia due to the repeated unwitting inhalation of animal or mineral oils medicinally (usually as laxatives or nose drops; liquid paraffin is the most common culprit). The inhaled oil causes patchy areas of pneumonia and collapse which may be widespread or localized, varying or relatively constant. Granulomatous lesions may develop which can mimic carcinoma. Cough is almost always present but there may be few other clues to suggest pulmonary disease. The diagnosis may be suspected when a chest X-ray reveals bizarre opacities in a moderately ill, elderly individual who is found to be using an oily preparation. Microscopic examination of the sputum (or sometimes of biopsy material) shows 'foamy' macrophages which contain abundant globules of oil.

Note. The term lipoid pneumonia is also used to describe cholesterol and fat deposition in incompletely resolved pneumonic areas accompanying a variety of pulmonary diseases. The lipid here is of endogenous origin.

Chapter 11
Respiratory Disease in AIDS

Background

AIDS (acquired immune deficiency syndrome), the disease associated with the human immunodeficiency virus (HIV), first came to light in 1981 when a high incidence of Kaposi's sarcoma and later *Pneumocystis carinii* pneumonia was reported amongst male homosexuals in New York. HIV was identified in 1984. Infection is transmitted by sexual intercourse, particularly anal intercourse, and by contaminated blood products or needles and syringes. In the UK it is still rare outside of male homosexuals, intravenous drug abusers and those who have received contaminated blood products. The widespread use by haemophiliacs of Factor VIII concentrates derived from large numbers of donors led to a high incidence of infection with HIV. There is a high risk of transmission to babies born of infected mothers by placental transfer or breast feeding. The prevalence amongst heterosexual partners of infected persons is increasing. Where rates of infection in the general population are high, as in parts of Central Africa, the distribution between the sexes is more even.

The virus is a retrovirus which has a high affinity for the T4 (or CD4) 'helper' lymphocyte. The virus has RNA codes for the production of reverse transcriptase, which enables it to be incorporated within the cell's DNA. It is self-replicated when the cell is stimulated. Numbers of CD4 lymphocytes and their performance diminish and progressive immune incompetence is the consequence. Secondary impairment of CD8 lymphocyte function is seen. B lymphocytes are initially normal but with time they lose the capacity to generate an immunoglobulin response to newly encountered antigens.

Natural history

HIV infection is not accompanied by any immediately observable effects. Seroconversion occurs about 4–6 weeks later. Non-specific symptoms may occur at the time of seroconversion, which resemble glandular fever; with malaise, arthralgia and tender lymphadenopathy. A long symptom-free latent period follows seroconversion.

Within 10 years, about half of seropositive persons will have developed clinical manifestations of HIV infection. Intercurrent infection by other organisms accelerates the disease.

Persistent generalized lymphadenopathy

A proportion of HIV positive persons develop enlarged lymph nodes, in more than one site, which persist for more than 3 months. These individuals are more likely to go on to develop AIDS within a few years.

AIDS-related complex

This term describes a wide variety of phenomena which are due to HIV infection but which are not a direct consequence of recognized opportunistic infections. Symptoms include persistent generalized lymphadenopathy, weight loss, recurrent oral candidiasis, persistent malaise. There may be splenomegaly. Ordinary pathogens frequently cause infection.

AIDS

AIDS is diagnosed when there is a documented infection by a recognized opportunistic organism, which is not a pathogen of normal persons. Recognized infections in this context include *Pneumocystis carinii*, cytomegalovirus and opportunistic mycobacterial infection of the lung, oesophageal or bronchial candidiasis and a variety of others. The development of Kaposi's sarcoma, non-Hodgkin lymphoma or diffuse degenerative brain disease also results in a diagnosis of AIDS.

In the developed world, the commonest infection announcing AIDS is *Pneumocystis carinii* pneumonia. In undeveloped countries, florid tuberculosis may bring HIV infection to light.

Pulmonary infections

Pneumocystis carinii pneumonia (PCP)

Pneumocystis carinii is related to fungi rather than protozoa and is a motile unicellular organism. Infection is almost universal in childhood and is clinically silent. Infection arising in AIDS is thought to be a re-awakening of latent infection, previously controlled by lymphocytic activity.

Clinical features

Clinically, the features are of an individual usually belonging to one or other high risk group, who has a cough and, a little later, shortness of breath and a sense of chest discomfort. Fever and associated malaise is generally present. Usually clinical examination is unremarkable. There may be tachypnoea, particularly on exercise. The chest X-ray shows an abnormality in well-established disease, but may be normal in the presence of early symptoms. The most common pattern is of a fine hazy stippling, bilaterally. Other patterns of bilateral, patchy shadowing are seen, and unilateral disease has been reported.

Spirometry may show a minor degree of airways obstruction and blood gas estimation may show lowering of Pao_2. Lowering of Pao_2 on exercise has been shown to be a sensitive marker of the presence of PCP. Transfer factor may show progressive reduction. The diagnosis of a respiratory infection can, however, usually be assumed if there are symptoms, in which case elaborate investigation of pulmonary function is not indicated. It will usually be necessary to identify the organism by examination of respiratory secretions. Other investigations are not sufficiently reliable.

Confirmation of diagnosis

If there is difficulty in producing sputum, it can often be induced by inhaling hypertonic saline by nebulizer for 15 minutes. Careful mouth toilet precedes the inhalation. The sputum is examined by Giemsa or silver methenamine staining for the trophozoites of *Pneumocystis carinii*. If sputum induction fails, then bronchoscopy is necessary. The patient is examined under local anaesthesia (Chapter 23). Usually bronchoalveolar lavage is undertaken. The bronchoscope is advanced into a segmental or subsegmental bronchus until it wedges. About 60 ml of warmed sterile saline is then injected and gently aspirated. This is usually repeated twice, with the instrument in the same bronchus. Specimens are examined for PCP as above, cultured for bacteria and also examined for viruses by antigen immunofluorescence and sometimes tissue culture. Transbronchial biopsy may also be carried out but it carries a significant risk of pneumothorax or troublesome bleeding and is best avoided in the diagnosis of pneumonia in AIDS. Transbronchial biopsy increases the diagnostic rate, from about 40–90% with lavage to 90% of all cases eventually regarded as PCP. Diagnostic performance increases with experience of specimen collection and cytological examination. In specialist centres, most cases of PCP are now diagnosed from induced sputum specimens. Experience of sputum generation and cytology of PCP is important.

Treatment

Co-trimoxazole (Septrin) is given in high doses (about 4 times the conventional dose used in ordinary infections), orally or intravenously and continued for at least 3 weeks. Co-trimoxazole in high dose is not innocuous and can cause vomiting, rashes and marrow suppression. Pneumocystis may be found in secretions for a week or more after the start of effective treatment. Clinical recovery is not rapid, so that there is often doubt about effectiveness of treatment for some days after starting. Pentamidine is sometimes given intravenously and is effective. PCP tends to recur—more than half of cases relapse within 18 months. Pentamidine is now coming into routine use as a prophylactic given by inhalation weekly after recovery from the first attack of PCP. Dapsone given orally, once weekly, is also sometimes used. Ill patients need oxygen and aspirin or paracetamol. If respiratory failure develops, despite treatment, it is usually unkind to resort to artificial ventilation as survival is unlikely to be secured. The mortality rate in PCP is about 20%.

Cytomegalovirus infection

Cytomegalovirus (CMV) infection in AIDS causes retinitis, colitis and other non–pulmonary infections more often than pneumonia. When identified from respiratory secretions by culture or fluorescence technique, it may appear as a mixed infection with PCP. Ganciclovir is used in confirmed infections.

Opportunist mycobacterial infection

Opportunist (or 'atypical') mycobacterial infection is very common in AIDS, infecting up to a quarter of patients. Infection may be principally extrathoracic. In the chest, lymphadenopathy is as common as overt parenchymal disease. Symptoms are those of progressive AIDS with unexplained fever and worsening malaise and weight loss. Diagnosis may be made from lymph node biopsy or stool culture, rather than the sputum. Histologically there is little granuloma formation, but large numbers of acid-fast bacilli are seen. The most common opportunist mycobacteria are those of the *M. avium intracelullare* group. These are relatively resistant to antituberculous treatment and cure is never achieved. In patients who are still fairly early in the clinical course of AIDS, treatment is usually begun with rifampicin, ethambutol and isoniazid (INH) in the hope of retarding progress.

Tuberculosis

Tuberculosis is a common presenting infection in communities with a high prevalence. The illness is atypical and lung disease may be relatively unimpressive. Lymphadenopathy is pronounced and often very rapid in development. There may be abdominal involvement and miliary spread. Biopsy of nodes does not show prominent granuloma formation.

Other lung infections

Ordinary bacterial pneumonia may develop and run a dramatic, sometimes fatal course. *Legionella* infection is uncommon but a recognized hazard. Invasive aspergillosis and candidiasis have been described.

Kaposi's sarcoma and related neoplasia

Kaposi's sarcoma appears to be a malignancy associated with altered immunity. In AIDS patients it occurs almost exclusively in homosexuals. It generally involves the skin, or mucosal surfaces such as the mouth.

If it involves the lungs there may be non-specific symptoms of cough, shortness of breath and pleural pain. The chest X-ray may show pleural effusion or irregular nodular shadowing in the lung fields. Sometimes there is haemoptysis. The diagnosis is usually made because of evident skin involvement, but is sometimes made from the visual appearances on bronchoscopy. The bronchial mucosa shows very characteristic bright red patches which bleed easily. The biopsy of such patches is unhelpful and inadvisable. Sometimes there is spread to the pleural cavity, but pleural biopsy is generally unhelpful in diagnosis.

Management
Opinion is divided on the best form of treatment. The outlook is very bad and strenuous antineoplastic chemotherapy, causing marrow depression and even worse predisposition to overwhelming infection, carries its own risks.

Interstitial pneumonitis accompanying AIDS

Patients with AIDS may develop either a lymphocytic infiltrate of the lung parenchyma or a non-specific infiltration of lymphocytes and plasma cells, with associated inflammatory changes in the alveolar lining cells and interalveolar septa. Infiltrations are a relatively common manifestation of HIV infection affecting children and uncommon in adults. These infiltrations are poorly understood and are mainly diagnosed either post-mortem, or in the process of trying to diagnose presumed intercurrent infections.

Treatment of AIDS

Treatment with zidovudine has been shown to retard development of AIDS if given regularly to HIV positive individuals. It can also prolong life in symptomatic patients with AIDS. It is an unpleasant treatment and causes marrow suppression and other side-effects. It is extremely expensive.

Chapter 12
Respiratory Disease in the Severely Immunocompromised Patient (non-AIDS)

General causes of immunodeficiency

Interference with immune mechanisms occurs in a number of disease contexts. These include processes such as severe undernutrition, diabetes, uraemia, alcoholism and long-term administration of high doses of corticosteroid.

Severe immunodeficiency

This chapter is primarily concerned with severe disorder of the immune system, such as is encountered in the following states:

Primary immunodeficiency syndromes
These include hypogammaglobulinaemia, severe combined immunodeficiency syndrome, thymic aplasia.

Chronic lymphatic leukaemia and multiple myeloma
These disorders are characteristically associated with deficient immunoglobulin production. Treatment may compound the immunosuppression.

Myeloid leukaemia
This is generally associated with impaired granulocyte function.

Lymphomas
Impaired lymphocytic function is the rule. During chemotherapy there is comprehensive immunosuppression.

Antineoplastic chemotherapy
Neutropenia and impaired lymphocytic function occur in varying degree.

Immunosuppressive treatment for organ transplantation
This is of course designed to impair lymphocytic function.

Where there is a mixture of the general causes of immunodeficiency and one of the predisposing illnesses, lung infection is extremely likely.

Many patients with these disorders have organ failure of greater or lesser degree and are extremely ill. Some have coagulation defects or thrombocytopenia. When lung disease occurs in this context there is often a difficult differential diagnosis (Fig. 12.1):

Causes of respiratory disease in the immunosuppressed

1 Lung infection
See below.

2 Non-infectious pulmonary disease

Haemorrhage

This is usually in the presence of severe thrombocytopenia and there is likely to be bleeding elsewhere. Lung shadows tend to develop suddenly rather than gradually. There may be associated blood streaking of the sputum.

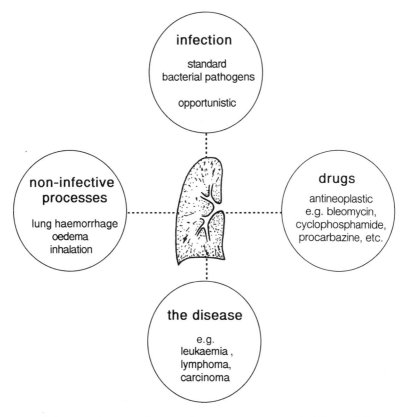

Fig. 12.1. Lung disease in the severely immunocompromised: differential diagnosis in the non-AIDS patient.

Lung oedema

This may accompany renal failure, excessive fluid infusion or heart failure. Some non-haemodynamic forms of pulmonary oedema occur and adult respiratory distress syndrome may develop (see Chapter 26) particularly where there is septicaemia.

Other processes

These include aspiration, transfusion reaction, radiation, pulmonary embolism and, rarely, alveolar proteinosis—an ill-understood condition in which thick, mucoid protein-rich material accumulates in alveoli, causing respiratory distress and patchy diffuse X-ray shadowing, sometimes notably perihilar in distribution. It is potentially treatable by alveolar lavage. It may be due to impaired scavenging of surfactant by macrophages.

3 Adverse lung reaction to drugs

Some forms of pulmonary reaction to drugs cause radiological lung shadowing which may mimic infection. These take the form of acute pulmonary oedema, rapid fibrosis or eosinophilia. Most antineoplastic drugs have been recorded as causing parenchymal pulmonary reaction (see Chapter 30).

4 Pulmonary extension of underlying disease

Lymphomas, leukaemias and other malignancies may extend in the lung causing radiological shadowing which may be difficult to distinguish from pulmonary infection.

Infections encountered

Bacteria

Pyogenic bacteria

These constitute the main threat in the severe immunodeficiency states which produce neutropenia.

Severe pneumococcal infections are particularly likely to occur in multiple myeloma and in splenectomized individuals; lifetime penicillin prophylaxis is advised in the latter group.

Infection by *Legionella* may cause overwhelming infection and be difficult to diagnose.

Tuberculosis is especially likely in disorders interfering with lymphocyte function and may present in generalized form without the usual characteristic histological appearances. Constant vigilance is necessary, and sometimes treatment needs to be started on just slight suspicion if the patient is deteriorating in a way which could be explained by tuberculosis. In pyrexia of unknown orgin (PUO), where the patient's condition is not desperate, a therapeutic trial may be appropriate and here the agents employed should be specifically antimycobacterial in their effects (like isoniazid, pyrazinamide and ethambutol) rather than broad spectrum agents such as rifampicin.

Where there is evidence of previous TB infection, prophylactic chemotherapy may be required during periods of severe immunosuppression.

Atypical mycobacteria (see Chapter 13)

These agents are occasionally revealed later, on culture, when the working diagnosis is tuberculosis.

Viruses

Viruses are particularly likely in circumstances where lymphocytes are primarily impaired.

Cytomegalovirus

A member of the herpes virus family, this infection is widespread and poses particular problems in treatment of patients who have undergone organ transplantation. Some infections may be introduced with the donor organ. Previously uninfected CMV antibody-negative recipients are at risk and many centres aim to match CMV status between donor and recipient. Diagnosis is either by microscopic examination of secretions for inclusion bodies or by demonstrating a rising titre of antibody to CMV—especially IgM. Some patients who are infected are unable to mount an antibody response. Treatment is by reduction of immunosuppressive treatment in mild disease, where graft survival is not a problem, and by use of novel agents such as phoscarnate phosphonoformate or ganciclovir in severe cases and those with a fragile graft (e.g. bone marrow graft).

Herpes simplex

Pneumonia due to herpes simplex may be diagnosed by immunofluorescence microscopy of secretions. Generalized disease and especially encephalitis may result. Treatment is with vidarabine or acyclovir.

Herpes zoster

Pneumonia and severe shingles or chickenpox may occur. Herpes zoster infections in the immunosuppressed are dangerous, and all possible contact with chickenpox or shingles in family, staff or other patients must be avoided. Treatment is with acyclovir, initially usually intravenously.

Measles virus

Infection with measles virus is particularly likely to cause pneumonia when associated with childhood leukaemia or lymphoma. The histological appearances have led to the description of giant cell pneumonia.

Pneumocystis carinii

This is dealt with in Chapter 11 in the context of AIDS. *Pneumocystis carinii* pneumonia is a regular cause of obscure fever and respiratory symptoms in the severely immunosuppressed—particularly in transplant recipients.

Fungi

Candida albicans is commonly troublesome in the oropharynx and oesophagus, but pulmonary infection is rare except as a near-terminal event in leukaemia or lymphoma. The association of progressive lung changes and positive blood cultures may lead to diagnosis and treatment. Sometimes the infection is only evident post-mortem. Treatment of severe infections is with amphotericin.

Aspergillus fumigatus is the most troublesome fungal agent. A rapidly invasive form of the infestation may occur in severely immunosuppressed individuals, with lung destruction occurring over a week or so followed sometimes by the development of a crescentic shadow, indicating the acute formation of an aspergilloma (see Chapter 17) in the necrotic lung. Severe disease is usually treated with a combination of amphotericin and flucytosine.

Other agents

In the tropics a common nematode parasite, *Strongyloides stercoralis*, may become rampant and invade the lung in large numbers, producing pneumonia with larvae in the sputum and leading to profound illness, with septicaemia and intravascular coagulation. *Toxoplasma gondii* infection may also be a problem.

Diagnosis of lung infection in the immunocompromised

The diagnosis of infection may be clear from the features of the illness (sudden fever, new local pulmonary shadow, retrieval of a causative organism from blood or other body fluid). The diagnosis of non-infective lung disease may be clear from clinical circumstances.

Where the diagnosis is not clear, or where treatment is not having the expected effect, bronchoalveolar lavage usually should be undertaken. Lavage is relatively non-traumatic and fairly well tolerated. Transbronchial biopsy may increase the yield, but carries a significant risk in these patients through the development of haemorrhage or a pneumothorax.

If the patient is unwell, not responding to treatment and in particular where there is already respiratory failure and the need for artificial ventilation is approaching, there are virtues in obtaining an open lung biopsy through a limited thoracotomy. Artificial ventilation may be precipitated in the process of this investigation. It is nevertheless important to have as clear a diagnosis of the lung condition as possible in this situation, as well as an indication of the likelihood of reversibility. The risk of open lung biopsy is a relatively small part of the overall risk borne by the immunosuppressed patient with serious lung disease.

Treatment

See individual agents.

Chapter 13
Tuberculosis

Tuberculosis is an infection due to *Mycobacterium tuberculosis*, characterized by necrosis and granuloma formation. It most commonly affects the lungs, but may involve other organs or be widespread.

Prevalence, incidence and mortality

One hundred years ago, more than 30 000 persons died from tuberculosis annually in the UK (about the same mortality rate as for bronchial carcinoma today). Ignoring the effect of war, the mortality rate in the UK has shown: (1) a steady decline to about 1940 (attributable to improved nutrition); (2) a much sharper exponential decline from 1940 to the present (attributable to the introduction of effective treatment). Death from tuberculosis is now rare in the UK, occurring mainly in the elderly, the diagnosis sometimes being unrecognized in life.

Notification of new cases has also declined progressively. Since the 1950s, notifications have included a higher and higher proportion of patients born in the Indian subcontinent. By the 1980s this proportion reached nearly half. The risk of an Asian immigrant developing tuberculosis is highest in the early years after immigration from a high prevalence area. The annual notification rate is about 5 per 100 000 in the White ethnic group and 150 per 100 000 in Asian ethnic groups. Surveys show a similar rate of decline in incidence in both groups.

In developing countries, tuberculosis is still responsible for a substantial mortality and much severe illness. Mortality and incidence rates may be more than 20 times those seen in developed countries, and the pattern of the disease resembles that seen in developed countries more than 50 years ago.

Tuberculosis occurs as an opportunistic infection in immunosuppressed individuals and the notification rate is increasing in some areas, as a consequence of AIDS.

Pathology

The elements of the typical tuberculosis granuloma are summarized in Fig. 13.1. Typically there may be central cheesy necrosis which, in time, commonly attracts calcium deposits. The epithelioid cells, forming layers around the central zone, probably represent transformed macrophages. Established lesions become surrounded by dense fibrosis. In the lung, foci of infection are commonly surrounded by small 'satellite' lesions, fibrosis is prominent and large foci become cavitated. The extent to which lesions proliferate or become caseated or fibrosed is related to the immunological status of the patient.

Evolution of the disease

Knowledge of the time course of tuberculous infection (summarized in Fig. 13.2) comes from the days before effective chemotherapy; the disease is no longer seen to evolve in this characteristic fashion in the UK.

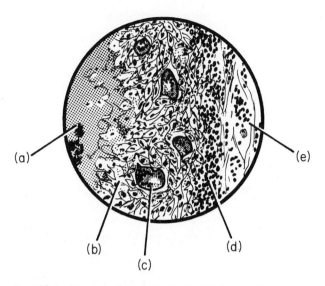

Fig. 13.1. Diagram of main histological features of tuberculous lesion. The centre of the lesion is to the left of the diagram. (a) Caseating central portion containing calcium deposits; (b) epithelioid cells; (c) giant cells of Langhans' type; (d) lymphocytic infiltration of the outer layers; (e) fibrous tissue. The appearances vary considerably depending upon the age of the lesions, its situation and the degree of immunoreactivity of the host.

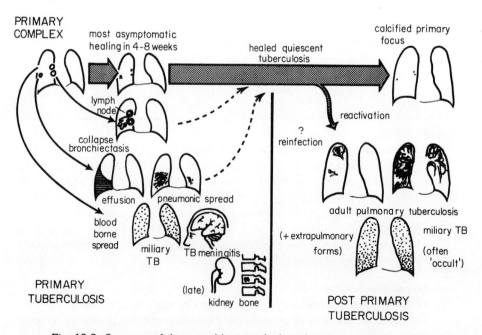

Fig. 13.2. Summary of the natural history of tuberculosis

Primary tuberculosis

Source of infection

The disease is always acquired from an infected individual who is excreting bacteria; usually the contact is close and the exposure heavy. None of the tuberculosis in developed countries is bovine in origin and this source will not be considered further here.

The primary complex

The primary complex comprises the reaction at the site of the initial infection together with that which develops in the regional lymph nodes. The most common example is the primary pulmonary focus accompanied by tuberculous hilar adenopathy (Fig. 13.2). This develops within 4 weeks of first infection and usually its progress is limited and there are few, if any, symptoms. Occasionally erythema nodosum develops at this stage. Healing then takes place, the tuberculin test becomes positive, a degree of immunity to the tubercle bacillus is developed and the lymph nodes subside. The peripheral lung lesion becomes reduced to a small nodule which may calcify and be evident on the chest X-ray indefinitely (Gohn focus).

Progression of pulmonay primary complex

In children, the lymph nodes may become much enlarged and cause pulmonary collapse by compressing lobar bronchi. Occasionally air-trapping causes over-inflation of an obstructed lobe. Diffuse areas of radiological hazy opacification may be assoicated with lymph node enlargement. This phenomenon is referred to as epituberculosis; it may be due to a parenchymal hypersensitivity reaction and it usually gradually subsides. In young adults, the parenchymal pulmonary reaction may enlarge and cavitate with progressive pulmonary spread. Small parenchymal lesions may present with a pleural effusion, identifiable by pleural biopsy.

Spread of infection

At any time in the course of tuberculous infection, spread may occur by several routes:

Bronchial tree

This leads to spread to other areas of lung or, via the sputum, to the larynx (causing ulcerations) and gastrointestinal tract.

Lymphatic system

This leads to regional lymphadenopathy or to blood, spread via the lymphatic duct, causing miliary spread.

Bloodstream

Pulmonary veins draining pulmonary lesions may carry infective material, leading to remote spread of the disease particularly to bone, kidney, adrenal gland, brain and meninges.

Post-primary infection

This term refers to any development of tuberculosis beyond the first few weeks of a primary infection and after the development of hypersensitivity. It includes cases of reinfection and reactivated primary infection even when this occurs years later. Re-activation tends to occur in old age and in the course of illness or drug treatment which impairs immunocompetence. The lungs are the most usual site of post-primary disease and the apices of the lungs are the commonest pulmonary site.

Clinical presentation

In developed countries, the diagnosis is usually suggested by the finding of compatible changes on chest X-ray during investigation of patients with:

1 *Persistent cough and purulent sputum.*

2 *Haemoptysis.*

3 *Unresolved pneumonia.*

4 *Non-specific symptoms.* Investigation of patients of beyond middle age with fever, malaise and weight loss may reveal tuberculosis. Immigrants from Asia and Africa may present unusual forms of tuberculosis with fever, malaise and splenomegaly associated with hilar or cervical gland enlargement.

5 *No symptoms.* Tuberculosis may be revealed during the course of routine clinical and X-ray examinations.

Physical signs

Almost any combination of physical signs may be found (e.g. consolidation, effusion, fibrosis, collapse). Quite often the signs are rather slight, even in the presence of advanced pulmonary tuberculosis.

Radiological features (Fig. 13.3)

These override the physical signs in importance. A great variety of appearances is encountered, including:

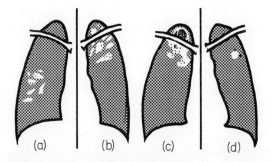

(a)   (b)   (c)   (d)

Fig. 13.3. Radiographic appearances in pulmonary tuberculosis. Tuberculosis can produce almost any form of pulmonary shadowing. Some common forms are indicated above. (a) Irregular mottled shadowing of any part of the lung especially (b) one or both apices. (c) Cavitation of an apical lesion is particularly suggestive but cavitation also occurs in carcinoma. (d) Solitary tuberculoma presenting as a 'coin' shadow. Calcification suggests tuberculosis but the diagnosis is generally only established at thoracotomy; the majority of such shadows is caused by carcinoma.

1   *Patchy solid lesions* of irregular shape, tending to be localized to one lung or part of a lung or to the upper lobes.

2   *Cavitated solid lesions.*

3   *Streaky fibrosis.*

4   *Flecks of calcification.* Calcification is always suggestive of tuberculosis but occurs in other conditions

All of these changes may be present together. Other patterns which may be encountered include:

5   *Solitary round shadows.* Less than a quarter of these shadows are tuberculous and the majority of the remainder are of neoplastic origin.

6   *Hilar gland enlargement.* The combination of hilar enlargement and a solid lesion which may be cavitated tends to resemble bronchial carcinoma.

7   *Pleural effusion.*

8   *Pneumothorax.*

9   *Miliary mottling* (see below).

Miliary tuberculosis

This term refers to the widespread dissemination of tuberculosis, usually with multiple (millet-seed size) nodules evident in the lung fields on the chest X-ray, which is generally believed to follow entry of a large amount of infective material into the circulation either via the lymphatic system or the veins draining a local lesion. Formerly this variety of the disease was most usually seen following primary infection in children, but it is now encountered more frequently in the older age groups. Usually the patient is ill, pyrexial and anorexic, but occasionally individuals appear to be active and fairly well. A low-grade fever is the most constant of the non-specific features. Sometimes anaemia is the most obvious clinical feature and the blood picture may show abnormal cells, suggesting a diagnosis of leukaemia. Occasionally these non-specific features are present without any miliary changes on the chest X-ray; the diagnosis may then be exceedingly difficult. Persisting fever in an elderly individual who is deteriorating may call for a therapeutic trial of specific antituberculous therapy, even if attempts to isolate the tubercle bacillus have failed.

Diagnosis of tuberculosis

The combinations of clinical and radiological features described will often make a diagnosis of tuberculosis virtually certain, but definitive diagnosis requires identification of the tubercle bacillus.

Sputum smear examination

Examination of a sputum smear stained by the Ziehl–Neelsen method, by adequately-trained individuals, is a vital step in diagnosis. Identification of acid- and alcohol-fast bacilli is presumptive evidence of tuberculosis and infectivity (in an untreated case). Repeated sputum examinations are indicated where suspicion of tuberculosis is high.

Sputum culture

The tubercle bacillus can be cultured *in vitro* on Dover's medium. This takes between 4 and 7 weeks. Assessment of *in vitro* sensitivity to antituberculous drugs may take a further 3 weeks after positive identification.

120 CHAPTER 13

Guinea-pig inoculation

This technique permits isolation of tubercle bacilli when they are present in very small numbers in the material. It is expensive and rarely required.

Biopsy

The diagnosis can sometimes be made from biopsy material and this is particularly the case with isolated pulmonary nodules, which require thoracotomy, pleural effusion and tuberculous cervical adenopathy.

Tuberculin testing (Fig. 13.4)

After 3 weeks or so from the time of the initial infection, hypersensitivity to a protein part of the tubercle bacillus is developed. Hypersensitivity can be

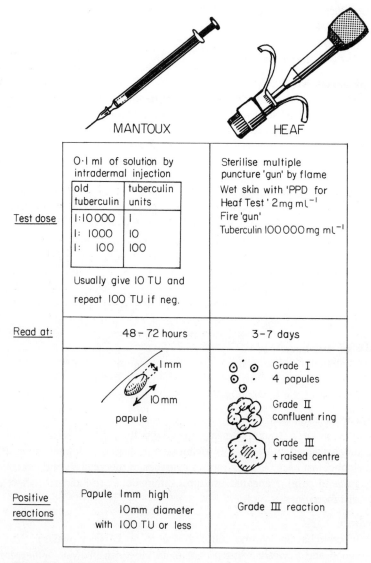

Fig. 13.4. Tuberculin testing.

detected by intradermal injection of a purified protein derivative (PPD) of cultured tubercle bacilli. The response is of the Type IV cell-mediated variety and takes the form of a raised area of induration and reddening of the skin.

Mantoux test

In the Mantoux test, 0.1 ml of tuberculin solution is injected intradermally (not subcutaneously). The test is read at 48–72 hours. A positive result is indicated by redness and induration at least 10 mm in diameter (the lesion is slightly oedematous and can be located by palpation with the eyes shut). If active tuberculous infection is very likely 1 TU (tuberculin unit, see Fig. 13.4) should be used, otherwise 10 TU is normally employed and the test repeated with 100 TU if the result is negative.

Heaf test

The Heaf test is widely used in the UK and very convenient. If properly sterilized, by dipping of the gun in alcohol which is subsequently ignited, there is no risk of HIV or hepatitis transmission. The test uses strong tuberculin at a strength of 100 000 TU ml^{-1}. It can be read at 3–7 days. Some patients can be issued with cards showing diagrams which allow them to make their own reading.

A positive Mantoux test using 1 : 100 strength (10 TU) and a grade III Heaf test are roughly equivalent.

Significance

A positive tuberculin test merely indicates previous tuberculous infection. A negative test virtually excludes active tuberculosis (except in rare cases of overwhelming disease or severe immunosuppression). A weak reaction to tuberculin (less than 10 mm induration; Heaf Grades I to II) may be non-specific and indicate hypersensitivity to other mycobacteria. Weaker responses tend to be seen in the elderly. Exceptionally vigorous reactions suggest currently active disease. The principal role of turberculin testing is epidemiological. Spontaneous conversion in childhood is presumed to indicate primary infection and treatment is usually advised. A source amongst adult contacts must be carefully sought. In the UK, the policy of BCG vaccination of tuberculin-negative children at about 13 years-reduces the usefulness of the tuberculin test above this age.

Case detection

The great majority of new cases of tuberculosis are detected by chest X-ray examination of individuals in the high-risk groups already mentioned. Mass miniature radiographic screening is important where the prevalence of tuberculosis is high. In the UK the yield of new cases from this source became so small that the service was abandoned.

Management of tuberculosis

The management of tuberculosis may be summarized as follows:

Curative chemotherapy. Achieved by ensuring that the patient receives:
1 at least two drugs to which his organism is sensitive;
2 in appropriate dosage;
3 for long enough.

Prevention of spread of infection. Achieved by:
1   rapidly sterilizing antituberculous chemotherapy;
2   identification of close contacts who have become infected or who may be the source of the infection. This remains very important;
3   isolation of infective cases (now rarely necessary);
4   chemoprophylaxis (may be recommended in certain high-risk susceptible contacts).

Curative chemotherapy

The aims stated above are simple, but treatment nevertheless demands expertise and attention to detail, and it should be supervised by doctors working as part of a health team with special experience of the problems involved.

Refinement of antituberculous treatment

Effective treatment for tuberculosis really began in 1947 with the introduction of streptomycin, given by daily intramuscular injection. This was given together with oral *para*-aminosalicylic acid (PAS) and isoniazid (INH) to discourage the development of resistance. For about 25 years this remained the standard combination of drugs. Three drugs were given for 3 months and PAS and INH continued for 9 months or longer. There were problems with: (1) hypersensitivity reactions to the drugs; (2) emergence of resistant organisms; (3) poor compliance because of long duration; (4) a relapse rate requiring long follow-up; (5) need for isolation of sputum-positive patients because of slow sterilization. Rifampicin replaced streptomycin about 20 years ago and ethambutol replaced PAS. Careful trials showed that resistance was now rare; courses could be shortened to 6 months and follow-up was not necessary as cure was almost 100% if compliance was perfect. In practice a 2% relapse rate was encountered. In the last few years, concern about possible rare ocular toxicity from ethambutol has led to its being dropped except where atypical organisms are grown or suspected.

Modern short-course treatment

Initial treatment

For 2 months the patient takes orally: rifampicin, INH and pyrazinamide, daily in the morning.

Continuation treatment

For a further 4 months rifampicin and INH are taken orally, daily in the morning.
To this simple schedule it is usual to add a small daily dose of pyridoxine to prevent the development of peripheral neuropathy due to INH. Tolerance is good, compliance is assisted by the relatively short duration. Results are excellent so far, so that continued follow-up is not thought necessary where there have been no irregularities with treatment. Resistance is a great rarity. Although treatment is now very simple, attention must be paid to encouraging perfect co-operation on the part of the patient and to some relevant points of detail. It is particularly important to ensure that patients, members of their families and all

health workers involved understand that the rifampicin and INH are both taken together in the morning—not as divided doses.

There are a number of other proved and effective regimens available for the treatment of tuberculosis but these will not be detailed here. It is worth noting that these include regimens in which treatment is given three times weekly. This allows supervision of each dose where there would otherwise be inadequate compliance with treatment.

Review of principal antituberculous drugs

Rifampicin

Rifampicin is a broad spectrum antibiotic which is outstandingly effective against *Mycobacterium* tuberculosis. It is taken by mouth in a single daily dose of 600 mg by individuals weighing 50 kg or more and in a dose of 450 mg by those who are lighter.

Adverse effects are uncommon. Itching of the skin and an erythematous rash may develop early. Withdrawal and re-introduction of treatment usually resolves the problem. Jaundice may appear early in treatment and a rise in serum transaminase is fairly common. If jaundice is evident, rifampicin is temporarily withdrawn until bilirubin levels are normal once more. The drug can then be re-introduced without further jaundice developing. Thrombocytopenia and haemolytic anaemia are rare adverse effects. Rifampicin is largely excreted by the liver but enough appears in the urine to colour it red and suitable testing is easily carried out to confirm patient compliance.

Isoniazid (INH)

Isoniazid is an effective, well-tolerated antituberculous drug, given orally in a single daily dose of 300 mg (for normal sized adults).

The acetylator status of the individual affects the rate of disposal of INH but the above doses are sufficient to allow for rapid disposal by fast acetylators, and concurrent treatment with pyridoxine affords adequate protection against neuropathy in slow acetylators, so that it is not essential to establish acetylator status in all patients.

Apart from peripheral neuropathy, side-effects are rare. Skin rashes and hepatitis are occasionally attributable to INH and it is one of the drugs known to cause a form of systemic lupus erythematosus.

Pyrazinamide

Pyrazinamide is an effective bactericidal antituberculous agent given in a single oral daily dose of 2 g in patients weighing 50 kg or more and 1.5 g in those who are lighter.

It appears able to kill mycobacteria inside cells and it penetrates the cerebrospinal fluid well. Together with rifampicin it ensures rapid reduction in infectivity of sputum-positive patients. Pyrazinamide may cause arthralgia or even frank gout. Hepatotoxicity is also seen. This is occasionally severe and pyrazinamide is not reintroduced if jaundice seems attributable to it.

Other drugs

Ethambutol

Ethambutol is bacteriostatic in action and is now usually given in a dose of 15 mg kg^{-1}. It has an important action in preventing resistance as cross-resistance with other agents is unusual. It is useful in the treatment of atypical mycobacterial infection (see below). Optic neuritis is a worrying, but very rare, side-effect. Mild impairment of vision is reversible if the drug is stopped by the patient. Isolated cases of permanent blindness have occurred. Pretreatment screening of vision and regular testing cannot warn of the development of the complication.

Streptomycin

Streptomycin is a bactericidal antituberculous aminoglycoside antibiotic, given by intramuscular injection once daily in a dose of 1 g in normal sized adults with normal renal function. Beyond middle age the daily dose is reduced by 0.75 g or 0.5 g daily.

The principal side-effect is vestibular damage, which may cause permanent disabling ataxia. Generalized rashes and fever may also occur.

Para-aminosalicylic acid (PAS)

This is now little used, as it is unpleasant to take and has a high incidence of adverse effects and relatively low effectiveness. It is cheap and finds application in undeveloped countries.

Thiacetazone

This is cheap, variably tolerated and only moderately effective. It is not used in developed countries.

Cycloserine, prothionamide, capreomycin, viomycin and kanamycin

These are expensive, little-used 'reserve' antituberculous drugs. Their main application is in the treatment of drug resistant disease. Drug resistance is now largely confined to patients treated with older regimens which do not include rifampicin and to those individuals who, for psychosocial reasons, have not proved able to take treatment properly. Rifampicin is the drug of choice in 'resistant' disease where it has not already been used.

Prevention of the spread of infection

Infectivity

1 For practical purposes, only persons with acid- and alcohol-fast bacilli (AAFBs) in the sputum on direct examination are infectious. In sputum-negative patients, even if a culture is subsequently positive, the numbers of bacteria must be so small as to make infection of others very unlikely.

2 Patients with sputum positive for AAFBs may be considered technically non-infectious after they have completed 2 weeks of a modern three or four drug regimen which includes rifampicin.

3 Admission to hospital is unnecessary except: (a) in the gravely ill; (b) in a few degenerated alcoholic patients, vagrants and others for whom it might otherwise prove impossible to initiate proper treatment. The patient's own family will already have been exposed to the risk of infection for some considerable time before diagnosis so that segregation at the time of diagnosis is irrelevant: the infectivity of the patient will diminish very rapidly indeed once treatment is started.

4   In the case of patients who require to be in hospital for some reason, those with sputum negative for AAFBs may be managed in the same way as any other patients. Patients with sputum positive for AAFBs should be nursed in a single room until at least 2 weeks of chemotherapy have been completed. Patients should not cough over other individuals and the sputum should be regarded as highly infectious. Staff should wash the hands on leaving the cubicle. More elaborate measures—masks, gowns, gloves, separate crockery and afterwards fumigation of the room—are all unnecessary.

5   At home, patients with sputum positive for AAFBs should remain in their homes until at least 2 weeks of short course treatment, containing rifampicin, have been completed. Young children from other families should not visit the house during this time.

6   Patients may continue to produce AAFBs in the sputum for many weeks despite taking effective chemotherapy. If treatment is being taken correctly these organisms may be regarded as killed after 2 weeks and cultures should prove negative.

Contact tracing

This is important. About 10% of all tuberculosis diagnosed in the UK is detected by examination of contacts of known cases. Persons living in the same household are those most at risk. About 10% develop active disease where the index case is sputum-positive. It is usual to limit contact tracing to household contacts, but the search is generally widened to include close family members who visit frequently and also to include any young children who visit. Close friends and sexual partners are contacts. Other casual contacts, including those encoutered at work are only rarely sufficiently close to merit tracing and examination. Particularly high rates of tuberculosis are found in the contacts of Asian immigrants with the disease.

Adult non-immigrant contacts

Adults should have a chest X-ray performed immediately. In contacts of sputum-negative patients this is all that is required. Contacts of patients with sputum positive for AAFBs should have a repeat chest X-ray 3 and 12 months after the patient starts treatment. In most UK communities, tuberculin testing of non-immigrant adults is unrewarding as a high proportion of the normal population give positive results.

Adult Asian immigrant contacts and all children under 16 who have not had BCG

Contacts should be Heaf-tested and those with a reaction of Grade III or more should be treated. Where there is no evidence of the disease process, treatment may amount to prophylaxis using INH alone for 6 months. Those who are Heaf-negative should be offered BCG vaccination. Those who are Heaf-positive should have a chest X-ray which should be repeated at 3 and 12 months. Asian contacts and ideally all household contacts of sputum-positive patients should have a further chest X-ray at 24 months.

Children who have definitely had BCG vaccination
These contacts require a chest X-ray which should be repeated at 3, 12 and, in the case of sputum-positive index cases, at 24 months.

Note
Heaf-testing of contacts is best deferred until 6 weeks after a sputum-positive index case has started effective treatment. Otherwise testing could take place before the development of skin hypersensitivity to tuberculin in a very recently infected individual (leading to a false negative Heaf test).

Prophylaxis

BCG vaccination
BCG (Bacillus Calmette–Guérin) is a live-attenuated strain of tuberculosis which confers a useful degree of immunity in some communities. It is still offered to all tuberculin-negative children at about 13 years in the UK. It is given by intradermal injection. A local skin reaction is produced at about 4 weeks and there may be regional lymphadenopathy. The tuberculin test is positive after this time in successful 'takes'. Its continued use as a universal prophylactic is being questioned in countries where the risk of tuberculosis is low.
　　BCG is given to babies and children in contact with known cases of tuberculosis.

Chemoprophylaxis
Treatment is normally advised when positive tuberculin tests are encountered in children who have not received BCG. This is particularly important in adolescent girls because of the possibility of occult genital tuberculosis and subsequent sterility. A modified regimen may be adopted using INH alone, in a single daily dose of 100–300 mg for a year. Prophylactic treatment may also be indicated in particular high-risk groups: for example, patients with evidence of 'healed' tuberculosis who undergo treatment with steroid or other immunosuppressive drugs.

Opportunistic mycobacteria (atypical mycobacteria)
About 2% of clinically diagnosed cases of tuberculosis turn out to be due to atypical mycobacteria. The most prevalent of these are *M. kansasii*, *M. avium intracellulare* (a group of organisms), *M. malmoense* and *M. xenopi*. The organisms are widespread in nature and can be found in rainwater pools, soil, etc. They act as low-grade pathogens which pose no risk to normal individuals.
　　Infection occurs in individuals with:
1 *Severely damaged lungs.* Usually patients are old and have advanced emphysema or a remote history of ordinary tuberculosis; pulmonary function is often severely impaired.

2 *Impaired immune competence.* Those who are suffering from AIDS, haematological malignancy or other forms of immune incompetence are at risk.

Clinical and radiological features

The features are essentially those of tuberculosis. Cavitation is virtually always present. Some infections cause cervical lymphadenopathy.

Diagnosis

The diagnosis is made in the laboratory on the basis of cultural characteristics and biochemical tests.

Treatment

Treatment has commonly already begun on suspicion of a diagnosis of ordinary *M. tuberculosis.*

Treatment is with rifampicin and ethambutol for up to 2 years. *M. kansasii* may be adequately treated by 9 months of treatment. If progress is unsatisfactory, streptomycin is added. *M. avium intracellulare* shows most resistance.

Sometimes surgical resection brings about satisfactory cure but most patients are too frail to stand thoracotomy.

Chapter 14
Bronchiectasis

Bronchiectasis is a state of dilatation of at least some of the bronchi. The bronchial wall is irreversibly damaged as a consequence of earlier inflammation and infection of the bronchus or neighbouring lung tissue, and the normal transport of mucus is impaired. In severe cases there is chronic lung suppuration. The condition is characterized by cough and the regular production of large amounts of purulent sputum.

Prevalence
The true prevalence is not known. Minor bronchiectasis is probably often classed as chronic bronchitis or ignored. More than 50 years ago bronchiectasis was common. Most cases derived from severe lung infection in childhood. As the population has become replaced by people who have grown up in the antibiotic era, the prevalence of bronchiectasis has undoubtedly fallen. Post-infective cases are becoming proportionately less common and the importance of other causes of bronchiectasis (e.g. ciliary defects and immunosuppression) is becoming apparent.

Pathological features
Bronchiectasis may be localized to just part of a lung if there is a local cause. Usually it is patchy in distribution. The form of dilatation varies but the shape of the distortion is of small significance only (Fig. 14.1).

The wall of the bronchus is thin and dilated. It has much reduced elastin and commonly heavy inflammatory cell infiltration. The epithelium is generally cuboidal rather than columnar, cilia are absent and there may be squamous metaplasia. The epithelium is infiltrated by inflammatory cells and may slough off during exacerbations. The lung supplied by the bronchiectatic airways may show patchy consolidation and scarring and be reduced in volume.

Pathogenesis
The essential steps in the evolution of bronchiectasis are:
1 Impaired mucociliary clearance leads to the accumulation of secretions.
2 Accumulation of secretions leads to infection by bacteria.
3 Infection by bacteria leads to increased mucus production. Infection by bacteria produces impaired ciliary performance. Infection by bacteria leads to inflammatory response.
4 Excessive inflammatory response causes tissue damage.
5 Tissue damage eventually produces dilated bronchi. Tissue damage includes loss of ciliated epithelium and impaired mucociliary clearance. Impaired mucociliary clearance . . . return to step 1.

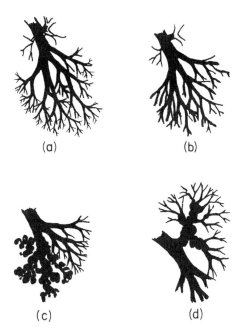

(a)   (b)

(c)   (d)

Fig. 14.1. Bronchiectasis. Diagram of appearances of bronchogram: (a), (b) and (c) left lower lobe; (d) left upper lobe. (a) Normal. (b) Bronchiectasis—the normal graceful tapering of bronchi is lacking; bronchi are crowded and the finer peripheral branches do not fill. (c) Gross saccular bronchiectasis. (d) Proximal bronchiectasis with normal peripheral bronchi accompanying allergic aspergillosis.

These steps form a closed loop or vicious circle which is illustrated in Fig. 14.2. Bronchiectasis could derive from a process which starts at any of the steps. For example if some major insult (say tuberculous damage) causes tissue damage to a bronchus, the sequence may start at step 5. If ciliary action is abnormal, the process can start at step 1. Immune globulin deficiency may result in excessive bacterial survival in the airway and the process start at step 3.

Underlying causes

Severe infection
1   Previous severe whooping cough (responsible for perhaps a quarter of present-day cases).
2   Previous tuberculosis (a small proportion in the UK).
3   Previous severe pneumonia.
4   Repeated infection from aspiration.

Bronchopulmonary aspergillosis
The damage here is a consequence of the intense immunological response rather than direct fungal invasion. Sometimes the bronchiectasis is striking, proximal and produces a glove-like pattern on bronchography (see p. 181 for more detail).

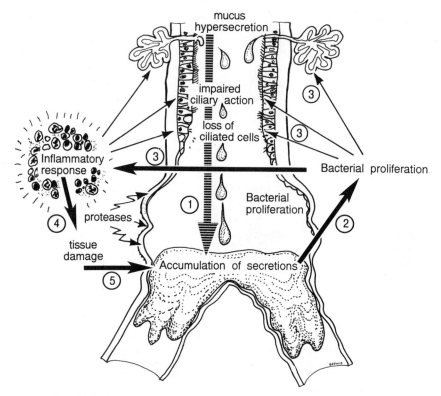

Fig. 14.2. Summary of the principal factors at work in worsening bronchiectasis.

Bronchial obstruction

Obstruction due to tumour, foreign body or external gland compression.

Congenital anomaly

Bronchiectasis develops in sequestered lobes—malformations in which the lung tissue has no proper connection with the airway and commonly has a systemic rather than a pulmonary blood supply.

The above causes may produce bronchiectasis limited to the abnormal area of lung.

Ciliary dyskinesia

This term covers a number of syndromes, in which there is a genetic defect responsible for impaired cilial beating, which were formerly lumped together as 'immotile cilia syndrome'. They include Kartagener's syndrome in which dextrocardia and situs inversus is associated with bronchiectasis. Dyenin arms (p. 7) are found deficient on electron microscopy. In Young's syndrome, ciliary dyskinesia is accompanied by male infertility and by blockage of the epididymis. This form is probably the commonest dyskinesia and has a very high incidence of associated sinusitis. In primary dyskinesia, symptoms are almost always present from early life. The diagnosis of ciliary dyskinesia may be assisted by the assessment of nasal ciliary clearance. In this test, saccharin is placed gently on the anterior end of the inferior turbinate and the time taken for the patient to notice a sweet taste is recorded. In ciliary dyskinesia this may take more than 30 minutes. More specialized tests involve examination of ciliary beating by microscope photometry and of ciliary ultrastructure.

Hypogammaglobulinaemia

Hypogammaglobulinaemia may become evident in childhood or the first half of adult life. Bronchiectasis may be the most prominent manifestation and can be steadily progressive and fatal. Patients tend to have other disorders such as chronic diarrhoea from abnormal intestinal colonization, e.g. by *Giardia lamblia*. The progress of bronchiectasis and other manifestations can be controlled by regular 3-weekly injections of gamma globulin. Children or adults with progressive bronchiectasis should all be screened for hypogammaglobulinaemia.

Clinical features

The cardinal clinical feature of bronchiectasis is longstanding, easy, frequent coughing up of green sputum. Assuming that the chest X-ray does not show obvious lung abscess, tuberculosis or other local disease and the patient does not have cystic fibrosis, this feature is virtually diagnostic. There is considerable variation in severity of bronchiectasis. Severe disease is nowadays uncommon because of the effect of more intensive use of antibiotics.

Mild

Rattly cough and green sputum after colds only.
Changing position may produce sputum.
Occasionally small haemoptysis.
Patient generally very well; normal pulmonary function.
Normal chest X-ray.

Moderate

Rattly cough all the time.
Able to produce a specimen of sputum at any time—usually green, rarely mucoid. Occasional haemoptysis.
Patients or relatives may notice hallitosis.
Patient usually generally well; pulmonary function usually normal.
Rarely clubbing. Crackles commonly audible.
Chest X-ray usually near normal.

Severe

Very large volumes of khaki-coloured sputum.
Occasional pneumonic illness with haemoptysis and pleural pain.
Clubbing very common.
Particularly if associated with airways obstruction, dyspnoea, cyanosis and respiratory failure may develop.
Patient often generally unwell, off work frequently, may vomit during expectoration.

Pyogenic skin and ocular infections common.

Gram-negative bacteria commonly present in sputum.

At risk from pneumonia, septicaemia, remote abscess formation and (rarely) amyloidosis.

Widespread coarse crackles audible.

Chest X-ray may show increased bronchovascular markings and sometimes multiple cysts containing fluid levels.

Investigation

Sputum examination

Naked-eye inspection of the sputum is essential to confrim the patient's account. Direct smear examination and culture for tuberculosis should be included in the initial assessment. Bacteriological examination is often unhelpful despite the obvious purulence of the sputum. *Haemophilus influenzae* and staphylococci are commonly isolated, but more often no pathogens are recovered. More advanced cases tend to harbour *Ps. aeruginosa* or *Klebsiella* species. Anaerobic culture techniques carried out in specialist laboratories have shown that there are usually very many different saprophytic organisms present in sputum which appears sterile on standard culture.

Radiography

A chest X-ray is necessary in order to exclude obvious localized lung disease but the appearances are often normal. In severe disease there may be peribronchial thickening, which is evident as parallel tramline shadowing or unusually prominent small circular shadows near the hila, where bronchi are seen in profile or end-on, respectively. Sometimes severe cystic bronchiectasis is directly visible. There may be associated consolidation, collapse or feature suggestive of the cause, such as oesophageal disease, aspergillosis or sequestrated lung (usually a collection of cysts at one base).

Computerized tomography (CT) is a useful tool for the confirmation of moderate to severe bronchiectasis. Minor degrees may be missed by CT but are detectable by bronchography.

Bronchography (see p. 84)

This investigation is expensive and uncomfortable and need not be carried out where the diagnosis is clear and management is satisfactory. It may be necessary where the diagnosis is in doubt: for example, in the investigation of haemoptysis or recurrent regional collapse. It may also be necessary where management is unsatisfactory and there are grounds to suspect that the condition might be localized and treatable by resection.

Occasionally major saccular or varicose bronchiectasis is revealed, but more usually the appearances are less dramatic and comprise: disturbance of the normal tapering pattern of part of the bronchial tree, abrupt failure to fill small bronchi in these areas and crowding of bronchi reflecting a degree of collapse in the part of the lung supplied (Fig. 14.1). The condition is generally patchy, basal and bilateral. Occasionally only one lobe is involved; left lower lobe and lingula are the most common sites for localized disease. Allergic bronchopulmonary aspergillosis has been shown to be accompanied sometimes by proximal bronchiectasis (see p. 181). In general, however, the pattern of the bronchial abnormality is not helpful in suggesting aetiology.

Management

The most important elements in the management of the patient with bron-chiectasis are generally explanation and reassurance. The patient is usually anxious about such things as: whether they are infectious to others, whether frequent cough damages their lungs, whether they will become disabled by breathlessness, or die prematurely—perhaps from haemoptysis. Reasonable reassurance can be expressed on all of these points in most patients.

Active treatment aims to interrupt the vicious circle (Fig. 14.2) and comprises:

1 Postural drainage to combat the accumulation of secretions (1 in Fig. 14.2).
2 Antibiotic treatment (and gamma globulin where relevant) to combat infection by bacteria (2 in Fig. 14.2).
3 Anti-inflammatory treatment with low dose corticosteroids. This may be needed in exceptionally severe disease to modulate the intensity of damaging inflammatory response.
4 Surgical treatment (rare).

Postural drainage

The patient should be encouraged to 'tip' for at least 10 minutes up to three times daily, if by doing so additional sputum is produced. In mild cases this will apply for a week or two after colds and in severe cases it will be necessary indefinitely. Intelligent patients will discover the most productive position by trial and error. Usually a steep head-down position is most satisfactory. Exercise and 'huffing'—forced expiration continued to residual volume—may also be very helpful in encouraging sputum production.

Antibiotic and chemotherapy

Mild cases require an antibiotic after a cold and this will usually render the sputum mucoid (clear coloured). Some moderately severe cases require an antibiotic at intervals, as this is found to render the sputum clear for useful periods.

In some, more severe, patients the sputum becomes purulent again as soon as the antibiotic is stopped. In these patients a judgement needs to be made of the benefits and snags of continuous treatment. Where the disease is distressing it is now common to recommend long-term, high dose treatment with a well tolerated antibiotic such as amoxycillin. This may be used in doses of 500 mg to 3 g twice daily. The treatment at high dose is usually effective, whatever the microbiological content of the sputum. Additional antibiotic can be administered by nebulizer driven by a powerful compressor. Continuous antibiotic treatment offers some protection against the important progression seen in a few patients. Difficulty due to the emergence of important resistant stains of pathogenic bacteria is not a common problem.

Some patients beyond middle age have good pulmonary function and have felt perfectly well for years, despite permanently purulent sputum; these individuals may not feel benefit from long-term antibiotic treatment.

In addition to amoxycillin, co-trimoxazole is effective and may be used long term with little difficulty. Augmentin may be used if β-lactamase producing *H. influenzae* is thought to be important. If a staphylococcus is regularly produced, flucloxacillin is used. Metronidazole can be used to control foetid unpleasant sputum. Some clinicians prefer a rotating sequence of antibiotics, e.g. amoxycillin, co-trimoxazole, tetracycline or oral cephalosporin.

When a patient with bronchiectasis becomes severally ill, the possibility of pneumonia or septicaemia from *Staphylococcus, Pseudomonas or Klebsiella* should be considered.

Anti-inflammatory treatment

Corticosteroid treatment is indicated exceptionally, to control severe malaise, anorexia, arthritis or vasculitis.

Surgical excision

This may be indicated in rare instances of distressing bronchiectasis which has been shown to be confined to one lobe. In practice, most cases of bronchiectasis are patchy and bilateral.

Complications

Haemoptysis

This is common and only very rarely threatening. It may happen at any time—not necessarily during a striking exacerbation. The bronchial circulation is much increased in bronchiectasis. Severe unceasing haemoptysis is uncommon and may require bronchial artery embolization (by an expert), using tiny wire spirals introduced by a special catheter passed up the aorta from a femoral puncture. If this is not available, or fails, then emergency lung resection may be required.

Septic complications

Cerebral abscess and other systemic spread of sepsis is very uncommon in the developed world. Secondary amyloidosis is now rare because of the more active control of chronic sepsis by antibiotics.

Respiratory failure

This is uncommon. Usually there is associated airways obstruction or previous severe lung destruction from pneumonia or tuberculosis. Heart–lung transplantation may be a relevant option.

Prognosis

This is obviously related to the severity. The vast majority of patients are able to lead normal lives and have a life expectancy which is nearly normal. The oulook is much less certain in those with extensive lung destruction or airways obstruction.

Chapter 15
Cystic Fibrosis

Cystic fibrosis (CF) is caused by a defective gene, which is responsible for compiling a protein important in the transport of ions across cellular membranes. Abnormally high concentrations of sodium and chloride ions are found in the secretions of all exocrine glands in the body. The main clinical effects of the disease are secondary to the alteration of the physical characteristics of the secretions in the lungs and gastrointestinal tract. These are the development of chronic suppurative bronchiectasis with lung destruction, pancreatic failure and intestinal obstruction.

Inheritance

The gene for cystic fibrosis is the most common inherited abnormality and one of the most common in the world in European societies. It is carried by about 1 in 25 of the population and is recessive. Affected individuals are homozygous for the abnormal gene. The chance of two heterozygote carriers mating is 1 in 25 $\times$ 25 —that is 1 in 625. Only 1 in 4 of the offspring of two carriers would be affected. This accords with the observed frequency of cystic fibrosis—about 1 in 2000–2500 live births.

A family history of CF is usually lacking. There is a 1 in 4 chance of a sibling being affected, a 1 in 50 chance of a half-sibling being affected and a 1 in 2000 chance of a first cousin being affected.

The basic defect

The abnormal gene is located on the long arm of chromosome 7. It was identified in 1989. The protein derived from the gene has been described and is named CF transmembrane regulator (CFTR), reflecting views on its function. There appear to be several deletions in the sequence of base pairs, close together on the DNA molecule. This may help to explain the puzzling variation in severity of cases of CF which is quite independent of treatment measures. The gene is expressed in epithelial elements in the lungs and gastrointestinal tract but not in some other tissues such as fibroblasts. Work on human sweat glands has shown that the fluid produced deep in the gland is normal in composition, but that there is a failure of reabsorption of sodium and chloride ions in the more distal parts of the gland, so that the sweat has abnormally high concentrations of these electrolytes. Similar effects probably occur in the pancreas and in glands and glandular cells of the respiratory tract. Altered electrolyte concentrations in the sol layer in which the cilia beat and alterations of hydration of the mucus gel layer probably interfere with the delicate process of mucociliary clearance so that secretions accumulate and infection can become established.

The term 'mucoviscidosis' has been in use for many years and is potentially misleading. The end result of severe disease in the lungs, pancreas, intestine and liver, may be that the secretions become thick and viscid but there is no evidence of any defect in the mucus itself.

Pathology and natural history

The main effects are seen in the lungs and pancreas. The untreated progress of individuals severely affected by the disease evolves through the sequence shown in Fig. 15.1.

Pulmonary effects

The pulmonary lesion is characterized by bronchiectasis. There is dilatation of bronchi with perpetual inflammation in the walls of the airway and neighbouring lung. The secretions become permanantly colonized by bacteria and are constantly purulent. Sputum is produced in greatly increased amounts. Some comes from hypertrophied mucous glands. Initially, commensal organisms and relatively harmless anaerobic bacteria are present. In time, colonization by *Staphylococcus aureus* commonly occurs and in those with substantial bronchial damage *Pseudomonas aeruginosa* becomes resident. Mucociliary transport is impaired by products from many bacteria, especially *Pseudomonas* species. Damage from the toxic effects of these organisms is believed to occur during exacerbations of infection and inflammation, which may be occasioned by superadded viral infection. In severe disease, small lung abscesses develop and cause focal lung destruction. Purulent sputum contains high levels of proteolytic enzymes—elastases and collagenases derived from cells (particularly neutrophils) and bacteria. Antiprotease activity may be overwhelmed, leading to structural damage and the development of patchy emphysema.

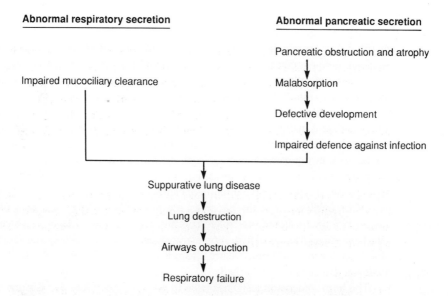

Fig. 15.1. Sequence of effects of cystic fibrosis in untreated individuals.

Gastrointestinal effects

The pancreas is almost always affected, even though about 10% of patients have no clinical evidence of pancreatic insufficiency. Obstruction of small ducts occurs; the glandular tissue atrophies and the pancreas becomes scarred and cystic. The term cystic fibrosis was originally introduced to describe the characteristic pancreatic lesion rather than the lung appearances.

Pancreatic failure leads to malabsorption and steatorrhoea.

Other disorders

Biliary cirrhosis

The quality of biliary secretion may be altered and one-third of patients have either abnormal liver function tests or histological abnormalities. Rarely this progresses to cirrhosis and sometimes to the development of portal hypertension with varices and hypersplenism.

Nasal polyposis

The mechanism of nasal polyposis in cystic fibrosis is obscure.

Gonadal dysgenesis

Males are virtually always sterile because of a defect of development of the Wolffian system so that the epididymis and vas deferens are rudimentary and obstructed. This defect is present from earliest childhood.

Clinical features

The principle clinical features are set out in Table 15.1.

Infants and young children

Meconium ileus

About 10% of affected children present in this way. The meconium is inspissated, dark and sticky. Intestinal obstruction is evident within the first few hours after birth. Factors other than simple pancreatic insufficiency seem to underlie the condition. True meconium ileus is restricted to the first day or so, but a related disorder occurs in older children and adults, which is sometimes referred to as meconium ileus equivalent or MIE (see distal intestinal obstruction below).

Failure to thrive

More than half of affected children have obvious malabsorption by the age of 6 months. They show growth retardation and are underweight despite a large appetite. There is abdominal distension and the stools are copious and highly offensive. Some children have rectal prolapse.

Respiratory illness

First respiratory symptoms may develop at any age. The main features are: persistent cough, recurrent respiratory infections with cough after colds and

Table 15.1. Features of cystic fibrosis.

Major or common features	Less common features
Childhood CF	
Respiratory features	
Cough	Nasal polyps
Frequent infections	Asthma
Airways obstruction	
Gastrointestinal features	
Meconium ileus	Rectal prolapse
Malabsorption	Liver disease
Steatorrhoea	cirrhosis
Failure to thrive	hypersplenism
Malnutrition	Diabetes
Adult CF	
Respiratory features	
Bronchiectasis	Asthma
Airways obstruction	Pneumothorax
Respiratory failure	Allergic bronchopulmonary aspergillosis
	Opportunistic mycobacterial infection
Gastrointestinal features	
Steatorrhoea	Liver disease
Low body weight	gallstones
	portal hypetension
	varices
	Distal intestinal obstruction syndrome
	(DIOS or MIE)
	Peptic ulceration
Reproduction	
Male sterility	
Delayed puberty	
Inheritance stress	
Stress of pregnancy & child	
rearing	
Other	
Employability stress	Diabetes
Life expectancy stress	Arthritis
	Vasculitis
	Salt depletion

retching and vomiting associated with coughing. Small children do not produce sputum but the cough sounds rattly and productive. Wheezing is common in smaller children.

Older children and adults

Respiratory illness

Persistent cough producing copious purulent sputum is characteristic. The sputum is initially pale yellow, but with advancing bronchiectasis becomes green or khaki in colour.

Suppurative lung disease

The progress of bronchiectasis is accompanied by finger clubbing and, sometimes, intermittent haemoptysis (which may be severe). Infective exacerbation tends to be accompanied by malaise, anorexia and sometimes pleuritic pain. Advanced disease is accompanied by dyspnoea and examination shows overinflation and the presence of crackles and wheezes on auscultation.

Other lung changes

Pneumothorax occurs in about 5–10% of individuals and can be a dangerous development in advanced disease. Prompt tube drainage may be needed. Previously, prompt surgical closure and pleurodesis was advised but this is now avoided because it may prevent later transplantation surgery.

Haemoptysis is common in established disease. Rarely this may be torrential and require embolization of dilated bronchial arteries.

Some patients develop asthma and as a group have increased levels of serum IgE.

Bronchi and abnormal lung spaces may become colonized by *Aspergillus fumigatus* and the features of allergic bronchopulmonary aspergillosis (p. 180) may be added to those of cystic fibrosis.

Pulmonary function

Airways obstruction is the universal pattern. The name cystic fibrosis describes the pancreatic lesion; the lung disease does not resemble fibrotic lung disease. Serial measurement of FEV_1 gives a reliable indication of the severity and progress of the disease. Peak flow is less sensitive and less repeatable. When FEV_1 is reduced below about 0.5 litre in a fully grown individual, ventilatory failure soon supervenes. Hypoxia is the rule. Full-blown cor pulmonale may develop and this is not usually survived for more than a few months.

Radiographic features

These are highly characteristic. The chest X-ray will be of a young person. The earliest features are small scattered irregular marks in the upper and mid zones accompanied by features of bronchial wall thickening (prominent ring shadows and parallel 'tram line' shadows). There is usually overinflation, reflecting the adaption to airways obstruction. With increasing severity of disease, small areas of consolidation with shaggy outlines occur, varying in prominence from time to time but remaining constant in position. Small abscess cavities may develop. Streaky shadows may be added in advanced disease and there may be enlargement of the pulmonary artery and features of aspergillosis.

Gastrointestinal illness

Malabsorption

The effects of pancreatic insufficiency vary in severity in older children and adults. All but about 10% will have steatorrhoea with frequent bulky offensive stools, unless they receive adequate pancreatic replacement therapy.

Distal intestinal obstruction syndrome (DIOS)
Also referred to as meconium ileus equivalent (MIE), this disorder is character-ized by colicky abdominal pain, constipation and occasionally vomiting. On examination there may be general abdominal distension or, more usually, merely a palpable mass of fullness in the right iliac fossa. There may be a history of neglect of pancreatic supplements to cover unusually high fat intake.

Less common disorders
Liver failure is very rare. Bleeding from varices is rare. Splenic enlargement is occasionally seen and may be accompanied by thrombocytopenia. The perpetual immunological response to bacterial colonization of the lungs may lead to disorders related to circulating antigen/antibody complexes, such as vasculitic skin rashes, mononeuropathies and arthritis. These effects are reduced by intensive antibotic treatment.

Failure of development
Failure to grow causes distress in childhood, as does failure to achieve secondary sexual development. The effects are proportional to the severity of both lung disease and nutritional inadequacy. Mildly affected individuals grow and mature normally.

Reproductive problems
Male sterility is irreversible surgically. It causes anxiety and depression and reduces the chances of attracting a life partner, although marriage (and equivalent) is still quite common.

Females with advanced disease have reduced fertility. Mildly affected females are fertile. Pregnancy is not entered into lightly. Firstly, pregnancy is sometimes accompanied by significant and permanent deterioration in respiratory health. Possible explanations are the nutritional stress and sometimes reluctance to take treatment and maintain bronchial clearance. Secondly, the demands of rearing a child are physically stressing and can distract the patient from her own treatment needs.

In females, there is always concern about producing an affected child. The initial probability is 1 in 50 if the father's carrier status is unknown. If DNA analysis shows him not to be a carrier of any of the known genetic variants there is virtually no risk of an affected child although all offspring will be carriers. If the father is a carrier, half of offspring will be affected and half carrier.

Social and emotional stresses
In addition to stresses related to reproduction, the patient with cystic fibrosis has concerns about long-term outlook for survival, outlook for employment, problems about insurance and security for house purchase. Treatment can be costly and some treatment is demanding and time-consuming. Throughout life, the patient with cystic fibrosis will have a socially embarrassing loud rattly cough, which can turn disapproving heads at any gathering.

Serious emotional problems may arise in teenage, when anxieties over failure of sexual development and retarted growth may be added to the frustrations of ill health and impaired job prospects, at a time when patients are struggling for independence. Rejection of medical aspects of care is common and this is sometimes accompanied by rapid progression of disease.

Diagnosis

DNA analysis

DNA analysis is now the only satisfactory diagnostic test, where it is available. The reliability is high but not perfect. There are several related deletions which can make up the abnormal gene. The test can also be undertaken on chorionic villus biopsy material, to achieve antenatal diagnosis of high reliability in the first trimester.

Older tests

The principal test was the sweat test, which relied on demonstrating that the sweat of affected individuals had an abnormally high chloride and sodium ion content (normally about 20 mmol litre^{-1} and in CF usually >70 mmol litre^{-1}). This was simple in concept, but technically difficult because of the small samples and the tendency for results to be spoiled by evaporation. Extreme attention to detail was required. In recent years there has been interest in the finding that patients with cystic fibrosis show a higher potential difference across respiratory epithelium than normal. This can be detected by measuring the potential difference between a nasal probe and an indifferent electrode elsewhere. The test is convenient but not wholly reliable and not in wide use. Investigation of pancreatic function is now less often indicated to resolve diagnosis. Formerly, duodenal intubation and the urinary detection of ingested *para*-aminobenzoic acid (PABA) were in regular use.

Screening

Early diagnosis may carry advantage. Infants with cystic fibrosis have elevated serum immunoreactive trypsin activity. This can be measured by a filter paper test on a single drop of blood. DNA analysis is more accurate. Screening babies for cystic fibrosis is undertaken in a number of centres. The public is thought to favour the theoretical idea of universal screening of young adults considering child rearing, but it is not known whether this would be welcomed in practice.

Management

The basic elements of treatment comprise: bronchial clearance, antibiotics, pancreatic extract and diet. Management includes much more than this; it includes education and continuous encouragement. Skills from several disciplines are needed.

Respiratory disease

Bronchial clearance

At all stages of the disease, measures to encourage bronchial drainage are important.

Postural drainage is the most effective procedure. It involves lying in a steep head-down position for at least 10 minutes twice daily. Postural drainage is carried out more frequently and in various positions if this is shown to yield more sputum. Prolonged forced expiration (huffing) may release secretions in distal bronchi, where it is not produced by standard coughing. Huffing and postural drainage can be combined beneficially. Frappage and other vibration seems to have little effect, but participation by a partner in clearance measures encourages the performance of the patient.

Antibiotic treatment

Oral antibiotics
No universally agreed policy for antibiotic use has emerged. Some children are given long-term flucloxacillin if the sputum is known to contain staphylococcus. Some children and adults follow a regimen of long-term, continuous, broad spectrum antibiotic treatment, e.g. with amoxycillin. There is probably no point in frequent sputum culture with a view to starting treatment based on these results alone. Oral antibiotic treatment is, however, always started in the event of an exacerbation; previous culture results can guide antibiotic choice. Amoxycillin, erythromycin, co-trimoxazole or an oral cephalosporin are commonly used in the UK. If *Pseudomonas aeruginosa* is known to be present, ciprofloxacin can be useful as a first measure, but if response is delayed beyond a few days or disease is advanced, intravenous treatment will be required without delay. Very high dose regular treatment with amoxycillin is increasingly popular. It can produce prolonged sputum clearing and well-being, even when sputum culture shows that there are organisms present which are not sensitive on laboratory testing (e.g. *Ps. aeruginosa*).

Intravenous antibiotics
In severe disease, *Ps. aeruginosa* is almost always present and intravenous antibiotic treatment is needed in exacerbations. It is impossible to eradicate *Pseudomonas* once established. Either a modified penicillin such as azlocillin or modified cephalosporin such as ceftazidime is given, together with an aminoglycoside antibiotic such as gentamicin or tobramycin. Treatment is often conducted at home by the patient. There is interest in the practice of giving regular elective treatment, say at 3 month intervals, even in the absence of frank exacerbations. This may defer the development of important lung damage. Where venous access is difficult, a 'Port-a-cath' or 'Lifeport' system can be implanted, comprising a subcutaneous diaphragm connected to a central venous cannula. Using special needles, repeated injections can be given easily through the same diaphragm. Intravenous treatment is expensive: depending on drug combination, dose and duration, a 2 week course can cost up to £1000 sterling.

Inhaled antibiotics
In advanced disease, antibiotic treatment can be given twice daily by inhalation using a nebulizer and a strong compressor. Gentamicin and sometimes carbenicillin or amoxycillin have been used alone, or in combination, and evidence

suggests that exacerbations and need for hospitalization are reduced. Treatment is inconvenient and time-consuming.

Treatment of associated respiratory disease

Pneumothorax and severe haemoptysis are referred to above. Allergic broncho-pulmonary aspergillosis may require low dose steroid treatment. Opportunistic mycobacterial disease is treated in standard fashion (p. 121). Many patients obtain useful benefit from bronchodilator treatment with β-agonists by aerosol. Patients with frank asthma usually benefit from inhaled steroid treatment.

Management of advanced disease

In addition to antibiotic treatment, severe pulmonary suppuration may be helped by low dose corticosteroid treatment, by reducing the damaging level of pulmonary inflammation. Anorexia may be helped at the same time.

Respiratory failure and cor pulmonale indicate the need for lung transplantation where this is an option. Over 100 transplants have been carried out in the UK, with generally good results. The donor lung does not develop characteristics of cystic fibrosis. The treatment is problematic because of shortage of donors, problems with rejection and obliterative bronchiolitis and the fact that not all patients with cystic fibrosis are suitable. Unsuitability usually arises through severe suppuration and severe respiratory disability contributing to the cachexia of malabsorption and anorexia, so that body weight and muscular strength are inadequate for the challenge of transplantation. The advent of transplantation has placed greater emphasis on the nutritional aspect in advanced disease. Tube feeding and gastrostomy feeding may be employed.

Where transplantation is not an option, all possible palliative measures to ease the terminal stages are relevant. Long-term oxygen treatment by concentrator (p. 301) may extend survival and improve well-being, but experience is not encouraging. Patients generally know when death is approaching and need opportunities to talk about this and about specific fears that they harbour with people they know and trust. Death is usually peaceful, after a short coma due to profound ventilatory failure and hypoxia.

Nutrition

Pancreatic extract

Pancreatic extract derived from pig or cow is taken by mouth. The extract is destroyed in the stomach: the most effective presentation comprises enteric-coated microspheres ('Pancrease', 'Creon'). Patients may need to take 2–10 capsules per meal. Other simple coated preparations are less effective. The patient should have only one normal inoffensive stool per day. Effectiveness can be improved by reducing gastric acid production with H_2 blockers.

Diet

The diet should be full, normal and balanced; hearty eating is to be encouraged. Fat avoidance is counterproductive since it leads to calorie restriction. The aim is to cover with pancreatic extract whatever fat intake the patient prefers.

Patients who tend to be underweight need snacks between meals and supplements in the form of polymerized carbohydrate (e.g. 'Caloreen'), milk-based protein-fortified proprietary drinks such as 'Build Up' and may benefit from medium-chain triglyceride preparations, which are easily incorporated.

Overt vitamin deficiency is very rare, but levels of fat soluble vitamins have been shown to be low and supplementation is usual in patients with more than mild disease. Oral vitamin A, D and sometimes E are usually given. Vitamin K analogue is given if a prolonged prothrombin time is encountered.

In advanced disease, nasogastric or gastrostomy feeding may be needed for short-term objectives.

Management of distal intestinal obstruction syndrome (DIOS)

Full-blown obstruction is managed initially by nasogastric suction and intravenous fluid replacement. Three treatments are in use: one comprises flushing the bowel with a high volume of balanced electrolyte solution; another comprises administration of sodium diatrizoate ('Gastrographin'); the third involves administration of N-acetyl cysteine by mouth and sometimes by enema. Distal intestinal obstruction syndrome (DIOS) is best avoided by adequate pancreatic supplementation together with H_2 blockers. Occasional minor relapses can be self-treated with Gastrographin.

Information, guidance and support

Continuity of care and consistency of advice is crucial. Cystic fibrosis is a chronic disabling and threatening condition of young people, generating considerable stress in patients and families. Controlling worry takes time. Patients need free access to staff with experience in cystic fibrosis and care is increasingly concentrated in regional centres. Care may be shared between the regional centre and a local hospital—prompt treatment being available locally and visits being made to a centre for problem discussion and to ensure that progress meets desirable targets.

The Cystic Fibrosis Trust co-ordinates fund raising for research and acts as a focus of information for families by organizing meetings and publishing leaflets and books. The CF Adults Association provides information and opportunities for mutual self-help.

Prognosis

In the 1950s, survival beyond 10 years was unusual. Before the 1970s survival beyond late teenage was unusual. Now most patients survive to late teenage and many reach their late twenties. With time, it is likely that more will reach 40 years and beyond. Although attention to nutrition and more intensive use of antibiotic treatment probably explains the overall improvement, many long survivors have not had unusual care; it is likely that genetic variation underlies this paradox.

Chapter 16
Lung Abscess

This term is customarily reserved for localized suppurative lesions of the lung parenchyma which are not obviously due to tuberculosis or other specific infections.

Aetiology

Aspiration
This is the commonest cause of lung abscess. Inhalation of food, vomitus, sputum or other material is particularly likely to occur in association with:
1 States of impaired consciousness.
2 Alcoholism.
3 Incompetence of the larynx due to paralysis or sensory impairment (myasthenia gravis, bulbar palsy, local anaesthesia, etc.).
4 Oesophageal obstruction.
5 Persistent vomiting.
6 Severe bronchiectasis.
7 Infection in the mouth or sinuses (particularly dental sepsis in the elderly).

Bronchial obstruction
Partial or complete bronchial obstruction leads to retention of sputum and subsequent pyogenic infection. Common examples are bronchial carcinoma and foreign body (especially peanuts and extracted teeth).

Post-pneumonic
The centre of an area of destructive pneumonia may break down to form a lung abscess particularly when the pneumonia is due to *Staphylococcus aureus* or *Klebsiella pneumoniae*.

Tumour
Cavitation is quite common in bronchial carcinoma and this results in what is effectively a lung abscess lined with tumour tissue.

Embolic infection
This may result from secondary infection of a pulmonary infarct, or from embolization of infected material from other sites of sepsis in the body or from contaminated intravenous infusion fluids and catheters. Intravenous injection of unsterilized material by drug addicts is especially likely to cause lung abscesses. Some thrombotic pulmonary emboli cause infarction which becomes secondarily infected.

Other causes

Trauma to the lung may rarely cause a haematoma which may become infected. An amoebic abscess may develop in the right lower lobe following trans-diaphragmatic spread from an amoebic liver abscess.

Clinical features

Fever and obvious systemic upset are present at least in the initial stages and a leucocytosis is almost invariable. Later when the abscess opens into a bronchus there may be a cough with expectoration of large amounts of foul material which is variably bloodstained at first and later brown or green. Fever and malaise may recede as the abscess becomes chronic.

Investigations

Chest X-ray

The diagnosis of lung abscess is almost always confirmed by the chest X-ray, which shows one or more round lesions of almost any size which with time cavitate and may contain fluid levels (Fig. 16.1). Abscesses due to inhalation most commonly develop in the apical segments of the lower lobes (especially the right) and the lateral and posterior parts of the upper lobes (especially the right).

Sputum

Culture may yield *Staphylococcus aureus* or other common respiratory pathogens. Anaerobic bacteria may predominate in foul sputum which commonly yields no growth on standard culture. The tubercle bacillus must always be sought. Cytological examination for malignant cells is unrewarding when sputum is largely pus.

Bronchoscopy

When carcinoma or a foreign body is suspected bronchoscopy may be relevant.

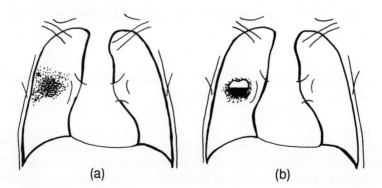

Fig. 16.1. Lung abscess. Typical X-ray features. Initially a zone of consolidation (a) gives way to cavitation (b), in which there may be a fluid level due to the presence of liquid pus.

Diagnosis

Most lung abscesses develop during the course of serious disease and the mechanism of their causation may be evident. Fine-needle aspiration or thoracotomy may be necessary to exclude a cavitated carcinoma where such evidence is lacking or where the abscess increases in size. If a cavitated abscess is due to tuberculosis the sputum almost invariably contains acid-fast bacilli on direct smear.

Management

Management comprises:

1   Postural drainage.
2   Antibiotic and chemotherapy.
3   Surgical excision or drainage (rare).

Postural drainage

The most satisfactory position will be evident from the radiological localization of the abscess.

Antibiotic and chemotherapy

In the initial phase of acute illness, therapy will be guided by bacteriological examination of the sputum and the results of blood culture. *Staphylococcus, Pseudomonas* and *Klebsiella* will require special measures. Later, penicillin in large doses orally, perhaps with the addition of probenecid to block renal excretion, will generally show gradual healing. When the patient is no longer seriously ill, there is less call to treat Gram-negative organisms recovered from the sputum, as they are unlikely to be responsible for the persistence of the abscess. As an alternative to penicillin, co-trimoxazole may be found satisfactory empirically and should be continued for several weeks if improvement occurs. Metronidazole is also useful. Flucloxacillin should be added if *Staphylococcus aureus* is regularly recovered. The great majority of lung abscesses heal with medical treatment, but this commonly takes many weeks.

Surgical treatment

Surgical excision is only occasionally required except in the case of suspected carcinoma or where healing is delayed beyond about 4 months. Occasionally complications such as empyema or bronchopleural fistula require surgical intervention.

Chapter 17
Asthma and Allergic Disorders of the Lung

Definition

Asthma is a disease characterized by variable dyspnoea due to widespread narrowing of the peripheral airways in the lungs, varying in severity over short periods of time, either spontaneously or as a result of treatment.

Extrinsic/intrinsic asthma

Much emphasis has been laid upon the distinction between extrinsic and intrinsic asthma. In practice the distinction is rather blurred and of limited value. In extrinsic asthma hypersensitivity to an external allergen is known or strongly suspected on the evidence provided by the patient's history or response to skin-testing. In intrinsic asthma such evidence is lacking.

Atopy

IgE (tissue-fixed, immediate reacting antibody, also called reagin) is normally produced in very small amounts and only in response to substantial exposure to an external allergen. Certain individuals possess a constitutional tendency to produce important amounts of IgE following mere trivial exposure to everyday antigens. Such individuals are referred to as atopic and they tend to exhibit asthma, hay fever and other forms of allergic rhinitis, urticaria and eczema. Usually the atopic diathesis is evident from an early age, a family history is common and skin-tests to common antigens are positive (extrinsic asthma).

Sometimes the term atopy is used merely to indicate that the individual has positive reactions to two or more common inhaled antigens on prick skin-testing.

Prevalence

Asthma is common. It is estimated that more than 5% of the population has recognizable asthma in the course of a lifetime. Prevalence is greatest amongst children. There is evidence that prevalence may be increasing.

Mortality

Until comparatively recently, asthma was regarded as a fairly minor complaint which did not cause death. Asthma is, however, responsible for about 2000 deaths annually in the UK and many of these occur in young people. For many years the mortality has remained remarkably constant. During the 1960s there was a striking increase in the death rate, particularly amongst young people. The possible cause of this 'epidemic' has been the subject of protracted debate (see discussion of treatment, this chapter).

Most deaths from asthma occur outside hospital. In many the apparent period of worsening before death is very brief—from minutes to a few hours—although confirmatory measurements of well-being shortly before death are lacking. Characteristically, deaths occur in individuals who were not thought by their family doctors to be suffering from severe asthma (actual measurements of ventilatory performance are rare in such individuals). There is strong evidence that those who die are, as a group, relatively undertreated, particularly with respect to steroid treatment. Deaths occur most commonly at night or in the early hours of the morning. Mortality in the UK is significantly increased in the summer.

Pathological features

In fatal cases, the main changes are found in the bronchial wall and these are summarized in Fig. 17.1. The lungs are hyperinflated and do not deflate on opening of the chest but otherwise they appear normal. Eosinophilia of the bronchial wall, sputum and sometimes blood is characteristic of asthma. Interestingly, a lesser degree of the same changes is seen incidentally in individuals with apparently mild, well-controlled asthma (for example at post-mortem after death from a traffic accident).

Mechanisms underlying the asthmatic process

Major features of the process are:

1   Bronchial hyperreactivity (greatly increased responsiveness to non-specific stimuli).

2   An inflammatory process in the bronchus in which eosinophilic infiltration is a prominent feature.

The factors controlling bronchial smooth muscle contraction, the nature of the inflammatory process and the interrelationships between these and other elements are still incompletely understood. Intensive research, especially during the past decade, has greatly increased knowledge and a complicated network of inter-

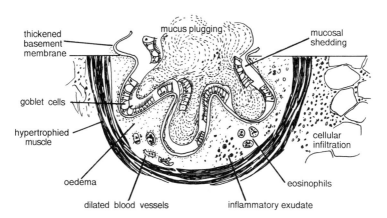

Fig. 17.1. Summary of the pathological features of asthma. Half of a cross-section of a bronchiole is shown. Although these features are characteristic of appearances after death from asthma, identical appearances are present patchily in patients who are apparently untroubled by their asthma at the time.

related immunological, cellular and biochemical processes has been revealed. The reader is referred to the 'Further Information' section (p. 304) for directions to a detailed review.

Bronchial hyperreactivity

An important characteristic of asthmatic bronchi is their tendency to respond very actively to a variety of physical and chemical stimuli, in circumstances in which normal bronchi would show little or no response. This can be assessed by observing the fall in FEV_1 when the subject inhales an aerosol of histamine or methacholine. Measurements are made after each of a series of inhalations of increasing concentration. Reactivity or responsiveness can be expressed as the concentration of the agent which will induce an agreed standard fall in FEV_1. Various expressions are used but the most common is the PC_{20} which is the provoking concentration (of histamine or methacholine) which will cause the FEV_1 to drop by 20% from the starting value. Various other challenges are sometimes used experimentally—e.g. water aerosols, cold air hyperventilation and vigorous exercise. Bronchial hyperreactivity varies in severity, roughly in parallel with the clinical activity of the asthma, but it is wrong to regard tests of hyperreactivity as tests of asthma severity or of the effectiveness of treatment.

Bronchial hyperreactivity of abnormal degree is also seen in other conditions—notably after acute upper respiratory tract infections; in cigarette smokers; in some cases of chronic obstructive pulmonary disease, bronchiectasis and cystic fibrosis; and after accidental heavy exposure to irritating chemical vapours or smoke (although the reactions are usually more subdued than in asthma).

Autonomic nervous control

Adrenergic control

Surprisingly there seems to be no sympathetic innervation of the airways in man. Nevertheless, bronchial smooth muscle carries receptors which are stimulated by circulating adrenaline. Stimulation of β-adrenergic receptors on bronchial smooth muscle causes bronchodilatation. Stimulation of α-adrenergic receptors causes bronchoconstriction.

Cholinergic control

Cholinergic receptors are also present in bronchial smooth muscle and vagal stimulation causes bronchoconstriction.

NANC nerves

There is now good evidence for non-adrenergic–non-cholinergic (NANC) nerves supplying human bronchial muscle. The transmitter appears to be a vasoactive intestinal peptide which is known to be of importance in the gut. It exerts a bronchodilator effect.

Cellular components of the reaction

Several cell types are known to participate in the reaction and most liberate mediators which act on other cells and tissues.

Mast cells

Mast cells are present in slightly increased numbers. They have high affinity for IgE which attaches to the surface. When the specific antigen is encountered, changes take place in the membrane of the mast cell which result in release of preformed mediators from granules (histamine, eosinophil chemotactic factor (ECF-A), bradykinin, neutrophil chemotactic factor (NCF), adenosine and others). There is also release of mediators manufactured in the cell membrane of the mast cell—leukotrienes which are highly active, long-acting stimulants of bronchial smooth muscle contraction, derived from metabolism of arachidonic acid. Prostaglandins are also produced, which are further products of arachidonic metabolism (by the cyclo-oxygenase pathway).

Eosinophils

These may be recruited by ECF-A released by other cells and platelet activating factor (PAF) produced by other eosinophils. Eosinophils can release leukotrienes and prostaglandins. They contain a substance known as major basic protein, which when released seems to cause disruption and shedding of the surface epithelium. Eosinophils may be stimulated to release mediators by an IgE–antigen reaction. This may reflect the evolutionary origin of the eosinophilic reaction—it could be related to a gut mechanism for rejecting parasites.

Neutrophils

Neutrophils are attracted to the asthmatic reaction probably by NCF, which can be detected in the serum in asthma and during antigenic challenges. Neutrophils are less numerous than eosinophils and, although they are rich in destructive enzymes, it is not known what part they play.

Macrophages

These abundant cells seem to be activated in asthmatic reactions and produce potent mediators such as platelet activating factor.

Mediators

Some mediators are discussed below.

Histamine

Asthmatic patients are very sensitive to histamine and may produce more than normal during worsening asthma. Its role is uncertain; antihistamines have only a very weak effect in asthma.

Platelet activating factor

This causes marked and sustained bronchoconstriction. It also causes microvascular leakiness and mucosal oedema. It is produced by mast cells, eosinophils, neutrophils, macrophages and platelets themselves.

Prostaglandins

Asthmatic subjects show very striking bronchoconstriction in response to prostaglandin $F_{2\alpha}$. The role of this and related prostanoids is not clear. Prostaglandin

E_1 seems to have a bronchodilator effect. Aspirin-like suppressors of prostaglandin synthesis have unpredictable effects in asthma.

Leukotrienes

There are a range of leukotrienes known to be produced as a product of arachidonic acid metabolism. Some have very intense and protracted bronchoconstrictor properties and others act as chemo-attractants for neutrophils and eosinophils.

Clinical features

The main features are wheezing dyspnoea, a sense of chest tightness, cough and an increase in sputum volume and viscosity. Sometimes the patient describes a sensation of choking in the neck, or tightness in the chest, rather than wheezing. Sometimes the cough is given more emphasis than wheezing, particularly when it occurs at night.

Age of onset

Asthma may occur for the first time *at any age*. Males predominate in childhood and females in later life. In childhood, extrinsic factors and associated atopy are much more likely to be encountered than later in life. When asthma occurs for the first time in the elderly it is commonly misdiagnosed.

Patterns of variability in asthma

The acute attack

Distressing wheezing of more or less acute onset is the hallmark of asthma. The majority of patients have such attacks at some time and often refer to them as 'spasms'. Some patients with asthma do not have abrupt attacks and suffer more or less persistent symptoms.

The patient sits or stands, bracing the shoulders with the hands on the knees or on the arms of a chair. The expression is one of preoccupation with the business of breathing, breath by breath. Inspiration is snatched and expiration prolonged; both are wheezy. Examination reveals overinflation of the chest, use of accessory muscles of respiration and marked recession of the lower part of the chest during inspiration. There is a tachycardia and usually pulsus paradoxus; cyanosis may be present. Auscultation usually reveals universal inspiratory and expiratory rhonchi. Sometimes, in very severe acute asthma, wheezing is unimpressive or absent, despite obvious distress and laboured chest distortion. This is a sign of dangerously severe airways obstruction.

Most attacks subside spontaneously in minutes but some are prolonged for hours despite treatment.

Unconsciousness is occasionally encountered in an acute attack. Sometimes this is brief and suggestive of cough syncope; sometimes actual asphyxia, accompanied by impairment of venous return due to overinflation, seems a more probable explanation. Attacks of unconsciousness suggest very severe asthma and inadequate treatment.

Sometimes an acute attack is totally unheralded in a completely symptom-free patient, but more usually attacks occur on a background of less severe symptoms.

Exacerbations of intermittent asthma

One of the most common patterns comprises long periods of relative freedom from symptoms, interrupted by exacerbations which follow upper respiratory tract infections. These exacerbations can last from several days to a few weeks.

Chronic asthma

Some patients have persistent symptoms which may be mild or severe. There is virtually always a characteristic diurnal variability.

Diurnal variation

Diurnal variation in symptoms is one of the most important diagnostic features of asthma; it is seen in chronic asthma as well as during exacerbations. The characteristic pattern is illustrated in Fig. 17.2. The main elements are:

Morning tightness

The patient notices tightness and wheezing usually within seconds of waking and this may take minutes or hours to subside. Coughing exacerbates symptoms.

Nocturnal attacks

Attacks at night are also characteristic of asthma. The patient generally wakes between 2 and 3 a.m. with tightness, cough and wheezing dyspnoea. He or she

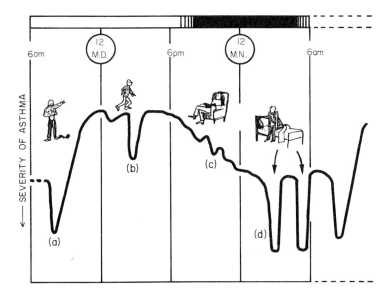

Fig. 17.2. Diurnal variation in symptoms in asthma. The most striking features are usually: (a) chest tightness and wheezing dyspnoea on waking, improving during the morning and (d) nocturnal attacks. In addition there may be exercise-induced asthma (b) and worsening of symptoms whilst resting in the evening (c).

may sit up or rise to sit by an open window. Nocturnal attacks may be prolonged or repeated. Such episodes are commonly misdiagnosed as 'paroxysmal nocturnal dyspnoea due to left ventricular failure'. One of the most useful features which distinguishes this last type of nocturnal attack is the lack of morning tightness.

Seasonal variation

Marked seasonal variation is characteristic of extrinsic asthma. In the UK, aggravation of asthma in the months May–July is typical of grass-pollen sensitivity. Aggravation in the winter months is common and probably due to two factors—frequent upper respiratory tract infections and house dust mite sensitivity. Patients with sensitivity to mould spores are generally worst in the autumn.

Trigger factors

A number of factors are known to aggravate asthma although they are not regarded as primary causes of the condition:

1   Exercise.
2   Non-specific irritants.
3   Infection.
4   Drugs.
5   External allergens.
6   Emotional factors.

Exercise-induced asthma

Severe exercise may provoke asthma especially in young subjects. Wheezing and tightness are experienced a minute or two after the end of exercise and are quite different from the hyperpnoea of the effort. If exercise is prolonged, asthma may come on whilst it is still in progress. In some patients, especially children, exercise-induced wheezing is the only expression of asthma.

The underlying mechanisms of exercise-induced asthma are the subject of much research. It has been shown that the hyperpnoea of exercise may cause cooling of the trachea and perhaps bronchi. If respiratory heat loss is prevented by breathing warm humid air, then exercise-induced asthma may be prevented. There is uncertainty over whether cooling itself or evaporation of secretions (and local osmotic change) may be the trigger. After an episode of exercise-induced bronchoconstriction there is a refractory period, during which it is much harder to induce the phenomenon. The discharge of mast cells may be one part of the reaction. Exercise-induced asthma can be blocked by prior medication with a β_2-agonist drug or disodium cromoglycate.

Provocation by non-specific irritants

Patients with asthma demonstrate hyperreactivity by developing bronchoconstriction in response to non-antigenic dusts, smoke, histamine and acetylcholine, in concentrations which produce no detectable effect in normal individuals. Asthma may also be provoked by laughing, coughing and forced expiration.

Provocation by infection

It is doubtful whether asthma is caused by specific allergy to common respiratory infective agents, but it is certainly aggravated by viral and bacterial infections.

Provocation by drugs

A full account of drug-induced asthma is given in Chapter 30. Particular note should be made of the importance of **aspirin hypersensitivity**. A proportion of asthmatic individuals may develop sudden, very severe asthma after consuming aspirin. The following points are relevant:

1 Aspirin sensitivity should be considered whenever sudden severe asthma develops, within a few minutes, on a background of very good control of symptoms (symptom-free nights and mornings).

2 Patients are commonly unaware of the relationship between aspirin and attacks of asthma.

3 The association of intrinsic asthma and nasal polyposis increases the likelihood of aspirin sensitivity.

4 Susceptible individuals should be warned never to take aspirin again and taught how to recognize preparations which contain it.

5 The hypersensitivity extends to other non-steroidal anti-inflammatory agents such as indomethacin, ibuprofen, etc.

6 Susceptible individuals also react to tartrazine which is used to give yellow colouring to foods and some drugs.

Other drugs causing aggravation of asthma include beta-blocking agents, cholinergic drugs, radiocontrast media, anaesthetic agents and muscle relaxants.

Provocation by external allergens

Airborne allergens, in minute quantities, may provoke asthma. In the UK, the most common airborne allergens are grass-pollen and the house dust mite. Other pollens, moulds, animal danders, etc. may also provoke asthma but these are numerically relatively unimportant.

Acute exposure to the airborne antigen in a hypersensitive individual generally produces an almost immediate onset of cough, chest tightness and wheeze. This may improve over some minutes, or hours, if exposure is modest. Some individuals develop a delayed reaction (Fig. 17.3) reaching its maximum 6–8 hours after

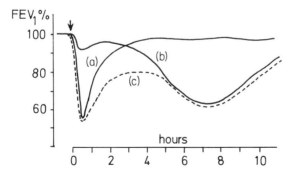

Fig. 17.3. Immediate and delayed responses to bronchial challenge. FEV_1 as a percentage of the resting value plotted against time after antigen inhalation (arrow). Stylized representations of three different types of response from three individuals: (a) immediate response; (b) delayed response; (c) biphasic response. Most individuals with a later response show some immediate reaction. Cromoglycate pretreatment typically blocks both immediate and delayed reactions. Steroid pretreatment blocks only the delayed response.

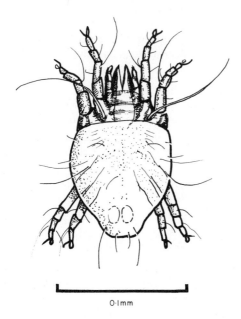

0·1mm

Fig. 17.4. *Dermatophagoides pteronyssinus:* the house dust mite.

exposure. Occasionally a biphasic response is seen in which early and late phases are both present. Early reactions tend to be IgE-mediated and late reactions may be accompanied by the presence of circulating precipitins against the antigen in question, but this is by no means invariable. The delayed response is particularly important in the investigation of occupational asthma, because the relationship between symptoms and work may be complex. Patients with grass-pollen sensitivity, as well as experiencing seasonal asthma, commonly have hay fever and are aware that proximity to grass, particularly when newly cut, is likely to induce symptoms. Camping is especially likely to provoke an exacerbation.

The house dust mite (*Dermatophagoides pteronyssinus*) and its close relative the kitchen mite (*D. culinae*) are minute eight-legged arthropods about 0.15 mm in length (Fig. 17.4). They are almost universally distributed and are responsible for the antigenic properties of house dust. *D. pteronyssinus* is found in highest concentration in the superficial layers of mattresses where it finds ideal requirements of warmth, moisture and its principal foodstuff—desquamated human skin scales. Subjects sensitive to the house dust mite tend to suffer aggravation of their asthma:

1 at night, though not all nocturnal asthma is due to house dust;
2 during bed-making and household cleaning;
3 at weekends (but excessive smoking, beer and wine may cause aggravation at this time);
4 in the early winter.

Occupational asthma
See p. 282.

Allergy to foodstuffs

This is relatively uncommon but hypersensitivity to beer, wine, shellfish, eggs, etc. is occasionally encountered.

Provocation by emotional disturbance

The relationship between psychogenic factors and asthma is complex but the following points may be made.

1 Severe asthma is frightening and chronic *severe* asthma is, in addition, depressing. It commonly results is chronic loss of sleep which aggravates symptoms of anxiety. In chronic childhood asthma in particular, very great strains are put upon parents and child. Emotional disturbance in this situation is as likely to be a consequence of the asthma as it is to be the cause.

2 Psychogenic factors may undoubtedly aggravate the severity of established asthma and may provoke actual attacks. Anger, frustration and acute anxiety are particularly potent in this context.

3 It is widely believed that asthma is 'due to nerves' and this sometimes results in patients being rather unsympathetically treated by friends and relatives.

4 Some asthmatic patients are undoubtedly able to self-induce attacks. Usually this is brought about by repeated forced expiration near residual volume and this appears to produce reflex bronchoconstriction. This may sometimes be done more or less subconsciously to attract sympathy, or avoid unpleasant tasks.

5 Patients with asthma are generally very appreciative of a straightforward 'organic' approach to the management of their disease. If asthma is adequately treated and if patients understand their treatment 'psychogenic factors' almost always subside.

Asthma in children

Most of the discussion above refers equally to asthma in childhood. Treatment in children is covered on p. 176.

Diagnosis

One of the most important aspects of childhood asthma is the extent to which it is underdiagnosed. There is a strong tendency for children with recurrent cough and wheeze to be labelled as suffering from 'bronchitis'. Where cough and wheeze really are recurrent the diagnosis is virtually always that of asthma. Cough is often much more prominent as a symptom in childhood and it may be the only complaint offered by the parent. The eliciting of diurnal variation, exercise-induced attacks, co-existent features of rhinitis, eczema or of a family history may provide useful additional evidence pointing towards the correct diagnosis. Simple spirometry or peak flow measurement may provide further support by comfirming airways obstruction, but a formal demonstration of exercise-induced asthma may be even more useful in suspended asthma. Peak flow rate is measured before, and at intervals after, a 6 minute spell of very vigorous running free, out of doors. The characteristic post-exercise bronchoconstriction—and its relief by bronchodilator aerosol—provides valuable objective support for a diagnosis of asthma, particularly when the presentation has been atypical.

Wheezing under the age of 3 years

Not all babies who have important wheezing go on to show features of asthma later. Acute rhinorrhoea, cough and obstructed breathing in the first year may be due to bronchiolitis secondary to the respiratory syncytial virus (or sometimes other viruses). Only a proportion go on to develop asthma. Where there is a persistent or recurrent tendency to wheeze with severe exacerbations, very young children (under 2 years) show a resistance to most bronchodilator treatments which are effective later.

Progress of asthma

Childhood asthma

About 70% of those who develop asthma during childhood develop symptoms before the age of 5 years. The majority of children with asthma improve as puberty approaches. About 75% of children who suffer only occasional episodes, related to simple upper respiratory infections, will be free from symptoms by the age of 15 years. Those with the most persistent symptoms, the earliest onset and the most impressive atopic features show the least, and most postponed, improvement.

Adult asthma

Adults with a long history of chronic asthma tend to develop a degree of fixed airways obstruction, the severity of which is related to the severity and duration of their earlier asthmatic experience. In most adults it is reasonable to predict a varying degree of severity.

It is reasonable to suggest to patients that they will always have a tendency to asthma, that this will vary in intensity spontaneously, but that with adequate attention to the details of treatment, reasonable control of symptoms can be expected.

Tests for specific hypersensitivity

Skin-testing

Skin-testing is of limited value. It is undertaken for a variety of reasons:

1 To provide confirmation of immediate hypersensitivity to external allergens with a view to their subsequent exclusion so far as this is possible, or (in exceptional circumstances) with a view to subsequent specific desensitization.

2 To provide an indication of atopic status or to allow classification into extrinsic or intrinsic groups. This may not be of great importance to the individual patient but it may be relevant when comparing the results of treatment in different groups of patients.

There are two methods:

Intradermal method

This method may reveal immediate and delayed reactions but tends to produce a high incidence of positive results of doubtful significance. In very allergic individuals, severe local reactions, asthma or even anaphylaxis may be induced. It is now rarely used.

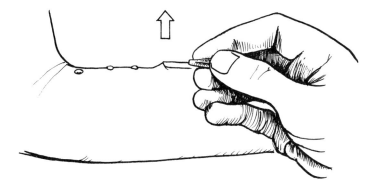

Fig. 17.5. Modified prick skin-test. Drops of antigen extracts and antigen-free control solution are placed on the flexor surface of the forearm. Each drop is pricked with a fine needle. The needle is held parallel to the skin surface, advanced slightly and a tiny fold of skin lifted briefly as shown. Deep stabs and bleeding should be avoided. Wheal and flare are measured after 10–20 minutes. Vigorous preparation of the skin is undesirable.

Modified prick skin-test

A drop of each solution to be tested is placed upon the skin and a prick made by the method illustrated in Fig. 17.5. There are fewer false positive results with this method and the results correlate well with circulating levels of specific IgE. The quantity of antigen introduced is minute and the method is safe. It is much more convenient in practice than the intradermal method. Delayed responses are almost never seen.

Note

Immediate skin-test responses are suppressed by antihistamines but not by steroid treatment. Delayed reactions are suppressed by steroid treatment. Patch-testing is not relevant to the assessment of immediate hypersensitivity.

Other tests for specific hypersensitivity

RAST test

The radio-allergo-sorbent test (RAST) is a means of measuring the level of circulating IgE which is specifically directed towards a particular antigen. It is performed on serum in the laboratory. It is expensive and of very little relevance to the management of patients with asthma. Exceptionally it may be useful where it is necessary to know whether an individual is highly sensitive to a particular substance and it is at the same time considered dangerous to try even prick skin-tests (e.g. in possible penicillin anaphylaxis).

Bronchial challenge

This too is of no relevance in the management of the great majority of patients with asthma. It involves the patient inhaling nebulized solution or a powder aerosol of the substance in question. Control inhalations on different days are generally required. In possible occupational asthma, it may be important to support clinical suspicion with a challenge test when decisions regarding employment are to be made. Bronchial challenge may be dangerous. Bronchoconstriction may be delayed; hospital admission is advisable where the level of hypersensitivity is not known.

Physiological changes in asthma

Airways obstruction

Reduction of FEV$_1$

FEV_1, vital capacity and FEV_1/VC ratio are reduced and there is reduction of peak expiratory flow.

Reversibility

Airways obstruction in asthma is often referred to as 'reversible' by bronchodilators. In fact, airways obstruction is usually only partly reversible by a bronchodilator aerosol and the degree of reversibility tends to vary from time to time and between individuals (Fig. 17.6)

1 Very large bronchodilator responses are virtually diagnostic of asthma; but they are seen in patients with very obvious asthma.

2 Absence of a response does not mean the diagnosis is 'not asthma'.

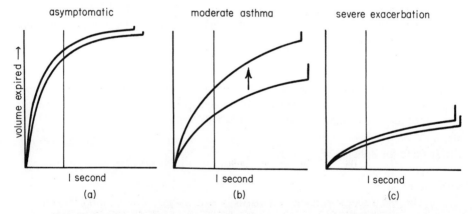

Fig. 17.6. 'Reversibility' of airways obstruction. Forced expiratory spirograms obtained from a patient with asthma on three different occasions. The upper of the two tracings was obtained some minutes after inhalation of a bronchodilator aerosol.

(a) When asymptomatic, performance is almost normal and the aerosol produces little improvement.

(b) During a moderate exacerbation of asthma the aerosol produces a major improvement.

(c) During a severe exacerbation there is relative resistance to sympathomimetic treatment and there is little or no response to a bronchodilator aerosol.

   Very large responses to bronchodilator aerosol such as shown in (b) are only encountered in patients with asthma. Lesser responses are seen in asthma and also in patients with airways obstruction related to chronic bronchitis and are thus of limited diagnostic value.

3   Moderate responses to bronchodilator are seen in airways obstruction associated with chronic obstructive pulmonary disease (COPD), bronchiectasis, etc.

Summary

Big responses indicate asthma when the diagnosis is obvious; any other response has little diagnostic content. The test is of little use if a proper clinical assessment has been made already.

Variability

The variation in peak flow diurnally—or from week to week—can itself provide valuable confirmatory evidence that asthma is present. Variability, like reversibility is most obvious in asthma of moderate severity; it may not be obvious in severe chronic asthma (Fig. 17.7).

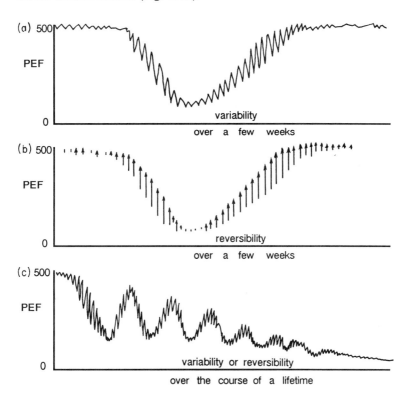

Fig. 17.7. Variability and reversibility in asthma—three diagrammatic views.

(a) In the course of an exacerbation and subsequent recovery, variability (diurnal variation) is most marked when asthma is moderately severe and may be absent when asthma is either very mild or very severe.

(b) In the course of an exacerbation and subsequent recovery, reversibility after an inhaled bronchodilator (arrows) is most marked when asthma is moderately severe and may be absent when either asthma is very mild or very severe.

(c) Over decades of chronic asthma, there is a general tendency for a decline in overall ventilatory performance, which is related to the duration and severity of the earlier experience. Accompanying this, there is a reduction in both variability and reversibility.

Prolongation of forced expiration time

This is generally evident, even in mild cases, with only slight reduction of peak expiratory flow or FEV_1/VC ratio.

Overinflation

This may be evident clinically and reflected by increase in total lung capacity, functional residual capacity and residual volume.

Ventilation

Asthma generates a very powerful drive to breathe, so that in exacerbations hyperventilation is the rule and the P_{CO_2} is found to be *low*. Only in critically severe exacerbations does the P_{CO_2} become elevated; this is a serious sign.

Chronic respiratory failure and cor pulmonale are rarely seen except in neglected, inadequately-treated cases of asthma or in people living at altitude. Hypercapnia, congestive cardiac failure and right ventricular hypertrophy can all disappear after treatment with corticosteroids.

Oxygenation

Hypoxia is an almost inevitable accompaniment of severe exacerbation of asthma owing to the presence of areas of underventilation. Cyanosis denotes severe asthma: it should be taken as an indication for hospitalization.

Management of asthma

Management of asthma is based firstly on the patient having a reasonable understanding of the nature of the disorder and, secondly, on the use of a very few highly effective treatments which, if used skilfully by the patient, can result in a very good measure of control of symptoms. Most patients with asthma can expect to be able to lead normal lives.

Education of the patient

Understanding the nature of asthma

Asthma is frustrating and frightening and the subject of myths and widespread misunderstanding. It is vital that the patient with asthma should have some reasonable concept of what asthma is. The terms in which this is presented and the detail of the description will obviously vary considerably, depending on the background knowledge and character of the patient. Time spent in this discussion is very worthwhile. Some patients feel guilty about suffering from asthma when they have been told that it is a 'nervous complaint'. When asthma has only recently developed, the patient may be hell-bent on finding a once-and-for-all cure which will restore him or her to the pre-existing state. Such an individual will not be sympathetic to the idea of carefully tailored treatment to suppress and relieve asthma, unless the practicability of the hoped-for cure is discussed fully. Many other entrenched attitudes may be revealed if discussion is unhurried.

Understanding the treatment

It is very desirable that patients with frequent or persistent asthma—and those who have acute severe asthma—should manage their own treatment as far as possible.

For this to be successful (and safe), the patient must understand the use of each preparation employed and must have a plan of action prepared for unexpected changes in his or her condition. A balanced understanding of the side-effects of treatment (and of neglected asthma) is also required. Just as in the management of diabetes, doctor and patient become involved jointly in an educational exercise which takes time—merely writing prescriptions is not enough. Quite a large number of items of information are required for self-management, and training requires fortification with written material. Experience has shown that a diagrammatic form is useful and that it helps if this is made out afresh in the presence of the patient rather than merely photocopied and handed out (see Brewis, Further Information).

Avoidance—control of extrinsic factors

In a small proportion of cases, where there is an identifiable extrinsic cause, it may be possible to treat asthma satisfactorily by merely reducing exposure to the allergen. Unfortunately, most patients with regularly troublesome asthma are unaffected by manipulation of the environment, even if specific allergens are identified. Complete avoidance of grass pollen is not possible, but exposure can be reduced. It is extremely difficult to avoid exposure to the house dust mite, although measures such as daily airing of the bed, frequent vacuum-cleaning of the bed and bedroom floor, discarding old mattresses, etc. may have some effect. On the whole, the result of these efforts is disappointing. It is very unwise to advise patients with asthma to move to a different house or climate, or to dispose of pets or to change employment on account of asthma, unless the indications are particularly compelling.

Desensitization

There is no place for desensitization in the routine management of asthma. The treatment comprises repeated subcutaneous injections of weak extracts of specific allergen; it appears to act by inducing 'blocking antibody' of IgG type. Response to treatment is variable and difficult to assess, because exposure may vary and the patient will usually be receiving a number of other treatments concurrently. It can cause fatal reactions and its use is limited to exceptional circumstances and to the hands of specialists.

Review of available treatments

The drugs used in the treatment of chronic or frequently recurrent asthma can be divided into three broad groups:

1   Treatment for **relief**. Bronchodilators by aerosol or, less effectively, orally.

2   Treatment for '**prevention**'. A steroid aerosol, cromoglycate or inedocromil by inhalation.

3   **Reserve** treatment. Oral prednisolone, preferably started by the patient on his or her own initiative, in the event of deterioration (see below).

Most patients with chronic asthma can be managed very satisfactorily with regular inhalation of a steroid aerosol to control the asthmatic process, a bronchodilator aerosol to reverse wheezing when this occurs and training to initiate emergency oral steroid treatment. The management of acute severe asthma will be considered separately after a review of the main groups of drugs.

Bronchodilators

Frequent or persistently troublesome asthma should *not* normally be managed exclusively with bronchodilator drugs. They are most useful when asthma is mild or already well-controlled and they lose effectiveness during exacerbations.

Bronchodilator aerosols

Aerosol preparations of β-adrenergic sympathetic stimulant drugs are extremely useful for the prompt relief of attacks of wheezing (Fig. 17.8). For example, their use may abbreviate a nocturnal attack to a minute or two, when it might otherwise last for half an hour or more; aerosol treatment is also particularly effective in curtailing symptoms of 'morning tightness'. Bronchodilator aerosols are best employed in putting the 'finishing touches' to asthma which is already well controlled. They should *not* be relied upon for the control of *severe* asthma when they are anyway ineffective. Salbutamol (Ventolin) and terbutaline (Bricanyl) are relatively selective β_2-agonists and cause little cardiac acceleration. They also have a longer action of around 5 hours. The usual dose is two puffs as required. If asthma is well controlled (spontaneously or because of other treatment) then bronchodilator

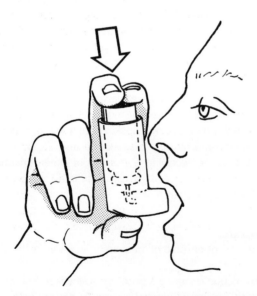

Fig. 17.8. Pressurized aerosol in use. The active preparation and an inert propellant gas solution are contained in a small pressurized canister which is housed in a plastic casing in an inverted position. Downward pressure on the base of the canister as shown releases a single standard 'puff' of aerosol. It is helpful if the inhaler is distanced slightly from the mouth, provided the aim is accurate. It is absolutely essential that the 'puff' is synchronized with inspiration (see text for note on technique).

usage will fall or cease. If more than about four puffs a day are required this indicates the need for regular prophylactic treatment with cromoglycate or a steroid aerosol preparation (see below). Salmeterol has a duration of action of about 12 hours and is best reserved for more severe chronic asthma, not fully controlled by aerosol treatment.

Cautionary note
During the early 1960s there was an alarming increase in the incidence of sudden death from asthma, which seemed to parallel the increasing use of isoprenaline aerosols. Extensive publicity led to reduction in consumption and this was accompanied by a decline in mortality. The relationship between isoprenaline aerosols and the sudden deaths was probably complex. Most deaths were unexpected and occurred in patients who had received no steroid treatment. Although it is possible that overdosage of isoprenaline may have caused some deaths through provoking dysrhythmia or by other mechanisms, it is now thought more likely that intensive use of the aerosols may have disguised the severity of the asthma, allowing patients to tolerate severe asthma which might otherwise have been recognized as intolerable and treated with steroids. There is concern that the increasing use of high dose bronchodilator treatment by nebulizer (see below) and the use of new, effective, long-acting oral and aerosol bronchodilators (e.g. salmeterol) might also distract patients from the need for suppressive anti-inflammatory treatment.

Experience with salbutamol and terbutaline in the high doses commonly employed in nebulizer therapy (see below) suggests that they are very safe drugs indeed. Nevertheless, a proportion of the general public sees inhalers as dangerous and initial refusal to countenance inhaled treatment is fairly common. Inhaled treatment is effective and important; unhurried discussion of the question of hazard is necessary so that it can be seen in proper perspective.

A note on technique—pressurized aerosols
It is important to ensure that the device is used properly; this requires a demonstration by the doctor who should also observe the patient's first attempts.

The patient first exhales and then positions the device in front of the open mouth (Fig. 17.8). An unhurried inspiration begins and during the inhalation the aerosol is discharged—the inhalation continuing to a position of almost full inspiration where the breath is held for about 10 seconds. The standard adult dose is two 'puffs'—each puff being delivered in a separate breath. If vapour is visible escaping from the mouth, nose, or the top of the device, then co-ordination is faulty and the puff should be repeated.

Problems with use—pressurized aerosols
Most patients find pressurized aerosols (metered dose inhalers or MDIs) convenient and effective. Problems with their use include:
1   *Poor synchronization.* Children and the elderly, in particular, may not breathe in at the same time as discharging the aerosol.
2   *Oropharyngeal deposition.* A high proportion of the dose is still in large particle size as it passes through the upper airway and droplets are impacted. In the

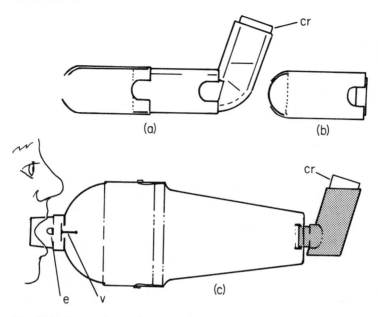

Fig. 17.9. Spacer devices for use with metered dose inhalers. (a) The Spacer-inhaler (Astra) is convenient and collapsible (b), and allows the patient to inhale after discharge of the aerosol; (c) the Nebuhaler (Astra) is a large-volume device, designed to allow even freer dispersal of the discharged material so that a high proportion of it forms particles small enough to be inhaled. It also allows large doses of aerosol to be inhaled relatively efficiently (see text). cr, canister of pressurized aerosol; v, valve which closes on expiration; e, expiratory port.

case of steroid aerosol this encourages candidal growth and huskiness.

3 *Use of fluorocarbons* . There is a move to eliminate fluorocarbon propellants because of concern about the atmosphere.

These problems have led to the development of spacer devices and dry powder inhalers.

Spacer devices
Examples are illustrated in Fig. 17.9. Distancing the inhaler from the mouth results in a fine aerosol of smaller particles. Upper airway deposition is less and lung dose is larger. Since the discharged aerosol is captured for some seconds in the device, inspiration need not be precisely synchronized. Spacer devices thus overcome problems 1 and 2 above. The spacer device has been found to be a convenient way of delivering a large dose of aerosol bronchodilator in an emergency. Repeated puffs can be discharged into the chamber. If high dose steroid aerosol treatment is required, a spacer device should be used with the MDI.

Dry powder devices
Examples are illustrated in Figs. 17.10, 17.11 and 17.12. In all of the available designs, the dispersal of the powder is achieved by the patient's inspiratory effort so that synchronization is guaranteed. Efficiency of use and particle size are

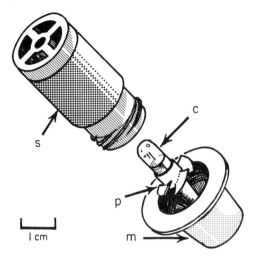

Fig. 17.10. Dry powder inhaler (Spinhaler: Fisons Pharmaceuticals) for administration of disodium cromoglycate. The mouthpiece (m) carries a central pin upon which a propeller (p) is free to rotate. The capsule (regular prophylactic treatment) is fitted into a recess in the propeller. The two parts of the inhaler are screwed together and the capsule is pierced by two pins which are operated by a sliding sleeve (s). The patient inspires vigorously through the inhaler causing the propeller to rotate. The powder is dispersed into the airstream.

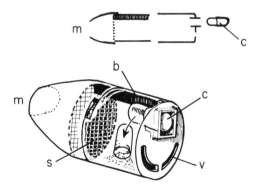

Fig. 17.11. Dry powder inhaler (Rotahaler: Allen and Hanbury). Both bronchodilator and topical steroid treatment may be administered in this way. The powdered aerosol is prepared in a gelatin capsule (c) which is inserted into the inhaler at the opposite end to the mouthpiece (m). The two parts of the inhaler (which are shown separated in the upper part of the diagram) are then rotated relative to each other and a bar (b) knocks off the inner end of the capsule (arrow), liberating the powder into the inside of the inhaler. A vigorous inhalation causes air to be drawn into the vent (v) and the resulting turbulence draws the powder into the inspiratory airstream. The free half of the capsule is retained within the inhaler by a perforated screen (s).

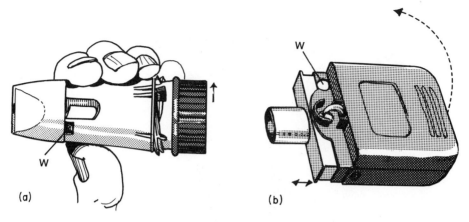

Fig. 17.12. Dry powder inhalers for administration of β-agonist or steroid aerosols. Two multidose non-capsule designs.
(a) Turbohaler (Astra). The inhaler is shown with the cover removed; the mouthpiece is to the left. Up to 200 doses of the powdered drug are stored in a reservoir through which the air channel passes. A dose of the dry powder is rotated into the air channel by turning the distal section (arrow) which moves a perforated disc through the reservoir. The dose is held in the perforations until the patient inspires. The internal design achieves very efficient dispersal. An indication of the number of doses remaining is given in a small window (w).
(b) Diskhaler (Allen and Hanbury). The inhaler is shown with the mouthpiece cover removed; the mouthpiece is to the left. The individual doses are contained in sealed 'blebs' on a disc which is placed on a 'carousel' assembly inside the inhaler. With an in–out movement of the front end of the inhaler (double arrow), the disc rotates and a new bleb moves into place. The bleb is perforated before inhalation by opening the top flap (interrupted arrow), which causes a curved 'claw' to pierce the top and bottom of the bleb. When the patient inspires, air is directed through the pierced bleb and the powder is dispersed into the airstream. Eight doses are carried in each disc and the number of unused doses remaining is indicated in a window (w).

determined by the design of the inhaler and the formulation of the powder. Correctly used dry powder devices may overcome all three problems above. Some may be less convenient, particularly when large doses are required.

Nebulizers

The most usual type of nebulizer takes the form shown in Figs 17.13 and 17.14, where the mechanism is incorporated in a face mask and operated by a source of compressed air or oxygen. In the home, the usual pressure source is a small, electrically driven compressor (cost about £120; not available via UK National Health Service). The medication (which can be bronchodilator, cromoglycate, antibiotic, etc.) is added in liquid form to the reservoir. Sometimes, instead of a mask, a mouthpiece is fitted to the nebulizer via a T piece.

The usual application of nebulizers is in the administration of a bronchodilator for acute asthma, in the home or in hospital, where the usual relieving dose of bronchodilator has failed to bring relief. Some patients with severe chronic asthma benefit from regular use. Bronchodilator treatment using a nebulizer is very effective. This is not due to special properties of the apparatus but to the

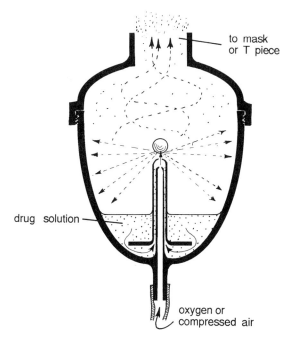

to mask
or T piece

drug solution

oxygen or
compressed air

Fig. 17.13. Nebulizer. Diagram of a typical mechanism. Oxygen or compressed air enters from below and escapes at high velocity from a pinhole, creating a local negative pressure as it does so (Venturi effect). The vicinity of the pinhole is connected to the drug solution which is drawn upwards by the negative pressure. When the fluid reaches the escaping oxygen or air, it is sheared off and passes with the stream through a larger second pinhole which directs the fluid/gas mixture on to a small sphere (a fixed part of the plastic moulding). The impact shatters the mixture into tiny droplets, the smallest of which are of a dimension sufficient to float freely as a true aerosol and be carried into the airway. Larger droplets hit the side wall and return to the reservoir at the bottom. The aerosol is commonly administered by mask (Fig. 17.14) or by breathing from a T piece fitted across the top of the nebulizer.

large dose of bronchodilator employed. In practice, between 10 and 50 times as much bronchodilator is used in nebulizer treatment as is used in the standard 'relieving' dose of two puffs of a salbutamol pressurized aerosol (see Fig. 17.15).

Indications for use of nebulizers
Nebulizers have a valuable place in the management of more severe asthma in childhood, where proper co-ordination of pressurized aerosols is often lacking. Only a few adults really need nebulizers. This is because: (1) the same effect can be obtained with an ordinary pressurized aerosol if an equivalent dose is used efficiently—for example, 12 puffs used with a large volume spacer; (2) patients who appear to have a requirement for large doses of bronchodilator are often found to be having insufficient (or inefficient) inhaled steroid treatment; attention to this may remove the apparent requirement for nebulizer treatment.

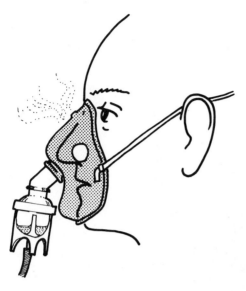

Fig. 17.14. Nebulizer mask. Mask for administration of high dose bronchodilator or antibiotic by inhalation. See mechanism described in Fig. 17.13.

Dangers of nebulizers

The danger of nebulizer treatment lies in the fact that it is usually extremely effective, it is popular and it fits in with what the patient and relatives perceive as being appropriate for the management of difficult breathing. Preoccupation with this form of treatment may, however, allow severe asthma to be tolerated until a stage where further deterioration may be suddenly critical. It follows that where nebulizer therapy is in use, it is important to ensure that regular suppressive therapy is being properly exploited, rather than neglected.

Nebulizer bronchodilator treatment itself seems to be safe. Important increase in pulse rate is unusual even with the high doses of bronchodilator used. There does not seem to be an important drop in Po_2 so that in ordinary use it is all right to give bronchodilators using air, rather than oxygen, as the driving gas.

Oral bronchodilator drugs

Inhaled prophylactic and bronchodilator treatment for asthma is so effective that, in most patients, oral bronchodilator treatment is unnecessary.

The main indications for the use of an oral bronchodilator are :

1   Where asthma has been shown by measurement to be very mild and the patient is unable or disinclined to use inhaled treatment.

2   Where a tendency to nocturnal attacks persists, despite otherwise very good control of asthma—for example with steroid aerosol treatment.

3   In the small number of patients with very severe chronic asthma on high doses of inhaled or oral corticosteroid treatment.

Oral bronchodilators are thus used as 'finishing touches' in the management of asthma rather than as mainstream treatment.

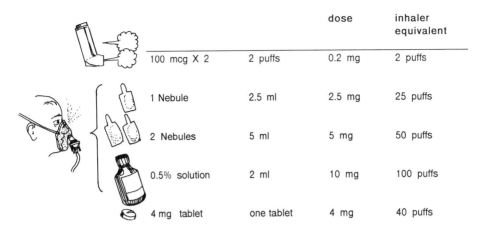

			dose	inhaler equivalent
	100 mcg X 2	2 puffs	0.2 mg	2 puffs
	1 Nebule	2.5 ml	2.5 mg	25 puffs
	2 Nebules	5 ml	5 mg	50 puffs
	0.5% solution	2 ml	10 mg	100 puffs
	4 mg tablet	one tablet	4 mg	40 puffs

Fig. 17.15. Nebulized salbutamol. Diagram to illustrate the relationship between doses of salbutamol commonly administered by nebulizer, those delivered by metered dose aerosol and those taken in tablet form. *Note.* All nebulizers retain some of the solution even when nebulization has ceased. This commonly amounts to about 0.5 ml. The amount of drug retained depends upon the dilution used. Other volumes of solution and other bronchodilators such as terbutaline are in general use (Nebule; Allen and Hanbury).

The most widely used oral bronchodilators are long-acting theophylline preparations, which can give therapeutic effect over 24 hours in twice daily dosage. There is a high incidence of intolerance of theophyllines, usually because of nausea, sometimes tremor. It is desirable to check the blood theophylline level to ensure that the optimum dose is being given. The conventional therapeutic range is 10–20 μg ml^{-1}, but useful effect is often seen at lower levels. Risks of overdosage include dysrhythmia and fits.

Oral preparations of β-agonists such as salbutamol and terbutaline are available in various formulations.

Steroid aerosols

Steroid aerosols form the hinge-pin of the management of chronic asthma. Highly active corticosteroids are delivered in low dosage, either by pressurized aerosol or by breath-activated dry powder device. The most widely used preparations are beclomethasone dipropionate (Becotide and Becloforte) and budesonide (Pulmicort). Improvement in chronic asthma is generally evident in a day or two and is often dramatic. Failure of steroid aerosol treatment to influence troublesome asthma suggests that some detail of the practical application of the treatment has been overlooked.

Distribution and absorption

Less than 20% of the dose actually reaches the respiratory tract, the remainder being swallowed. The two reasons why aerosol steroid treatment is safe, compared with the hazards of long-term systemic steroid treatment, are:

1 Low dosage is possible because of high topical activity and direct targeting of the bronchial tree.

2 First pass metabolism in the liver eliminates about 90% of the absorbed swallowed dose of the topical compounds (but not prednisolone).

Dosage

There is considerable variation in daily requirements. Many patients manage with 100 µg of beclomethasone dipropionate per day, but a few patients with severe chronic asthma may require 2 mg. The usual daily dose is about 400 µg. Inhalations need only be twice daily—morning and night—so that compliance is usually not difficult. Patients are encouraged to experiment by occasionally changing the dose in a systematic way to determine their requirements. If, on lowering the dose, morning symptoms are more than brief, or there are any nocturnal symptoms, then there is no point in trying to lower the dose further, as worsening asthma is virtually guaranteed.

Practical points

It is essential that patients grasp the preventative purpose of treatment, the need for regular dosing and the absence of any immediate relief.

Steroid aerosol treatment should not be started alone in a severe exacerbation. It may well be ineffective in this situation because of failure to penetrate and patients may conclude that the treatment is useless in their case. Patients with substantial asthma, which is well controlled by steroid aerosol, should understand how to start a short course of oral steroid in the event of worsening asthma (see below). This is because reduced efficiency of aerosol treatment, in the face of severe asthma, may result in striking deterioration and patients tend to put off seeking help from their doctors. Instructions on *when* and *how* to take a course of prednisolone should be given in written form.

Side-effects

A small proportion of patients develop pharyngeal candida. This is usually avoidable by using a spacer device and taking treatment before meals; it is easily treatable with antifungal lozenges such as amphotericin or nystatin.

Some patients complain of huskiness of the voice. This may be improved by use of a spacer device. It is not due to candida, but may be a direct effect on a tiny superficial muscle slip in the vocal cord itself.

At doses above about 1.6 mg, blunting of the adrenal response to tetracosactrin is seen. Apart from easy bruising in the elderly, clinical evidence of steroid side-effects is not seen. At doses above 2 mg, significant absorption probably occurs, equivalent to low dose systemic treatment. The few patients requiring these high doses would require oral treatment anyway, if they did not take the high inhaled dose.

Disodium cromoglycate (DSCG, Intal)

This inhaled treatment has a prophylactic effect. It is given either as a dry powder using a special inhaler (Fig. 17.10) or as a pressurized aerosol. A nebulizer solution is available. It is not a bronchodilator. Its actions are complex. One action is to oppose release of mediators from mast cells. It can inhibit the immediate asthmatic response to specific antigenic challenge if it is given before the challenge. It is effective in young persons, in whom treatment of asthma is, anyway, easier. It is effective in suppressing exercise-induced asthma, it is extremely safe and has no significant side-effects.

As in the case of steroid aerosols, patients need to understand the essentially prophylactic intent of treatment.

Nedocromil (Tilade)

This is an inhaled compound, with some similar properties to cromoglycate. It has been found to have steroid-sparing effects. It is relatively expensive.

Oral steroid treatment

Short-course treatment

A short course of oral steroid treatment is required in all cases of acute severe asthma (see below).

A short course is required at any time to regain control of asthma and enable prophylactic treatment (DSCG and steroid aerosols) to function again.

Self-administration

It is important not to delay the treatment of worsening asthma; patients with previously severe asthma should be taught how to start their own short course of oral prednisolone. They should understand the potential side-effects of long-continued treatment and the difference between this and infrequent short-course usage, which is safe.

Worsening of asthma may occur months after instruction of the patient and possibly away from home, so it is useful to provide a written list of circumstances in which a short course of prednisolone should be started.

When?

The following situations indicate unstable asthma and they are all easily recognized by patients:

1 *Bronchodilator aerosol not working* (see relationship between severity and response to bronchodilator described above).

2 *Bad night.* Protracted waking or repeated waking is a reliable hallmark of important worsening of asthma and poor control.

3 *Immobilizing asthma.* The patient has to sit for a time because of distressed breathing. Even brief episodes like this denote important unstable asthma, requiring prompt action.

4 *Morning tightness lasts till lunchtime* . Length of morning tightness is related to control of asthma and usually well known to the patient.

5 *Worsening day by day.* This suggests worsening penetration of prophylactic treatment and the need to restore airway patency and re-establish adequate suppression, so that aerosol treatment can be re-established.

6 *Intravenous injection needed.* Even if there is heartening, prompt improvement after intravenous treatment with β-agonist or aminophylline, oral steroid is required because asthma control must be poor and relapse is likely.

7 *Peak flow below pre-arranged level.* This level will vary according to the patient's known best achievable peak flow when well. A drop to half this level would normally signal the need for oral steroid treatment.

How much?

At least 30 mg of prednisolone should be given on the first day. The dose should not be reduced until obvious improvement has occurred. The length of a course is related to the severity of the attack; this is related to whether treatment was started promptly as soon as deterioration was obvious or deferred. Patients should continue aerosol steroid treatment during the short oral course or they may neglect to continue when they are improved afterwards. The reserve stock of prednisolone must be replenished.

Long-term treatment

The need for a long-term treatment with oral steroid only becomes clear when it is established that asthma cannot be satisfactorily controlled by other measures. Usually this means that short courses of prednisolone are required very frequently, despite the efficient and regular use of a steroid aerosol in above-standard dosage, together with supporting bronchodilator therapy. The aim is to maintain the dose at the lowest level compatible with reasonable (but not necessarily perfect) control of asthma; hence it is desirable that patients should control their own dosage. They must understand the compromise which is being attempted between disabling asthma on the one hand and the risk of side-effects on the other. There should be no hesitation in promptly increasing the dose in the event of progressive deterioration over hours or days. Peak-flow recordings will be found very helpful to patient and doctor when trying to adjust steroid usage to best advantage—avoiding high dosage and bad asthma. In titrating the dose, 1 mg tablets of prednisolone may be useful in combination with the standard 5 mg tablets.

Side-effects

The general public in the UK is very aware that steroids produce side-effects, and it is common for patients with severe asthma to put themselves at some risk through failing to restart or increase the dose of steroid because of fear of the consequences. A common fear is that use of steroid treatment will lead to 'resistance' and gradually escalating requirements. There is no evidence that this tendency exists. Blatant over-indulgence in too high a dose is uncommon. In many patients, worthwhile benefit is obtained with a regular dose of 5–7.5 mg of prednisolone daily, at which level serious side-effects are very rare. At doses up to 12.5 mg daily, some cushingoid redistribution of fat and facial fullness is seen. Most patients gain weight, but this can be controlled by dietary restriction. At higher doses, obvious cushingoid changes are seen and predisposed individuals may develop glucose intolerance, peptic ulceration, etc. Only a few severely incapacitated individuals can be shown to obtain worthwhile benefit from daily doses in excess of 20 mg of prednisolone daily. Probably the most sinister complication is vertebral collapse from osteoporosis, which is particularly likely to affect post-menopausal females.

Antibiotics

Antibiotics play a minor part in the management of asthma. Usually, adjusting the anti-asthma treatment is all that is required when asthma is aggravated by an intercurrent infection. It is difficult to decide what circumstances merit antibiotic treatment, but co-existing bronchiectasis, very yellow sputum, fever, or malaise-out of proportion to the asthma are commonly taken as indications. Bacteriological examination is not usually indicated. Amoxycillin (or erythromycin in penicillin sensitive individuals) is likely to be effective. Antibiotic treatment should not normally be given alone—it is generally ineffective and results in potentially dangerous delay whilst doctor and patient wait for treatment to work. Increase of anti-asthma treatment is virtually always required.

Assessment of progress in chronic asthma

Because of the striking diurnal and day-to-day variation in the severity of asthma, spirometric measurements made at infrequent intervals may not be particularly helpful in assessing progress (Fig. 17.16). It is relevant to make a note of:

1   Number of nocturnal attacks (for example, in a week).
2   The length of time taken for the chest to feel clear in the mornings.
3   Absence from work or school.
4   Consumption of bronchodilator preparations.
5   Peak flow recordings.

Improvement is usually accompanied by 'ironing out' of the morning and sometimes evening troughs.

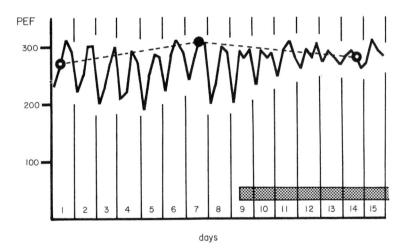

days

Fig. 17.16. Fallibility of isolated ventilatory tests in asthma.
Solid line: Record of peak expiratory flow (PEF) measured four times daily. The shaded area represents the start of new treatment (e.g. cromoglycate or steroid aerosol). Typical diurnal variation is present over the first 9 days. Thereafter there is progressive disappearance of the early morning 'trough', although values obtained later in the day remain similar to those recorded earlier.
Interrupted line: This line connects three isolated recordings of PEF made at three separate visits to a doctor. The doctor viewing only these results might have been tempted to conclude that at the second visit there was some improvement and that there had been deterioration between the second and third visits. The erroneous conclusion might have been that the new treatment was ineffective. In this situation adequate questioning of the patient would almost certainly lead to the clinician reaching the correct conclusion despite the PEF recordings he had obtained.

Treatment of asthma in childhood

Below the age of about 18 months β-agonist bronchodilators are ineffective whether given orally or by nebulization. In the 2–5 years age group, oral salbutamol may be useful. Regular asthma at this age can be suppressed by DSCG by nebulizer. More severe asthma in childhood requires regular steroid aerosol treatment, usually in adult doses. Children below school age are not usually good at using pressurized aerosols, whether for bronchodilators, DSCG or topical steroid treatment; either a dry powder device or a spacer will be required. These may become difficult to use during an exacerbation. One effective method of administering a bronchodilator aerosol is to fit a pressurized inhaler into the bottom of a polystyrene coffee cup and to give multiple puffs with the wide end of the cup near to the face as the child breathes normally.

Severe childhood asthma

An isolated severe exacerbation may be managed with a short course of oral prednisolone. Inhalation of salbutamol, terbutaline or equivalent by nebulizer is very effective in acute exacerbations in childhood—partly because of the relatively large dose delivered and partly because children find it particularly difficult to use inhalers when they are distressed. It is important that patient and parents do not

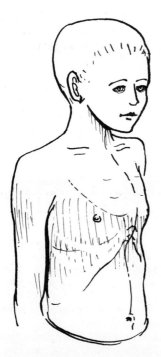

Fig. 17.17. Chest deformity in chronic childhood asthma. The sternum is pushed forwards (pigeon chest deformity) and there is a groove approximately in the position of the sixth rib (Harrison's sulcus). Deformity of the type shown is always indicative of severe asthma. It is, to a considerable extent, reversible if asthma is treated adequately and sufficiently early. It should be a rarity.

come to rely solely on a nebulized bronchodilator, when asthma could be treated more securely by suppression using steroid aerosol treatment.

Severe chronic asthma in childhood is sometimes not obvious. The usual marked fluctuations in severity and overt wheezing may be lacking and the parents and child may become accustomed to a limited level of activity. Stunting and chest deformity (Fig. 17.17) are indicative of severe asthma. As it may be difficult to judge the severity of asthma, spirometry is very important. A very small number of children are not adequately controlled by regular treatment with DSCG or aerosol steroids. In this situation, oral prednisolone or regular injections of ACTH or tetracosactrin may be necessary (the latter two on grounds of alleged lesser effect on growth).

Asthma in pregnancy

Asthma usually poses no particular problems in pregnancy. Occasionally exacerbations occur in the first few weeks, but the last two trimesters are often marked by unusually good control. It is common for exacerbations to occur 4–6 weeks after delivery.

Acute severe asthma (status asthmaticus)

A severe, progressive, prolonged attack of immobilizing asthma which is unresponsive to bronchodilator preparations is termed acute severe asthma. This is synonymous with status asthmaticus. Treatment may be started in the home, but hospitalization is indicated. Management is based upon giving large doses of bronchodilator and corticosteroid drugs and ensuring adequate oxygenation of the patient until the attack abates.

Note: the guidance below is adapted from guidelines approved by the British Thoracic Society. The full document covers the management of chronic as well as acute severe asthma, also giving step by step guidance to the handling of acute severe asthma in the Accident and Emergency Department. The reference is given in Further Information (p. 304).

Recognition of acute severe asthma

The severity of an attack is often underestimated by patients, relatives and doctors, largely because of failure to make measurements.

1 **Potentially life-threatening features:**
   (a) Unable to complete sentences in one breath or get up from a chair or bed.
   (b) Respiratory rate >25 breaths min^{-1}.
   (c) Heart rate persistently >110 beats min^{-1}.
   (d) Peak expiratory flow (PEF) <40% of predicted normal or of best obtainable if known (<200 litres min^{-1} where best obtainable value not known).
   (e) Inspiratory fall in systolic blood pressure >10 mmHg.

2 **Imminently life-threatening features**
The presence of any of the following indicates a very severe attack:
   (a) A silent chest on auscultation.
   (b) Cyanosis.
   (c) Bradycardia.
   (d) Exhaustion, confusion or unconsciousness.

3   Arterial blood gas markers of severity

Arterial blood gases should always be measured in patients admitted to hospital with acute severe asthma. The following are markers of a very severe (or life-threatening) attack:

   (a) A normal or high Pa_{CO_2} in a breathless asthmatic patient.
   (b) $Pa_{O_2} < 8$ kPa (60 mmHg) irrespective of oxygen therapy.
   (c) A low pH.

Immediate management

Oxygen
   The highest concentration available should be used; masks delivering 24% or 28% are not appropriate (see Chapter 31).

Nebulized β_2-agonist
   Salbutamol 2.5–5 mg or terbutaline 5–10 mg should be given immediately. In an emergency, multiple doses from a metered dose inhaler should be given with a spacer device.

High dose systemic steroids
   Prednisolone 40–60 mg and/or intravenous hydrocortisone 200 mg should be given immediately.

Intravenous bronchodilators
   If obviously life-threatening features are present, intravenous aminophylline (250 mg over 30 minutes) or β_2-agonist (e.g. salbutamol 200 µg or terbutaline 250 µg over 10 minutes). A β_2-agonist is preferred if the patient is already taking oral theophylline.

Reassurance
   Patients need to know that their mortal fears are understood and that they are now safe.

Continuing treatment
   Continued vigilance is required. Oxygen, high dose steroids and repeated nebulization of β_2-agonist should continue. If there is no improvement, ipratropium (atropine derivative) should be given by nebulization and an aminophylline infusion should be considered at a rate of 0.5–0.9 mg kg^{-1} hour^{-1}.

Investigation in hospital
   Very little investigation is usually necessary, apart from a chest X-ray, to reveal pneumothorax, consolidation or oedema.

Monitoring treatment
   Patients with features of life-threatening asthma require intensive monitoring by experienced staff. The following measurements are needed:
   1   Peak flow should be measured frequently in the first 24 hours and at least four

times daily throughout hospital admission. Some patients deteriorate surprisingly after 3–4 days. Nursing staff should be asked to seek help if peak flow falls to a pre-arranged level.

2 Blood gas measurement should be repeated within 2 hours of starting treatment if the initial Pa_{CO_2} was normal or raised, or if the patient deteriorates. Saturation measurement is also useful. If peak flow is improving, the blood gas status can be assumed not to have deteriorated.

3 Serum theophylline concentration should be measured if aminophylline is continued for more than 24 hours and infusion rate adjusted to achieve 10–20 µg ml^{-1}.

4 Serum potassium and blood glucose should be measured.

Unhelpful treatment

Sedatives and percussive physiotherapy are contraindicated. Antibiotics are rarely relevant.

Indications for intermittent positive pressure ventilation (IPPV)

IPPV is only rarely necessary and is used when there is:

1 Failure to achieve satisfactory oxygenation.

2 Exhaustion—as suggested by: rising P_{CO_2}, hopelessness and apathy, impaired consciousness, rising pulse rate (although pre-terminal hypoxaemia may be marked by bradycardia) and failure to produce sputum.

The purpose is to secure adequate oxygenation of the patient until other therapeutic measures bring the attack to an end.

With endotracheal intubation and a closed breathing system it is possible to administer higher concentrations of oxygen than with a mask and interruption of oxygenation is more easily prevented. The patient can be sedated and rested. Clearance of some of the more bulky secretions can be achieved by suction and small volume lavage. IPPV may be needed from as little as a few hours to as much as a week.

Management during recovery in hospital and following discharge

Patient education—prevention

The opportunity should be taken to improve the patient's understanding of asthma and its management and to provide written guidance on future management. Ways of improving the patient's response to worsening asthma should be identified. Most crises resulting in hospital admission are probably preventable. The importance of peak flow measurement in determining treatment changes should be explained. Possible precipitating factors should be identified.

Treatment on discharge

Patients should not normally be discharged until symptoms have cleared and lung function has stabilized or returned to normal or best levels.

Inhaled steroids should be started at least 48 hours before discharge. Nebulized bronchodilators should be changed to standard inhalers 24–48 hours before discharge unless the patient requires a nebulizer at home. Inhaler technique should be checked and performance recorded. If necessary, alternative inhaler devices should be used. In patients requiring oral xanthines, blood theophylline levels should be monitored.

Patients should be discharged taking:

1 Oral steroids (usually prednisolone 20–40 mg daily for 1 to 3 weeks, or longer in some chronic asthmatic patients). Treatment should not be stopped, nor the dose tailed, if the asthma is deteriorating.

2 On-going inhaled anti-inflammatory treatment (usually inhaled steroid).

3 Inhaled or nebulized β_2-agonists as necessary.

4 If required: bronchodilators or inhaled ipratropium.

Inhaled steroids and inhaled β_2-agonists should be continued in all patients, at least until the first out-patient hospital visit. Oral steroids can be stopped before the first hospital out-patient visit.

BRONCHOPULMONARY ASPERGILLOSIS

Principal patterns of disease

The clinical patterns of disease related to the ubiquitous mould *Aspergillus fumigatus* are illustrated in Fig. 17.18.

Allergic aspergillosis

In allergic aspergillosis, both immediate and delayed responses are usually demonstrable by intradermal skin-testing and by bronchial challenge (the latter is not part of routine diagnosis procedure). The recognition of allergic aspergillosis does not usually affect management; asthma is treated on its merits as outlined above. Asthma may well be more resistant to standard forms of treatment and a high proportion of individuals are found to have a requirement for regular oral corticosteroids. Desensitization is unhelpful and antifungal treatment has not been shown to play an important part in management. Steroid treatment, either by mouth or aerosol, is usually fairly effective.

Mucoid impaction

Episodes of lobar collapse due to 'mucoid impaction' may be treated by bronchoscopy and bronchial lavage. Usually the collapse resolves spontaneously or with the help of steroid therapy.

Mycetoma

Mycetomas (aspergillomas) have a characteristic radiographic appearance. They lie free within the cavity and there is a thin rim of radiolucency ('halo') surrounding the rounded mass. Mycetomas enlarge very slowly; some cause massive haemoptysis. Surgical removal is indicated if haemoptysis is threatening and lung function is not severely impaired.

Less common forms

Sometimes progressive spread of *Aspergillus* infestation is observed over days or weeks with progressive parenchymal shadowing. The term 'invasive aspergillosis'

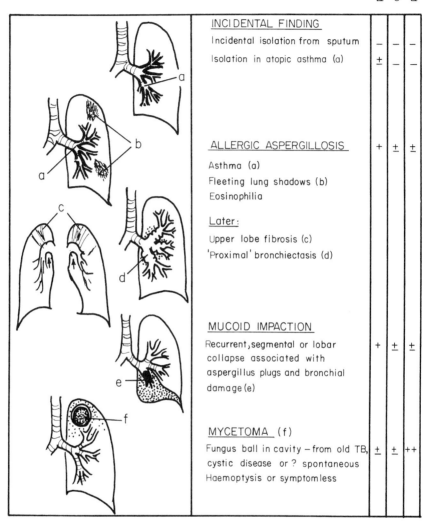

Fig. 17.18. Synopsis of bronchopulmonary aspergillosis.

may be used in this context. Usually this progression occurs in lungs which are already highly abnormal: for example, in cystic fibrosis or advanced fibrosing alveolitis.

Occasionally *Aspergillus fumigatus* may infect an area of necrotic lung: for example, after infarction. Generalized systemic infection by *Aspergillus* is, however, rare and is only seen in catastrophically immunosuppressed individuals such as those undergoing radical treatment for malignant disease.

Antifungal treatment becomes an important consideration in invasive aspergillosis and in generalized systemic aspergillosis. In the latter, the drug of choice appears to be intravenous amphotericin B. This may also be used in invasive pulmonary disease, but ketaconazole is an alternative oral treatment which has been shown to be effective in arresting progress, even though eradication may not be achieved. Early results with inhalation of ketaconazole are promising.

PULMONARY EOSINOPHILIA

This term is used to cover a variety of conditions in which radiological pulmonary shadowing is associated with a very high blood eosinophil count. The radiological shadows may be fluffy, wedge-shaped or reticulonodular in type.

Pulmonary eosinophilia with asthma

The majority of patients with fleeting isolated shadows and asthma have allergic aspergillosis, with supporting evidence in the shape of skin-test reactions and the presence of serum precipitins: regular recovery of the organism is commonly forthcoming. Other antigens (e.g. house dust mite) may be capable of inducing pulmonary eosinophilia. Sometimes no obvious association with an antigen can be found.

Simple pulmonary eosinophilia (Löffler's syndrome)

This term refers to a transient pulmonary reaction with reticular or nodular shadowing on the chest X-ray which may be produced by drugs (e.g. sulphonamides) and various intestinal parasites. The pulmonary changes very rarely last more than 3–4 weeks.

Tropical eosinophilia

Pulmonary eosinophilia occurring in the tropics, with or without asthma, is usually related to sensitivity to intestinal and other parasites. Filarial infestation is probably the principal cause and most cases respond to treatment with diethyl carbamazine or organic arsenicals.

Polyarteritis nodosa

Pulmonary eosinophilia, with or without asthma, may be a feature of polyarteritis nodosa. This is rare. The diagnosis will be suggested by features such as weight loss, skin rashes, peripheral neuropathy, nephritis, etc.

Churg–Strauss syndrome

This is uncommon. It is characterized by asthma and blood eosinophilia, together with eosinophilic vasculitis and associated granuloma formation affecting several organs (for example, skin, kidney, pericardium and lung).

Drug reaction

An eosinophilic reaction is rare. Sulphonamides and sulphonylureas are probably the most common causes.

Table 17.1. Some examples of extrinsic allergic alveolitis.

Name	Antigen responsible
Farmer's lung	Spores of thermophylic actinomycetes in mouldy hay
Bird fancier's lung	Avian antigens from dust from feathers, excreta, etc.
Pituitary snuff taker's lung	Porcine or bovine antigens associated with extracts of posterior pituitary
Mushroom worker's lung	Spores of thermophylic actinomycetes in mould
Maltworker's lung	Spores of *Aspergillus clavatus*
Lung disease of grain-handlers	Dust derived from the grain weevil *Sitophilus granarius*

EXTRINSIC ALLERGIC ALVEOLITIS

This term refers to hypersensitivity reactions affecting the lung parenchyma, which occur in response to inhaled organic dusts. Farmer's lung is the best-known example. Usually the exposure is heavy and occupational. The reaction is an expression of Type III hypersensitivity and precipitins can generally be demonstrated in the serum. Some examples of extrinsic alveolitis are listed in Table 17.1.

Where the condition is suspected but there is no recognizable occupational exposure to organic dust, a search for a cause should include investigation of humidifiers which may be part of a central heating or air-conditioning system. A variety of obscure bacteria may inhabit recirculated water used in humidification; these in aerosol form may induce systemic symptoms (humidifier fever).

Pathological features

The alveolar walls become thickened and infiltrated by lymphocytes, plasma cells and polymorphs. Small airways may show similar infiltrations. Advanced cases may show granuloma formation and variable degrees of diffuse lung fibrosis.

Clinical features

The most prominent complaints are often not related to the chest. They include muscular aching, malaise, headache and fever. The relationship of the illness to the dust exposure is often not appreciated.

The patient may notice immediate tightness in the chest with cough and sometimes wheezing on exposure to the dust concerned. This may, however, be mild and transient. Typically exposure is followed after an interval of about 4 hours by tachypnoea, tightness and cough. Soon after exposure there may be fine rhonchi audible on auscultation, but the most constant sign in all stages is the presence of persistent fine crepitations. In advanced cases, there may be constant dyspnoea and exercise limitation, accompanied by cyanosis and clubbing; the picture resembles that of cryptogenic fibrosing alveolitis.

Physiological changes

A restrictive defect of ventilation is the most usual finding, but variable degrees of airways obstruction may accompany this. There may be hyperventilation and arterial hypoxaemia. Transfer factor is usually significantly reduced.

Radiological features

In early cases there may be no abnormality. During regular exposure, fluffy or nodular shadowing may be seen. In advanced cases there may be areas of honeycomb change and condensed masses of granuloma and fibrous tissue, which may be particularly evident in the upper lobes.

Diagnosis

The diagnosis is made from the association of the total clinical picture with exposure to a suitable organic dust. Fever is an important clue. Identification of serum precipitins specific to the organic material may provide supportive evidence, but results need to be interpreted with caution. In the case of farmer's lung it should be noted that about 20% of unaffected workers handling hay have serum antibodies to the thermophylic moulds responsible for the disease.

Management

Avoidance of the responsible antigen is the most important measure. This may mean a change of job or control of the exposure. It is not sufficient to advise the use of masks, as these are unlikely to be used consistently by unsupervised workers. In the case of farmer's lung, improved methods of harvesting, aimed at reducing the moisture content of hay, are of importance. Sufferers are eligible for compensation under the Industrial Injuries Acts. Steroid therapy may be indicated on first diagnosis in a florid case, but such treatment must not be viewed as an alternative to control of exposure. Little benefit can be expected in cases with advanced fibrosis.

Chapter 18
Diffuse Lung Fibrosis

CRYPTOGENIC FIBROSING ALVEOLITIS
(Previously known as diffuse interstitial pulmonary fibrosis and Hamman–Rich syndrome)

This is a rather uncommon condition in which the lung parenchyma becomes involved in a diffuse fibrotic process causing progressive impairment of gas transfer and progressive dyspnoea. The cause of the condition is not clear. It is a disease of adult life, most common in late middle age.

Pathological features
The principal features are:

1 Thickening fibrosis and a variable degree of cellular infiltration of the interstitial tissue of the lungs, which is most obvious in the lung parenchyma.

2 'Desquamation' of large numbers of cells into the alveoli. These include macrophages and other mononuclear cells, some of which may be altered Type II pneumocytes.

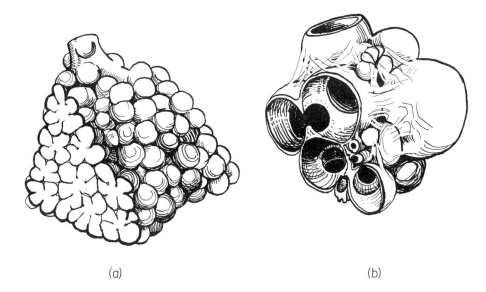

(a)   (b)

Fig. 18.1. Honeycomb lung. A three-dimensional impression of the structure of the normal lobule (a) and of the air-spaces in advanced lung fibrosis (honeycomb lung) (b). There is dense fibrosis with disappearance of normal lung architecture. The air-spaces are thick walled and much larger than alveoli. Most of them probably represent dilated terminal and respiratory bronchioles.

These changes may be irregularly dispersed within the lung and some individuals may show predominantly one form of change. As fibrosis progresses, alveolar tissue becomes absorbed within condensing cellular fibrous tissue; in large parts of the lungs no alveoli may be visible at all. Because the process tends to be widespread, complete collapse of large parts of lung is not generally seen; instead the lung remains aerated but the air-spaces are mainly made up of dilated bronchioles and the appearance is termed 'honeycomb lung' (Fig. 18.1). At autopsy, a characteristic peripheral distribution of the lung destruction and fibrosis is common.

Symptoms

In the earlier stages, the patient presents with an easy panting dyspnoea and symptoms of exhaustion on effort. Sometimes an irritating unproductive cough is a prominent symptom. With progress of the disease, dyspnoea can become frightening, even on trivial exertion. Additional symptoms may develop due to hypoxia, cardiac failure and bronchopulmonary infection and, terminally, features of respiratory failure and pulmonary embolism may be added to the clinical picture.

Signs (Fig. 18.2)

The patient is easily dyspnoeic, usually tachypnoetic, and may be cyanosed. Clubbing of some degree is seen in about two-thirds of cases. The chest appears

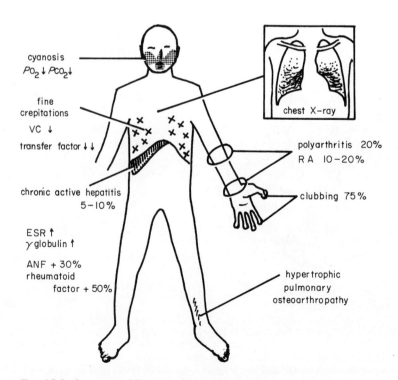

cyanosis
$Po_2 \downarrow Pco_2 \downarrow$

fine
crepitations

VC $\downarrow$

transfer factor $\downarrow \downarrow$

chronic active hepatitis
5-10%

ESR $\uparrow$
γ globulin $\uparrow$

ANF + 30%
rheumatoid
factor + 50%

chest X-ray

polyarthritis 20%
R A 10-20%

clubbing 75%

hypertrophic
pulmonary
osteoarthropathy

Fig. 18.2. Summary of features of fibrosing alveolitis.

normal and the costal margin moves upwards and outwards in the normal way (see Fig. 6.4), but in severe cases there is an inward movement of the lower sternum on inspiration. The most consistent finding is the presence of fine crackles on auscultation of the chest. These tend to occur throughout inspiration, being especially marked towards the end of inspiration.

Physiological changes

Spirometry

A restrictive ventilatory defect is almost always evident by the time troublesome symptoms are reported.

Lung volumes

All lung volumes are reduced but tend to maintain their relative proportions.

Lung compliance

This is reduced. Measurement is not essential to the diagnosis.

Blood gases

At rest, blood gases tend to be normal until the disease is well advanced, when arterial hypoxaemia and hypocapnia (low P_{CO_2} due to hyperventilation) are generally found. Exercise is limited by arterial hypoxaemia and exercise tolerance may be extended by breathing oxygen-enriched air.

Gas transfer

There is characteristically a pronounced impairment of transfer factor by the time the patient has troublesome symptoms (p. 75). Normal values for transfer factor show variation between different laboratories and are dependent upon age and stature. An average normal value might be in excess of 5.5 mmol min^{-1} kPa^{-1} (16.5), moderately severe symptoms would be expected below 3.0 mmol min^{-1} kPa^{-1} (9.0) and severe disability accompanies levels below 1.5 mmol min^{-1} kPa^{-1} (4.0) (values in brackets are traditional units: ml min^{-1} mmHg^{-1}). K_{CO} is always reduced. Traditionally, the defective gas transfer has been regarded as a 'diffusion defect' due to thickening of the alveolar membrane. This explanation is undoubtedly an oversimplification; it seems likely that other mechanisms are more important and these include:

1   A much extended range of ventilation/perfusion ratios throughout the lung due to irregularly-distributed stiffness (p. 22).

2   Replacement of alveoli by fibrous tissue resulting in overall reduction in alveolar surface and capillary blood volume.

Radiological changes

The appearances vary somewhat, depending upon the stage of the disease and its rapidity of onset. The most usual features are: (1) a 'ground-glass' haziness, especially at the bases; to this may be added (2) streaky wisps of shadow with elevation of the diaphragms, suggesting basal collapse; and (3) a generalized micronodular (miliary) mottling. The end-stage of the disease is characterized by

(4) the appearances of 'honeycomb lung' in which multiple circular areas of translucency 2–5 mm in diameter become evident within areas of opacification. Terminally there may be changes due to infection and pulmonary infarction.

Associated disorders

The ESR is usually elevated. Associated polyarthritis is common. About 10% of cases may have rheumatoid arthritis and a positive rheumatoid factor is found in the serum in about 50% of cases. Elevation of gamma globulins is fairly frequently found. A number of cases with co-existing chronic active hepatitis have been described and cirrhosis occurs more frequently than expected. Antinuclear factor (ANF) may be present and other non-organ-specific antibodies are found in about 30% of cases. A higher than expected incidence of thyroid disease has been reported. The relationship between cryptogenic fibrosing alveolitis and other collagen or autoimmune disorders remains conjectural.

Diagnosis

The diagnosis can usually be made on clinical grounds, with the support of radiological appearances and simple tests of pulmonary function including measurement of transfer factor.

In a typical patient, the diagnosis may be straightforward: a middle-aged individual with progressive panting dyspnoea and cyanosis, but with no evidence of cardiac disease or airways obstruction, is found to have clubbing and diffuse crepitations and a reticulonodular pattern of shadowing on the chest X-ray which is more pronounced at the bases. Spirometry reveals a much restricted vital capacity, but good early expiratory flow rate; transfer factor is found to be markedly impaired.

Differential diagnosis

In less typical cases, the differential diagnosis is potentially lengthy. Miliary mottling is discussed on p. 84. Some of the more important alternatives are:

1 *Extrinsic allergic alveolitis.* It is very important to differentiate this preventable form of alveolitis. Clinical, radiological and physiological features may be identical; points of difference are: (a) history of exposure to appropriate organic dust and presence of serum precipitins; (b) more prominent involvement of upper lobes in extrinsic alveolitis; (c) rheumatoid factor, ANF and elevation of gamma globulin are commonly found in cryptogenic fibrosing alveolitis.

2 *Bronchiectasis.* Basal crackles, clubbing and irregular basal shadowing on the chest X-ray may cause confusion. Points of difference are: (a) cough is longstanding and productive of large amounts of purulent sputum; (b) dyspnoea, if present, is usually a consequence of airways obstruction; (c) cyanosis is uncommon and generally associated with chronic ventilatory failure; (d) transfer factor is not usually reduced.

3 *Chronic left heart failure.* May rarely produce reticulonodular shadowing and dyspnoea; clinical, radiological and ECG changes of left heart disease will generally be present.

4 *Sarcoidosis.* Differentiation may be difficult without a positive Kveim test or other features of sarcoidosis, particularly in the skin and eye. In diffuse

sarcoidosis of the lungs, the defect in transfer factor is often more modest than would be expected from the radiographic changes.

5 *Lymphangitis carcinomatosa*. This may produce progressive dyspnoea with striking impairment of transfer factor. Deterioration is inexorable over a comparatively short period of a few weeks or months. There may be past or present evidence of carcinoma—usually an adenocarcinoma.

6 *Pulmonary embolism*. This should rarely cause confusion, but repeated embolism should always be borne in mind in any patient with progressive obscure breathlessness and basal shadowing on the chest X-ray.

7 *Industrial lung disease*. Most especially diffuse pulmonary fibrosis due to asbestos (see asbestosis).

Lung biopsy

Biopsy confirmation of the diagnosis is not essential when the diagnosis, or a particular line of action, is clear. Sometimes, however, a therapeutic decision is impossible without a histological diagnosis.

Open-lung biopsy

This allows removal of a relatively large specimen, which can be selected from a moderately affected part of the lung. The disadvantages are the hazards of anaesthetic, thoracotomy and subsequent convalescence.

Closed-lung biopsy

A number of needle techniques have been developed for obtaining specimens of aerated lung. The Jack needle shears off a tiny fragment of lung, snagged by small hooks on the stylet. Steels's lung trephine is operated by a high-speed air drill and cuts a small core of lung tissue. In most instances the disturbance is slight; only about one-third of patients develop a pneumothorax, and of these less than half require pleural intubation. Transbronchial biopsy (Fig. 23.7), performed by fine biopsy forceps passed through a fibre-optic bronchoscope and wedged in a peripheral bronchiole, offers an alternative means of obtaining multiple samples of lung parenchyma in the diagnosis of diffuse lung disease. The main drawbacks of closed biopsy are the risk of haemorrhage and pneumotheorax, the small size of the specimen and occasional failure to obtain a specimen. Bronchoalveolar lavage may be used to assess activity but is not essential. The fluid shows an increase in neutrophils which contrasts with the lymphocytosis of sarcoidosis.

Course of the disease

The course is very variable. A small number of patients have a rapidly progressive course, over only a few months, and the illness may be accompanied by severe malaise and pneumonic features. A slower downhill course is more usual, over a period of years. In some elderly individuals the condition is discovered by chance and appears to be completely stationary.

Treatment

Corticosteroid treatment

Patients with disturbing dyspnoea or clear evidence of progression should be treated with corticosteroids. It is usual to use a large dose (40–60 mg of prednisolone daily), for a period of up to 2 months if the disease threatens to disable. If any improvement is to be achieved it will generally be evident by this time. The dose is then progressively reduced to the lowest level capable of maintaining the improvement.

Result

Improvement of some degree is seen in about two-thirds of cases receiving corticosteroid treatment. The more acute the mode of onset and the younger the patient, the more likely it is that there will be a worthwhile improvement. However, a worthwhile response may be seen, even in advanced disease with honeycomb change.

Immunosuppressive therapy

Azathioprine may have some effect on the disease and may be useful where there are especially compelling reasons for avoiding large doses of prednisolone. More recently cyclophosphamide has been used where the response to steroid treatment has been disappointing.

Oxygen

This may be useful in advanced disease, when even gentle exercise is poorly tolerated. An oxygen concentrator and long lengths of plastic piping may enable the patient to negotiate the stairs or take a bath, which might otherwise be impossible. A rechargeable portable cylinder may extend the range of activities out of doors.

Supportive measures

Measures to control infection, heart failure and exhausting cough are required as the disease progresses. Opiates may be necessary to control terrifying terminal dyspnoea.

DIFFUSE FIBROSIS DUE TO DRUGS AND POISONS

Drugs

Drugs capable of producing lung fibrosis include: busulphan, bleomycin, nitrofurantoin, cyclophosphamide and methysergide (see p. 293).

Paraquat

Poisoning with the weedkiller Paraquat induces a vicious accelerated form of diffuse lung fibrosis in which the whole range of fibrosing alveolitis, from the earliest changes to widespread honeycombing, may be condensed into a period of less than 3 weeks, by which time death from hypoxia has usually supervened. Very occasionally, individuals may escape with lung changes arrested at an intermediate stage. Fatal poisoning follows accidental consumption of only a mouthful of agricultural concentrate (Gramoxone). Accidental poisoning with diluted material, or the more generally available Paraquat/Diquat mixture in granular form, is almost unheard of. Intentional self-poisoning with various preparations accounts for about half of the fatalities.

Radiation

Therapeutic irradiation which involves the lung fields may lead to an acute pneumonitis which generally resolves within a few weeks. A variable degree of fibrosis may follow over subsequent months in the distribution of the irradiated areas.

Occupational causes

See p. 281.

RHEUMATOID ARTHRITIS

The pulmonary accompaniments of rheumatoid arthritis are summarized in Fig. 18.3.

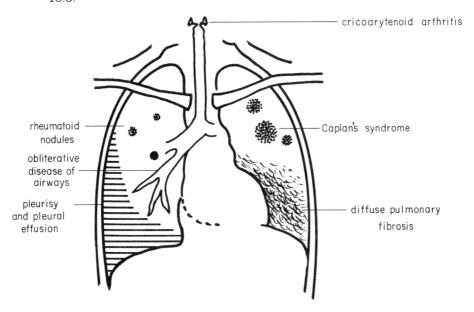

Fig. 18.3. Summary of pulmonary complications of rheumatoid arthritis

Pleurisy and pleural effusion

These are common in rheumatoid arthritis and may tend to be recurrent. Effusions are rarely large.

Pulmonary fibrosis

This is much less common, probably occurring in no more than 2% of cases. There is a definite but ill-understood relationship between rheumatoid arthritis and fibrosing alveolitis. The fibrosis accompanying rheumatoid arthritis may appear to be stationary for many years. If pulmonary fibrosis is disabling or progressive, treatment with corticosteroids may be indicated.

Pulmonary nodules

These are not common. The appearance is of several soft spherical nodules up to 1 cm in diameter, this may lead to the erroneous diagnosis of metastatic malignant disease. The nodules have the same histology as rheumatoid nodules elsewhere; they sometimes cavitate and may disappear spontaneously.

Caplan's syndrome

Rheumatoid arthritis occurring in association with coalworkers' pneumoconiosis may be marked by the occurrence of very large pulmonary nodules 2–3 cm in diameter. These may also break down and cavitate, sometimes leading to the suspicion of tuberculosis though tubercle bacilli are not found. Sometimes the rheumatoid arthritis is not clinically evident until years later. Other pneumoconioses may be associated with massive nodules in patients with rheumatoid arthritis.

Obliterative bronchiolitis

It has been recognized recently that a small proportion of patients with rheumatoid arthritis may develop rapidly progressive airways obstruction associated with obliteration of small bronchi.

Cricoarytenoid arthritis

This may lead to hoarseness or, occasionally, inspiratory stridor.

SYSTEMIC SCLEROSIS

This uncommon condition produces a number of pulmonary complications most of which only become evident when the disease is relatively advanced.

Diffuse pulmonary fibrosis

The clinical, radiological and physiological features of this are like those of fibrosing alveolitis, although there is some evidence that the alteration of fibrous tissue may be of a fundamentally different nature in systemic sclerosis.

Pulmonary hypertension

Right heart failure and syncope can develop in patients without advanced lung fibrosis.

Restriction of chest wall movement

This late complication may arise as a consequence of severe thickening and contraction of the skin of the trunk.

Inhalation pneumonia

Pneumonia and lung abscess may result overspill from a dilated oesophagus, secondary to stricture formation. Pneumonia is a common terminal event.

The diagnosis is made by recogniton of the characteristic changes in the skin and other organs. Where pulmonary fibrosis appears to be causing disability, corticosteroid treatment is generally tried—almost always with disappointing results.

SYSTEMIC LUPUS ERYTHEMATOSUS (SLE)
The pulmonary complications of this uncommon multi-system disorder are as follows:

Pleurisy
Pleurisy, sometimes with a small effusion, is common and may be the presenting feature. Pleurisy occurring in young female patients who are more ill than might be expected and who have a high ESR should lead to suspicion of SLE.

Pneumonia
Patchy recurrent pneumonia is a common feature of SLE in relapse. Usually the patient is ill and there may be a characteristic rash, arthritis and other features of the disease. The diagnosis will be supported by the finding of antinuclear factor, LE cells and DNA antibody in the serum.

'Small lung syndrome'
It is uncertain whether true diffuse pulmonary fibrosis occurs in association with SLE, but patients may complain of dyspnoea associated with a sensation of restriction within the chest. There may be no definite physical signs of radiological features, but spirometry may reveal a restrictive ventilatory defect and transfer factor may be moderately impaired. The syndrome tends to resolve fairly promptly with steroid treatment. One factor in its causation may be impaired action of respiratory musculature.

BRONCHOALVEOLAR LAVAGE (BAL)
This is a fairly new technique with limited clinical applications, which has given interesting new information about cellular activity in diffuse inflammatory lung disease. A fibre-optic bronchoscope (Fig. 23.4) is introduced under local anaesthesia and the tip is wedged in a segmental bronchus of suitable size. Several 20 ml aliquots of warm saline are then introduced and aspirated. The aspirated material is filtered, centrifuged and resuspended and then subjected to cytological examination.

Normal cell content
In non-smoking normals, more than 90% of cells are alveolar macrophages, about 7% are lymphocytes (of which three-quarters are T cells, only a small proportion of which are activated) and polymorph leucocytes are about 1% of the total. In smokers, about 3% of cells are polymorphs, mostly neutrophils.

Fibrosing alveolitis
In this condition and others associated with collagen–vascular diseases, there is a striking increase in the proportion of neutrophils. Eosinophils and lymphocytes may also be present in increased numbers. These changes may reflect intensity of inflammatory activity, but they are not diagnostically helpful.

Sarcoidosis

In sarcoidosis there is characteristically an increase in the lymphocyte percentage. There may also be an increase in neutrophils and eosinophils. Apical fibrosis disease is associated with an increase in neutrophils rather than lymphocytes. The clinical usefulness of the lavage fluid changes is still being assessed.

Other diseases

Bronchoalveolar lavage can be diagnostic in alveolar proteinosis (special staining of the secretions) and in *Pneumocystis carinii* pneumonia (microscopic identification of the organism). It can also produce evidence of unsuspected intrapulmonary haemorrhage (haemosiderin-laden macrophages). Lavage of localized lesions suspected of being due to tuberculosis sometimes results in the culture of mycobacteria when sputum culture has failed.

Chapter 19
Sarcoidosis

Sarcoidosis is a condition characterized by the presence, in all affected organs, of non-caseating granulomatous lesions, which may resolve or be converted into hyaline fibrous tissue.

The diagnosis is made primarily by recognizing the characteristic distribution of organ involvement; in practice, histological support for the diagnosis is not always required.

The histological picture

The characteristic cell is a largish epithelioid cell with a pale staining nucleus, arranged in clumps or whorls of varying size and bounded by a sparse zone of lymphocytic infiltration. The clumps of typical cells all look strikingly the same in the various affected tissues. Caseation is not seen, even in the centre of quite large masses; but hyaline degeneration may merge with areas of fibrosis. Occasional giant cells are present and some may be seen to contain concentric inclusion bodies (Schaumann bodies).

Although the histological appearances may contribute to a diagnosis of sarcoidosis, the granuloma is not sufficiently characteristic for a confident diagnosis to be made exclusively on histological grounds.

Aetiology

The aetiology is not known. It is no longer regarded as a neoplastic type of reticuloendothelial proliferation akin to Hodgkin's disease; discussion centres on the possibility that it represents an atypical response to the tubercle bacillus (and possibly other agents which are capable of producing granulomata), or that it may be due to an unidentified transmissible agent. Exposure to beryllium has in the past produced granulomata indistinguishable from those of sarcoidosis (exposure is now very strictly controlled).

Altered immune response in sarcoidosis

Accumulation of T4 (CD4) helper lymphocytes and of monocytes in the affected tissue is an early feature (Fig. 19.1). The initial inspiration for this is unclear, but once present, a cycle of: T4 cell activity – interleukin 2 secretion – further T4 accumulation is set up. Other interleukins encourage further monocyte attraction. These monocytes become transformed to macrophages, which eventually form part of the epithelioid cell arrangement in the granuloma. There is constant turnover of these elements.

There is an excess of T4 (CD4) lymphocytes in the affected tissues, especially in the lungs, and a corresponding shortage in non-affected tissues of the body, generally. The T4 to T8 (killer cell) ratio in sarcoid lesions is about 10 : 1 whereas

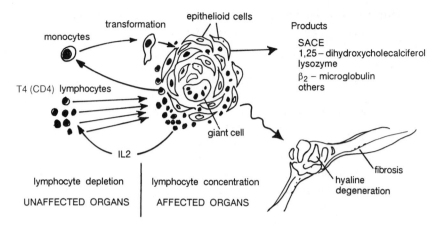

Fig. 19.1. The sarcoid granuloma. Summary of some of the better established elements of the development of the typical granuloma. IL2, interleukin 2. SACE, serium angiotensin converting enzyme.

it is about 2 : 1 in normal tissues. The relative shortage of T4 cells in the body, generally, probably underlies the partial impairment of cell-mediated immunity which is characteristic of sarcoidosis. There does not seem to be a serious predisposition to viral and fungal infection, as there is in AIDS, but there is a failure to express some forms of immune response, e.g. to tuberculin even when the subject is known to have had previous exposure or immunization against TB. It is difficult to evoke cell-mediated skin sensitization with application of dinitrochlorobenzene (DNCB). There are other examples.

Humoral immune performance seems to be normal or increased in activity. Serum Ig levels tend to be high; rheumatoid factor is sometimes positive. Circulating antigen–antibody complexes may be encountered in erythema nodosum (see below).

The granulomas themselves produce serum angiotensin converting enzyme (ACE), 1,25-dihydroxycholecalciferol (activated vitamin D), lysozyme, β_2-microglobulin and probably other substances.

Epidemiology

The precise prevalence is unknown, because mild acute sarcoidosis is often unnoticed unless discovered by chance. Probably about 15 per 100 000 individuals in Great Britain have some manifestation of the disease. The incidence of new cases in young adults is about 2 per 100 000. It is more common in immigrants from the West Indies and the Indian subcontinent, in a ratio of about 10 : 1. Its frequency is fairly constant in most parts of the world, but relatively less common in the Far East. There is a link between some manifestations of the disease and certain HLA patterns, but the genetic element in determining the disease is not felt to be very strong. Geographic or community clustering has been noted in some special studies, offering support for the idea that a transmissible agent may be the cause. Sarcoidosis is more common in non-smokers, which is consistent with the exlstence of a suppressive effect, of some sort, exerted by smoke on lymphocyte function (for which there is other evidence).

Clinical features

Sarcoidosis can be considered under two headings (Fig. 19.2).

1   Acute sarcoidosis. Here features develop abruptly in the young and almost always subsequently disappear. The most common form is characterized by bilateral hilar lymphadenopathy (BHL) accompanied by erythema nodosum. Sometimes acute uveitis is also present.

2   Chronic sarcoidosis. Chronic indolent features are found in an older age group. There is involvement of many tissues of the body and often extensive infiltration (and sometimes fibrosis) of the lungs.

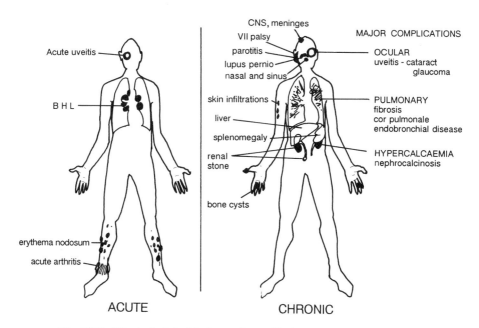

Fig. 19.2. Principal clinical features of sarcoidosis.

Acute sarcoidosis—BHL and erythema nodosum

This is by far the most common manifestation of sarcoidosis.

Bilateral hilar lymphadenopathy

Bilateral hilar lymphadenopathy (BHL) is sometimes found incidentally on a chest X-ray, but often the X-ray was taken due to the development of erythema nodosum or acute eye symptoms. It is usually symmetrical. There are no signs on examination of the chest and no disturbance of pulmonary function.

Erythema nodosum

The appearance of erythema nodosum is typical. Large round reddish raised areas appear, typically over the shins but occasionally elsewhere (e.g. thighs, upper arms). The patches become swollen and raised over about a week, becoming very painful and tender. After a few more days, the lesions darken and subside. The later appearances resemble those of fading bruises, which last 1 or 2 weeks. The skin may peel over the fading lesions. Sarcoidosis is the commonest cause of erythema nodosum in the UK. Streptococcal infections are the next largest group. Occasional cases are related to tuberculosis or to drugs, such as those containing sulphonamides, but about 40% of erythema nodosum is not attributable to known causes.

Other features

Other accompaniments are: acute arthritis of ankles, knees or wrists, with marked oedema, reddening, parotid enlargement and acute anterior uveitis.

Diagnosis

Bilateral hilar lymphadenopathy accompanied by erythema nodosum is always due to sarcoidosis and no further investigations are really necessary. Where BHL is found without any helpful clues, there is still rarely real difficulty in diagnosis. If BHL is slight, there may be difficulty in distinguishing the appearances from those of unusually prominent pulmonary arteries. Lymphoma is sometimes suspected, but this almost never shows the striking symmetry of the BHL of sarcoidosis and it is exceedingly rare for hilar adenopathy to be the sole manifestation of lymphoma. In cases of serious doubt, tuberculin and Kveim tests may be helpful (but not infallible) and lymph node biopsy or mediastinoscopy may be necessary. Patients with BHL and radiologically clear lung fields probably all have microscopic granulomata in the lung parenchyma. Granulomata can be retrieved in about 80% of cases by transbronchial biopsy; this finding can be useful when there is serious diagnostic doubt.

Course

The prognosis is excellent. Erythema nodosum and arthralgia subside within a month and uveitis rarely persists much longer. Radiological signs of BHL may persist for 2–3 years, but generally resolve over about 18 months. Occasionally some flecks of pulmonary infiltrate are seen to come and go during this time, but only a very small percentage of cases go on to develop the more indolent forms of sarcoidosis.

Treatment

As a rule no treatment is necessary. Particularly severe arthralgia or erythema nodosum may be helped by aspirin, or even prednisolone, in modest dosage for 2–3 weeks. There is usually no call for hospitalization or intensive follow-up, both of which foster concern and neurosis, which may be potentially more disabling than the condition itself.

Chronic sarcoidosis

Cases of chronic indolent sarcoidosis have not necessarily passed through a stage of acute sarcoidosis; indeed this sequence is rare.

Pulmonary involvement in chronic sarcoidosis

Although microscopic parenchymal involvement of the lung is present in acute sarcoidosis, and sometimes there are limited infiltrations evident on the chest X-ray, major involvement of the lung parenchyma with progressive permanent change is a feature of chronic sarcoidosis. It tends to be encountered when there is already other evidence of sarcoidosis, in other tissues of the body.

There may be an alveolitis accompanying the granulomatous infiltration. Bronchoalveolar lavage in sarcoidosis produces large numbers of lymphocytes, with T4 (CD4) cells predominating. In active sarcoidosis, lymphocytes make up more than 30% of the cells present (normally less than 10%).

Radiological appearances

Lung mottling, rather than hilar adenopathy, is the characteristic appearance in chronic sarcoidosis. It may take the form of fine stippling (miliary mottling—for other causes see index), or of a coarser irregular pattern. In advanced disease, where permanent fibrosis is well developed, streaky radially-arranged shadows are evident, often accompanying lung shrinkage, especially affecting the upper lobes.

The radiological changes in sarcoidosis are often classified into four crude groups or stages as follows:

Stage 0: clear chest X-ray.
Stage 1: hilar lymphadenopathy only.
Stage 2: hilar adenopathy and pulmonary infiltration.
Stage 3: pulmonary infiltration without hilar adenopathy.

The staging is an accepted, convenient, descriptive shorthand, but has no profound significance. There is no necessary progression from 1 to 3. In advanced disease, the chest radiographic changes may show a degree of resolution.

Physiological changes

These are often surprisingly modest, compared with the dramatic appearance of the chest X-ray, and the contrast is clinically useful in the early stages of diagnosis. The reverse impression of severe functional disturbance and moderate X-ray changes would tend to suggest a process like fibrosing alveolitis. The changes are not of a diagnostic pattern. There may be moderate reduction in vital capacity in a restrictive pattern; there may be moderate accompanying diffuse airways obstruction; there may be moderate reduction in transfer factor and K_{CO}. Features of large airways obstruction, from endobronchial or laryngeal disease, are sometimes seen.

Progress of pulmonary involvement

Infiltrations often remain stationary for years. Perhaps a quarter of patients with extensive infiltration develop some fibrosis, which may also remain constant for long periods and may not be associated with severe symptoms. Probably less than 10% with such infiltrations become disabled; a smaller proportion actually die from pulmonary involvement.

Pulmonary fibrosis

This is rare; representing an end stage following granulomatous infiltration and alveolitis. It usually involves the mid and upper zones most severely. X-ray changes are of contracture and spider's web-like linear shadows, with areas of condensed shadowing which may enclose honeycomb spaces or larger cysts. Lung volumes are by this stage small. Exercise is limited; there may be cyanosis; minor respiratory infections cause severe disturbance. Clubbing is rare in sarcoidosis, unless there are suppurative complications in seriously disorganized lungs.

Endobronchial sarcoidosis

Plaques of granuloma may occur, either scattered throughout the bronchial tree or as a localized deposit. Localized or, occasionally, diffuse airways obstruction may be produced. With the increased use of fibre-optic bronchoscopy in suspected sarcoidosis, for purposes of lung biopsy or bronchoalveolar lavage, endobronchial sarcoidosis has come to be recognized as quite a common accompaniment of chronic disease.

Extrapulmonary sarcoidosis

Some of the more common sites are indicated diagrammatically in Fig. 19.2; a few deserve special mention.

Ocular sarcoidosis

Anterior uveitis (iridocyclitis) is the most common manifestation. It may be obvious because of pain, misting vision and the presence of ciliary injection, but sometimes it is only revealed by slit-lamp inspection. Posterior uveitis (perivenous sheathing and chorioretinitis) is much less common. Uveitis occurs in about a quarter of all patients with sarcoidosis and sarcoidosis accounts for about 5% of uveitis presenting to ophthalmologists. Keratoconjunctivitis sicca and lacrimal gland enlargement may complicate chronic sarcoidosis.

Uveoparotid fever

This is the name given to a syndrome of uveitis, parotid gland enlargement and sometimes facial nerve palsy (usually temporary).

Central nervous system involvement

Facial nerve palsy is the most common feature. It may be due to meningeal involvement, which may also produce a variety of other obscure neurological syndromes and epilepsy. Hypophyseal involvement occurs rarely, producing diabetes insipidus.

Skin involvement

Lupus pernio is a chilblain-like lesion, occurring in violaceous, slightly raised patches; particularly involving the nose, cheeks, ears and sometimes the limbs. It is generally accompanied by pulmonary involvement. Nodules of sarcoid granuloma may occur in the skin, particularly in old scars.

Lymph node involvement

This is common, as is splenomegaly, which occurs in about a quarter of patients. Silent spleen involvement seems very common.

Liver involvement

This is very common indeed, but usually clinically silent, apart from occasional minor derangement of function tests. Biopsies produce about 90% positive granulomas in acute sarcoidosis and 60% positive in chronic disease.

Bone involvement

Bone cysts are the hallmark of established indolent sarcoidosis. Digits are commonly involved. Abnormal nail growth may occur when the terminal digit is involved. If affected, the digit is swollen; there is no point in routinely X-raying the hands in suspected sarcoidosis.

Calcium metabolism

Abnormal calcium metabolism is due to abnormal vitamin D activity. Activated macrophages, making up the epithelioid component of the granuloma, seem to act as conversion sites changing 25-hydroxycholecalciferol (vitamin D) to the active metabolite 1,25-dihydroxycholecalciferol (a reaction normally limited to the kidney). The result is increased calcium absorption, which is accompanied by high excretion (hypercalcuria). Almost all cases show a large calcium flux, but actual hypercalcaemia is relatively rare, unless there is co-existent renal failure. The high excretion can lead to renal stones or nephrocalcinosis and renal failure from this cause. The increased absorption, and any hypercalcaemia, is very responsive to corticosteroid treatment, even in low dosage.

Cardiac involvement

Involvement of the heart is uncommon and may be silent. It may present with heart failure or cardiac arrhythmia, such as heart block. Very rarely, sudden death is attributable to cardiac involvement.

Diagnosis

Where a number of features occur together, the diagnosis may be straight-forward; it is by no means obligatory to obtain supporting histological evidence. Where diagnosis is in doubt and needs to be resolved, biopsy of lymph nodes, liver or lung may be undertaken. Peripheral transbronchial biopsy is useful, particularly in uncertain acute sarcoidosis. Bronchoalveolar lavage may produce supporting evidence, in the form of lymphocytic fluid. Histological evidence amounts to demonstration of the presence of granuloma and is not diagnostic taken alone. Mediastinal lymph nodes, adjacent to invasion by carcinoma, some-times show a granulomatous response indistinguishable from that of sarcoidosis.

Tuberculin tests

There are negative results in over three-quarters of all patients with sarcoidosis.

Kveim test

An intradermal injection of suspension of an extract of human sarcoid spleen is made into the skin and the site marked (e.g. by tattooing). After 6 weeks the site is inspected and biopsied. A positive result is indicated by the presence of sarcoid granuloma. Individual extracts have differing records of reliability, but generally over three-quarters of patients give positive results. 'False positive' results may be found in Crohn's disease and a number of disorders associated with enlargement of lymph nodes.

Treatment

The great majority of patients with sarcoidosis require no treatment at all.

The most common cause of morbidity is anxiety. This is brought about by the knowledge that the person has an unusual disease with a sinister sounding name, which most general practitioners are unfamiliar with. Accordingly, explanation and reassurance are needed from a specialist and follow-up should be limited to that which is strictly necessary. In the usual form of acute sarcoidosis there is no need for follow-up after clinical recovery, and early discharge is important if neurosis is to be avoided.

The generally accepted indications for treatment with oral steroids are:

Progressive pulmonary changes

Where there is clinical, radiological and physiological evidence of deterioration, it is usual to start treatment with oral steroids. X-ray signs of infiltration often resolve promptly, with little change in physiological function, but sometimes with improvement in dyspnoea and cough. There is no convincing evidence that protracted control of radiological infiltrations with steroid treatment averts development of fibrosis.

There is no easy way to determine whether active, and progressively damaging, pulmonary inflammation or granulomatous infiltration is taking place in sarcoidosis. The following indices have been examined: serum ACE activity; gallium scan uptake; serum β_2-microglobulin level; cell content of lavage fluid; urinary hydroxyproline excretion. None are specific. The extent to which they reflect activity is uncertain. There is no evidence that giving treatment, so as to normalize the indices, influences eventual outcome.

Severe uveitis

Where uveitis cannot be adequately controlled by topical steroid treatment, oral prednisolone may be necessary, and this is the most common indication for such treatment.

Hypercalcaemia

Carries the threat of progressive renal failure; it is usually controlled by a modest dose of oral steroid.

Important neurological involvement

Epilepsy or meningeal involvement are usually regarded as indications for steroid treatment.

Skin manifestations of sarcoidosis may be amenable to local treatment by steroid creams or local steroid infiltration, which is worthwhile in cosmetically strategic areas.

Chapter 20
Smoking

Background

Tobacco smoking is the single most important cause of preventable premature death and suffering in the Western World. It was introduced to Europe from North and Central America around 1500 and became commonplace from about 1600. From about 1900, manufactured cigarettes were introduced; by 1940 this form of tobacco comprised 80% of the total smoked. The risks to the lungs are much greater from cigarette smoking than from life-long cigar or pipe smoking and only cigarette smoking will be referred to here. Cigarette smoking by women became increasingly common from about 1920 and the pattern of smoking, and of smoking related disease, has continued to show a lag of about 20 years behind the pattern seen in men.

Trends in tobacco consumption and smoking

The total number of cigarettes smoked by the population increased steeply in the UK to peak in the early 1980s. By about 1948, 65% of all men in the UK and about 35% of women smoked. Since then there has been a slow decline, so that in the second half of the 1980s about 30% of men and women were smokers (Fig. 20.1). The reduction in the proportion of people smoking has been greater in the higher socio-economic bands than in the lower ones. Smoking amongst professional groups decreased from 65% to about 28% between the mid 1950s and mid 1980s, whereas smoking in unskilled groups only decreased from 65% to 50%.

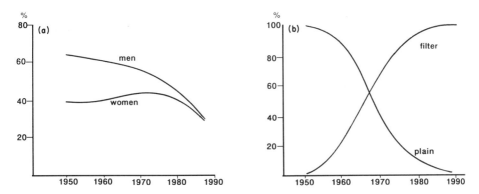

Fig. 20.1. Changes in cigarette smoking in the UK. (a) Percentage of men and women who smoke manufactured cigarettes. (b) Percentage market share of plain and filter cigarettes. For detailed information on smoking statistics see Wald *et al.*, Further Information.

From about 1955, filtered cigarettes began to replace plain unfiltered varieties and within 30 years virtually all cigarettes consumed were of filtered type (Fig. 20.1). The tar yield of the average cigarette smoked fell by about half between 1945 and 1985; the carbon monoxide yield changed little and the nicotine yield fell by about one-third. Over a similar period, the average number of cigarettes smoked by each smoker increased, from about 15 to 20 per day in men and from 7 to about 15 per day in women.

About 30% of smokers begin before the age of 16. About 85% of smokers have started by the age of 20 years.

For detailed statistics about tobacco consumption in the UK see Wald *et al.*, Further Information.

Smoke and smoking

Cigarette smoke has a very complex composition. The most important constituents comprise nicotine (for its pharamacological and addictive effect), tar (the carcinogenic fraction) and carbon monoxide (believed to be the atherogenic fraction). Tar itself is a very complex substance. There are numerous other products with harmful potential. The composition of smoke is assessed experimentally by analysis of the smoke from smoking machines. However, the nature of the smoke and the pattern of its deposition in the respiratory tract are importantly affected by the manner of smoking; the relevant variables are complex. One important finding is that when individuals change from a high strength cigarette to a lower strength, the pattern of smoking changes so as to tend to maintain the same level of nicotine intake.

Effects of nicotine

Nicotine, in the doses achieved in smoking, produces stimulant effects. Large doses produce depressant effects. The effects may differ between individuals and between different circumstances in the same individual. Animals have been found to self-administer nicotine in experimental circumstances and to make effort to maintain access if this is denied.

Nicotine is clearly addictive, but common experience shows that there is little to observe in the way of physical effects after abrupt withdrawal. Opinion varies on the length of the withdrawal symptoms after cessation. The decay is probably rapid—a matter of a few days. Smoking is pleasurable to smokers; the idea of an unconquerable physical addiction may be attractive to the smoker, who wishes to continue, but to be absolved from criticism on this count.

Risk to lungs

These are dealt with in sections on lung cancer and COPD. Smokers show higher than expected death rates in other categories of respiratory illness. Deaths from influenza and pneumonia are twice as common as in non-smokers; deaths from non-specified respiratory diseases, other than those already mentioned, are about five times as common in smokers.

Passive smoking and respiratory health

Measurement of smoking exposure by non-smokers is difficult, but measurable levels of smoking constituents are found in blood, urine and saliva of non-smokers in particularly heavily contaminated environments—theoretical extrapolations can be made to lesser exposure. The most common effects are short-term trivial reductions in pulmonary performance and sensations of irritation. There is a strong association between respiratory symptoms, such as cough, in children and parental smoking. Small and probably significant increases in incidence of lung cancer and of reduction in ventilatory performance have been found in non-smoking spouses of smokers.

Stopping smoking

The experience of attempts to stop smokers from smoking is disappointing. The reasons for failure are probably multiple and extend beyond simple pharmacological addiction. Despite government restrictions, the expenditure on advertising by cigarette manufacturers continues to be vast and continues to be projected in environments where sport and youth are in evidence. Price increases have been shown to be followed by reductions in smoking prevalence.

Validation of stopping smoking

Claims by previous smokers that they have stopped smoking have been shown to be completely unreliable. In many studies, only 10–20% of those claiming to have given up smoking are actually found to be telling the truth, as assessed by reliable biochemical means.

Smokers can be identified by obvious clues such as smell and finger-staining and by self-admission. Chemical tests include the following:

1   *Exhaled carbon monoxide concentration.* Greater than 8 ppm of CO is indicative of smoking. Levels in smokers are generally twice this.
2   *Blood carboxyhaemoglobin level* is less convenient. Exhaled CO level relates closely to it. The half-life of CO in the blood is about 4 hours.
3   *Cotinine levels.* Cotinine is a metabolite of nicotine and has a long half-life of about 20 hours. It can be measured in the urine or saliva.
4   *Thiocyanate level.* Salivary and urinary thiocyanate levels can be used to identify current smokers.

Results of attempts to stop smoking

Of those who cease smoking at the start of a campaign, or in response to advice, only about 10–20% are non-smokers at 6 months. The highest successes in smoking cessation are seen in sufferers from myocardial infarction. The initial intense period of care in hospital usually breaks smoking for at least a week, and powerful advice about risk to life is generally given. About 50% of smokers who are hospitalized with myocardial infarction stop smoking long term. In general, firm advice by a doctor to stop smoking has been shown to have a long-term validated success rate of about 5%. It seems clear that motivation by the individual is the key element determining success.

Nicotine replacement

The use of nicotine chewing gum is controversial. Some studies have found a small increase in the already small proportion of successful abstainers, but other studies, even of patients selected because of respiratory disease, have shown no effect. Nicotine craving may not be met by the gum (which achieves only slow delivery compared with the cigarette) and, where it is met, withdrawal must still be faced when the gum is stopped. Furthermore, the use of a prop may reinforce the idea that stopping smoking is dependent on factors other than personal determination. Patients should not lose sight of the fact that many people stop smoking successfully, and that a high proportion notice no effects from stopping. Well-meaning attempts to promote smoking cessation by anti-smoking groups, smoking clinics, Health Education bodies and some elements of the media may have the opposite effect by reinforcing rather than minimizing the idea that stopping smoking is complex, difficult and dependent upon factors outside the smoker's personal responsibility.

Prevention

Stopping starting

Due to the poor performance of attempts to stop smokers from smoking, and the early age at which the habit is started, attempts to accelerate the disappearance of the smoking habit are likely to exert most effect if concentrated on stopping teen-agers from smoking. Smoking prevalence in this group is lowest in Western countries with the most severe restrictions on advertising and sales, and the most severe taxes on smoking. It appears that young people are not greatly influenced by fear of fatal or disabling disease caused by smoking.

Developing countries

Of great concern is the rapid and largely unopposed increase in prevalence of smoking in developing countries. In these countries, large sums of money are put into advertising by international tobacco companies, which directly target young persons taking up the habit. Smoking is actively promoted as a characteristic of life in a modernized society. There is already evidence of increasing mortality from lung cancer and chronic obstructive lung disease in countries where smoking has increased markedly in the last 20 years. The pattern of an enormous epidemic of mortality and illness from smoking, seen in the past century in the Western world, may be repeated in the next century in the currently developing world. Complex economic issues underlie tobacco production (much of it in poor parts of the world) and tobacco taxation, which tend to maintain the industry. (See Nath, Further Information.)

Chapter 21
Chronic Obstructive Pulmonary Disease

Definitions

Chronic bronchitis: *Chronic cough with production of sputum on most days, for at least 3 months in the year, for at least 2 years.*

The term refers simply to the symptoms of cough and sputum (generally excluding that due to some localized lesion in the lungs). It is an indicator of mucus hypersecretion. Simple chronic bronchitis is not accompanied by shortness of breath.

Airways obstruction: *Diffuse airways narrowing causing increased resistance to airflow.*

The expression denotes a disturbance of physiology; airways obstruction is generally confirmed by physiological tests. Airways obstruction commonly accompanies chronic bronchitis and is generally responsible for the dyspnoea. Airways obstruction in chronic bronchitis is generally due to emphysema. Some individuals (almost always smokers) develop airways obstruction without ever having the symptom of chronic bronchitis or other evidence of mucus hypersecretion.

Emphysema: *Dilatation of the terminal air-spaces of the lungs, distal to the terminal bronchiole, with destruction of their walls.*

The term denotes a pathological lesion, not a clinical syndrome. Dyspnoea which occurs in association with chronic bronchitis is *not* necessarily due to emphysema. It is generally not possible to diagnose the presence of emphysema reliably in life, on clinical grounds alone. Generalized emphysema is always accompanied by evidence of airways obstruction.

Asthma: *A disease characterized by variable dyspnoea due to widespread narrowing of the peripheral airways in the lungs, varying in severity over short periods of time, either spontaneously or as result of treatment.*

As some patients with asthma present with chronic cough productive of sputum and as airways obstruction is a principal feature, it is to be expected that some patients with asthma may unintentionally be included in the group of diseases discussed here (see p. 216).

Response to bronchodilator is a poor discriminator. Response to corticosteroid, where this is clear-cut, is a generally accepted indication of the presence of asthma. Whatever criteria are used, there is inevitable overlap and patients may have both conditions.

Chronic obstructive pulmonary disease (COPD)

This term, and others rather like it, have grown into common use as a means of indicating the common clinical situation in which all of the above phenomena may be inextricably mixed. The term is convenient, but lacks precision and fosters the misconception that there is a single uniform disease entity in which all elements are necessarily present. Where it appears in this chapter, it should be taken to mean airways obstruction, probably due to emphysema, with or without the symptom of chronic bronchitis and which is not believed to be due to asthma.

Prevalence

1   In the UK, chronic bronchitis, as defined, occurs in about 15% of men and 5% of women. The ratio of males to females increases with age.

2   A huge amount of loss of work is attributable to chronic bronchitis and COPD (about 30 million working days each year).

3   The prevalence is higher in the UK than in other countries.

Mortality

1   In the UK about 30 000 persons die from COPD each year.

2   Mortality rises steeply with age but about a quarter of the deaths occur before retirement age.

3   The mortality from COPD is higher than in other countries.

Aetiology

It is not possible to identify a single cause of chronic bronchitis and COPD, but a number of factors are known to be involved.

Cigarette smoking

Cigarette smoking is overwhelmingly the most important factor in the genesis of chronic bronchitis and COPD.

Symptoms

Symptoms of simple bronchitis in the general population are:

1   common in smokers;

2   related to the number of cigarettes smoked per day;

3   exceptional in non-smokers.

Simple ventilatory tests

Smokers, as a group, have lower performance than non-smokers of comparable age, the severity of the impairment being proportional to the number of cigarettes smoked per day. Affected smokers show a more rapid decline in FEV_1 with age than normals. Some smokers remain unaffected.

Morbidity

Work-loss and hospital admissions are much more frequent in smokers and related to the number of cigarettes smoked per day.

Mortality

The mortality from COPD is much higher amongst smokers. The risk of death from COPD in a man smoking 15 cigarettes daily is 12 times that of a non-smoker. In a man smoking 30 cigarettes daily the risk is 20 times that of a non-smoker.

Atmospheric pollution

Long term

The effects of atmospheric pollution could easily be observed in studies carried out before the 1970s. A radical improvement in urban atmospheric pollution has taken place over the last 30 years, and now only the older adult population has lived for an appreciable period in high levels of pollution. In earlier years, mortality and morbidity were related to smokiness, SO_2 concentrations and degree of urbanization. Now the effect of urbanization in the UK is imperceptible. Chronic bronchitis and COPD is seen in non-smokers in cities in developing countries where there is heavy atmospheric pollution, for example in India and China. Chronic obstructive pulmonary disease is also prevalent in communities in which domestic cooking is done over interior fires—for example in Nepal and New Guinea.

Short term

Famous severe winter fogs associated with very heavy levels of smoke pollution (smog) in the 1950s in London and other major cities. Very high death rates from COPD occurred during and following the smog.

Other factors

In all UK studies, COPD has been found to be strongly inversely related to socio-economic status. In the UK, prevalence and mortality are higher in the North and West than in the South and East, even after allowing for other known factors.

Protease–antiprotease interaction and the development of emphysema

It is now thought likely that emphysema develops as a consequence of destruction of parenchymal lung tissue (particularly elastin) by proteolytic digestion. The demonstration that intratracheal instillation of the proteolytic enzyme papain in rats resulted in the development of emphysema, and the recognition that in humans, genetic deficiency of the principal antiprotease (α_1-antiprotease or α_1-antitrypsin) is associated with severe youthful emphysema, form the twin foundations for this theory.

The source of proteolytic enzyme in the genesis of human emphysema is thought to be the neutrophil. Very small numbers of neutrophils are normally present within alveoli, and in relation to small airways, but much greater numbers are present in smokers. Macrophages may play a part in bringing this about, as macrophages from smokers are more actively chemotactic to neutrophils. The turnover of neutrophils may become such that the released enzyme exceeds the local capacity to neutralize it and, over very long periods of time, emphysema may result. The mechanisms involved are likely to be more complicated than this outline suggests. For example, it is known that protease inhibitors other than α_1-antiprotease exist in the lung.

It seems quite probable that the performance of the inhibitors may be chemically impaired by local oxidant reactions. Macrophages are capable of such reactions as part of their antimicrobial activity and they are, moreover, capable of releasing elastase. Smoke has oxidant effects.

Clinical features and progress of the disease

Simple chronic bronchitis

The progress of simple bronchitis is generally insidious. Cough, which may be present initially only during the first part of the day in winter months, may, over several years, come to last all day throughout the year. Some patients relate the onset of symptoms to a single, severe respiratory tract infection.

Acute exacerbations

Particularly in relation to colds, patients with chronic bronchitis develop increased cough, productive of yellow purulent sputum, with mild symptoms of general malaise. The illness may last a few days or several weeks.

Development of airways obstruction

Symptoms

Not all patients with simple chronic bronchitis develop airways obstruction. Many who have never had chronic bronchitis develop airways obstruction. The cardinal symptom is dyspnoea, which may be accompanied by wheezing, and is generally related to effort. Dyspnoea is commonly noted for the first time after an acute exacerbation. Clinical and spirometric evidence of airways obstruction is common in patients who are quite unaware of any symptoms apart from cough. Airways obstruction is often already severe when medical attention is sought for the first time.

Bronchial hyperreactivity produces symptoms associated with airways obstruction and may help to distinguish dyspnoea due to this cause. The patient complains of sensations of tightness, choking or paroxysms of coughing when confronted by smoke, cold air, fog, car exhaust and other fumes. Symptoms are often related to particular weather conditions.

Signs

Clinical signs associated with the presence of airways obstruction are described at the end of the chapter. It is important to remember that these may be unreliable. In particular, the presence or absence of wheeze is not an indicator of the presence or absence of airways obstruction. It is very easy to overlook the presence of airways obstruction even when it is severe.

Measurement

Proper assessment of any patient with cough and breathlessness requires the use of a spirometer or at least measurement of peak expiratory flow, preferably as part of the examination. Although there is, in general, a relationship between severity of airways obstructions, as judged by the FEV_1 or peak expiratory flow on the one hand, and the severity of symptoms and disability on the other, there is wide individual variation. In adult males of normal stature, symptoms of exercise dyspnoea are not usually remarked upon when the FEV_1 is above 2 litres; disability is not usually critically severe above 1 litre. Some individuals are uncomplaining with an FEV_1 of under 1 litre. Most patients with an FEV_1 of 0.5 litre are very severely disabled indeed.

Progress of disability

There is generally a very gradual progression of disability extending over 10–40 years. It may become apparent through increasing absence from work, gradual limitation of exercise tolerance and a reduced range of activities. The prognosis is related to severity of exercise limitation; 40% of patients who are required to walk at a reduced pace on flat ground die within 5 years.

With time, acute exacerbations become more alarming and are accompanied by breathlessness at rest and difficulty in expectoration; admission to hospital may be required during these episodes.

Clinical patterns in severe chronic obstructive lung disease

Two patterns of disturbance may be discerned during the progress of advanced COPD, which differ mainly in the extent to which ventilatory drive is preserved in the face of increasing airways obstruction. The main features are summarized in Figs 21.1 and 21.2. Most patients do not fit either pattern completely, but have some features of both.

Type A ('pink puffer')

In this group, ventilatory drive is well preserved, even in the presence of very severe airways obstruction. Dyspnoea may be intense. Blood gases are maintained in the normal range at rest, until terminally.

Type B ('blue bloater')

Individuals meeting this description have poor respiratory drive and easily drift into respiratory failure, with elevation of P_{CO_2}, hypoxia and heart failure, particularly during infective exacerbations (see Cor pulmonale, p. 255).

In simple terms, 'pink' puffers can be regarded as 'doing their best' to breathe enough to keep the P_{CO_2} down, often in the face of great difficulties, whilst 'blue bloaters' 'give up' at a relatively early stage and settle for poor blood gases, when they could breathe more 'if they tried harder'.

The reasons for the early ventilatory failure of Type B patients are not clear. The prognosis for the group is poor: about 70% die within 5 years. Patients with severe day time hypoxaemia are subject to even more severe nocturnal dips in oxygen saturation during REM sleep. Many deaths occur at night. Long-term near-continuous oxygen therapy may prolong life (see below).

Emphysema

The term emphysema refers to a form of parenchymal lung damage and not to a clinical syndrome. It is difficult to diagnose reliably. Whether or not a patient has emphysema is not clinically very important—the management of the patient will only exceptionally be affected by the diagnosis. As emphysema is untreatable, the diagnosis tends to foster an air of hopelessness in the management. Treatable aspects may be overlooked.

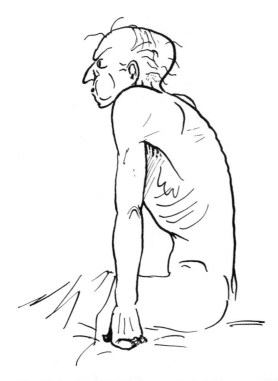

Fig. 21.1. Type A or 'pink puffer'—the picture of good respiratory drive. Individuals in this category tend to have the following features:
1   Intense dyspnoea often with purse-lip breathing.
2   Thin and often elderly.
3   Small sputum volume.
4   Rarely develop oedema or overt heart failure.
Investigations may show:
1   Near-normal blood gas values (until terminally).
2   Very severe airways obstruction.
3   Increased total lung capacity.
4   Radiological evidence of emphysema.
5   Impairment of transfer factor.

Pathological features

Two principal patterns are seen (Fig. 21.3).

1 *Centrilobular or centriacinar emphysema*

Distension and damage affect the respiratory bronchioles; the more distal alveolar ducts and alveoli tend to be well preserved.

2 *Panacinar emphysema*

Distension and destruction appear to involve the whole of the acinus.

Irregular emphysema

This term is used to describe the very common appearance of scarring and damage which affect the parenchyma patchily without particular regard for acinar structure.

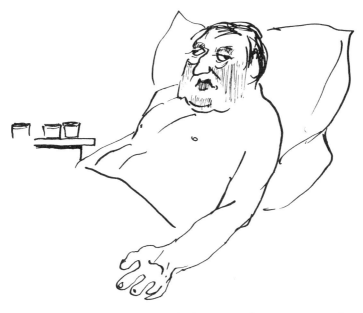

Fig. 21.2. Type B or 'blue bloater'—the picture of poor respiratory drive. Individuals in this category tend to have the following features:
1   Relatively mild dyspnoea.
2   Often obese.
3   Large sputum volume and frequent infective exacerbations.
4   Often oedematous and easily lapse into congestive heart failure.
Investigations may show:
1   Abnormal blood gases—hypercapnia, hypoxaemia with elevated plasma bicarbonate and polycythaemia, severe nocturnal hypoxaemia during REM sleep.
2   Sometimes only moderately severe airways obstruction.
3   Fairly normal total lung capacity.
4   No radiological evidence of emphysema.
5   Little or no reduction in transfer factor.

Clinico-pathological relationships

Centrilobular emphysema of modest extent is very common and not necessarily associated with disability. More severe degrees are associated with prominent bronchitic symptoms, disturbance of ventilation/perfusion relationships and hypoxia. This may be due to the relatively well-preserved blood supply to the badly-ventilated alveoli beyond the damaged zone.

Severe panacinar emphysema is less common. The elastic network of the normal lung is badly disorganized, the lung becomes floppy leading to a severe degree of airways obstruction, particularly during expiration. Changes in the blood gases tend to be less drastic, perhaps because the blood supply in damaged areas is reduced in proportion to the reduced ventilation to these areas. Ventilatory drive is generally better preserved than in cases with severe centrilobular emphysema. It is tempting to associate the 'pink puffer' with panacinar emphysema and the 'blue bloater' with centrilobular emphysema; available evidence suggests that this is an oversimplification but that some sort of loose relationship may exist.

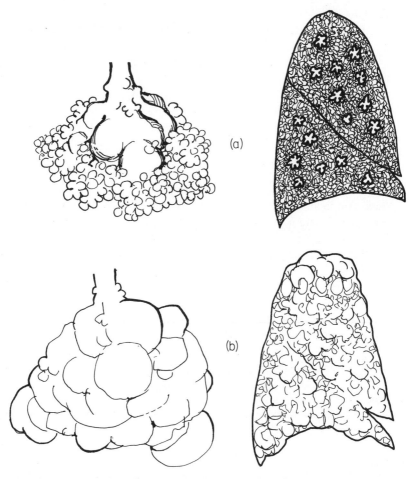

Fig. 21.3. Emphysema. Diagrammatic view of lobule and whole lung section in (a) centrilobular and (b) panacinar emphysema.

Which patients have emphysema?

Centrilobular emphysema

There are no helpful clinical or radiological features which allow the diagnosis of centrilobular emphysema although there are clinical situations in which its presence may be suspected.

Panacinar emphysema

Clinical

Most of the physical signs formerly thought to indicate emphysema are merely those of overinflation which may accompany airways obstruction of any sort. Emphysema may be suspected when the features of Type A are encountered (Fig. 21.1).

Radiological
The following features are strongly suggestive of severe panacinar emphysema:
1 Bullae evident on chest X-ray.
2 Deficiency of blood vessel markings in the peripheral half of the lung fields, in most areas seen on PA chest X-ray, compared with relatively easily seen more proximal vessels.

These features will often be accompanied by evidence of severe overinflation—low flattened diaphragms on the PA field and a large retrosternal air-space on the lateral film.

Note
1 When interpreting a reported radiological diagnosis of emphysema, it is important to know the criteria used by the radiologist. Many radiologists equate the signs of mere overinflation with the presence of emphysema; such signs can be completely reversible if the patient has asthma.
2 Radiological diagnosis of panacinar emphysema is only possible when the disease is advanced.
3 Widespread emphysema of any type may be present despite a normal chest X-ray.

Computerized tomography can be used to detect the presence of emphysema, but this is not a regular clinical indication.

Complications of emphysema

Pneumothorax
This can be particularly troublesome—protracted tube drainage or surgery are often required.

Giant bulla
Occasionally large bullae develop, which interfere with the ventilation of the remainder of the lung. Surgical removal is sometimes undertaken, with improvement in ventilator performance. Improvement is often slight and short-lived. Further large bullae may develop.

Weight loss
Some patients with extremely severe airways obstruction develop progressive weight loss which has no other obvious cause.

Management of chronic obstructive lung disease

Stopping smoking
Patients should always be urged to stop smoking, even when they insist that it helps them to produce sputum. Symptoms of simple chronic bronchitis may disappear, but there is often no change in the symptoms in the case of more advanced disease. Smokers with impaired ventilatory performance show more rapid deterioration in performance with age than normals. On stopping smoking, the rate of deterioration with age tends to return to approximately the rate experienced by

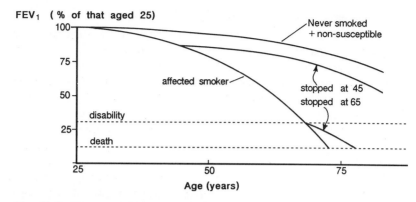

Fig. 21.4. Change in FEV_1 with age: effect of smoking and stopping smoking. Result of a long-term follow-up study of workers in London (Fletcher C. & Peto R. The natural history of chronic airflow obstruction. *Br Med J* 1977;**1**:1645). An important image for doctors (and smoking patients).

Several points are illustrated: (1) non-smokers show a small progressive decline in function with age; (2) by the time disability is noted, ventilatory function is seriously reduced to about one-third of predicted normal values; (3) many smokers are unaffected by smoking and show the same decline as non-smokers; (4) some smokers are affected and show a steeper decline; (5) those affected by smoking can be detected by measurement of FEV_1 many years before they become disabled, because they will already tend to show impairment; (6) stopping smoking is not accompanied by recovery although deterioration slows to about the rate shown by non-smokers of the same age; (7) stopping smoking carries more benefit if it occurs before the development of disability; (8) continued smoking by affected smokers is associated with continued accelerated decline in function.

normals (Fig. 21.4). Important improvement in performance is unusual, however, and patients should not be led to expect it, or ensuing disappointment may be followed by resumption of smoking.

Detection of unsuspected asthma

A proportion of patients diagnosed as having chronic bronchitis and airways obstruction may show dramatic improvement in respiratory symptoms when treated with corticosteroids—suggesting an unrecognized 'asthmatic' component. It is extremely important that such individuals should not be overlooked.

Trial of steroids

Prednisolone 20 mg daily for a fortnight is sufficient to determine whether or not there is responsive disease. Prednisolone in this dose for such a short duration is virtually devoid of harmful effects and minimal fuss should accompany the prescribing of the drugs; if there is no response then it may be stopped abruptly. A trial of steroid therapy should be carried out at a time when the patient is stable, rather than during recovery from an infective exacerbation.

Assessment

Sometimes the response to steroid treatment is dramatic and obvious and there is improvement in symptoms and simple ventilatory test (FEV_1 and PEF).

Sometimes the tests show no change, but enquiry reveals that exercise tolerance, nocturnal attacks and morning symptoms are improved. It is useful to give the patient a peak flow meter to record twice daily, morning and evening, PEF values before, during and after the trial period. Acute bronchial infection with purulent sputum may inhibit response to steroids. Where there is doubt it may be worth repeating the trial after an interval of a few weeks.

Who requires trial of steroids?

It can be argued that all patients who have chronic airways obstruction severe enough to interfere with their daily activities merit a therapeutic trial. It may be more practical to limit such a trial to those most likely to respond. Some obvious features which may suggest asthma are: onset in childhood, substantial periods of normality, a family or personal history of allergies (urticaria, eczema, asthma, nasal obstruction or operations for nasal polyposis), a family history of anything suggestive of airways obstruction. Some less obvious attributes of those who may respond are:

1 *Relatively short duration of dyspnoea.* Individuals dsypnoeic for 5 years are more likely to respond that those dyspnoeic for 25 years (except those with very early onset).

2 *Severe morning symptoms.* The more severe symptoms of tightness and breathlessness in the morning, relative to the remainder of the day, the more likely is a response to steroids. Equally significant is the tendency for these symptoms to persist for a perceptible period (usually stereotyped, well recognized by the patient and sometimes up to several hours)—longer than just 'the time it takes to get the phlegm up'.

3 *Presence of eosinophilia in blood or sputum.*

4 *Nocturnal cough and breathlessness.*

5 *Tendency to be worse in summer.* But a tendency to be worse in winter is of little help in forecasting responsiveness.

Pulmonary function tests

These are of little help in forecasting responsiveness to steriods in this group; huge responses to bronchodilator inhalation are only seen in asthma, but lesser degrees of 'reversibility' do not discriminate (see p. 160).

Antibiotic and chemotherapy

When?

1 All patients with chronic bronchitis should receive treatment with a broad spectrum antibiotic during infective exacerbations: that is, when the sputum is persistently purulent (yellowish or green) and increased in quantity above the usual. Antibiotic treatment shortens exacerbations and may prevent lung damage.

2 Treatment should be started promptly. It may be helpful for some patients to have a small stock of antibiotic at home so that there need be no delay in starting treatment.

3 There is no need to culture the sputum in an infective exacerbation unless the patient is gravely ill or the response to treatment is unsatisfactory. If the sputum

becomes purulent, it is generally safe to assume that the responsible organisms are the pneumococcus and *Haemophilus influenzae*.

4   If the sputum is mucoid in appearance, there is usually no need to prescribe an antibiotic, whatever the bacteriological results.

Which antibiotic?

Ampicillin, or one of its derivatives, is most widely used. Amoxycillin converts to ampicillin after efficient absorption and yields higher levels. Augmentin is a mixture of amoxycillin and clavulanic acid, which inactivates the β-lactamase produced by some strains of *H. influenzae*. A usual form of treatment in an ambulant patient who is not seriously ill might be amoxycillin 250 mg three times daily, but higher doses of double or four times this may be used in severe infections and disabled patients. High doses are only maintained for 1 or 2 days, as they are bactericidal for the organisms concerned. Sometimes *H. influenzae* is eradicated from the sputum for weeks after intensive treatment. Co-trimoxazole or tetracycline are well-tried alternatives. If the patient is prostrate, the possibility of staphylococcal pneumonia arises and flucloxacillin should be added.

Duration of treatment

Antibiotic treatment should be continued until the sputum is again mucoid and for not less than 5 days. There is little evidence that long-term treatment with antibiotics is helpful.

Bronchodilator treatment

Oral bronchodilator preparations (e.g. theophyllines) may bring about modest improvement in symptoms and are worthy of careful trial. Even slight amelioration of airways obstruction may be helpful in a disabled patient. There is no need for patients to take regular oral bronchodilators unless they can demonstrate benefit to their own satisfaction.

Aerosol bronchodilators usually produce more effective bronchodilatation. The response is much less marked than that obtained in asthma, but improvement in FEV_1 of 20% or so can commonly be obtained if higher than standard doses are used (for example, 600 µg or six puffs of salbutamol, instead of two). Regular ipratropium by inhalation is sometimes found to be helpful, either alone, or in addition to a β$_2$-agonist.

Mucolytics and expectorants

These agents play no significant part in the management of chronic bronchitis.

Management of more severely disabled patients

In this group, in addition to measures already mentioned, the treatment of heart failure and the encouragement of radical weight loss in the obese become important. Patients should be encouraged to be active and to regularly undertake such exercise as they are capable of. They may need to be reassured that 'overdoing it' is more of a theoretical risk than a real one and that it is not necessary to remain indoors 'to avoid catching a cold' during winter months. Practical measures such as provision of ground floor, single level accommodation (or a chair lift), central heating, regular visits by a home help and (in the very limited individual) a mobility allowance to allow regular use of a taxi may all make a difference to the quality of life.

Immunization of disabled patients against expected epidemic strains of influenza A virus is usually recommended.

Domiciliary oxygen therapy (see Chapter 31) may become relevant. Patients who have chronic hypoxia and severe airways obstruction and who have been proved to have stopped smoking may be candidates for long-term near-continuous oxygen therapy, which is most conveniently administered using an oxygen concentrator. This may improve well-being and survival.

Management of severely-ill patients requiring admission to hospital

Management comprises:

1 Antibiotic therapy.
2 Bronchodilator therapy.
3 Encouragement to expectorate.
4 Supervision of respiratory failure.

Parenteral antibiotic therapy may be necessary in desperately ill patients.

Intravenous bronchodilator therapy will be necessary in most instances. Aminophylline is effective and has stood the test of time. It may be given by continuous infusion, or slow intravenous injection over a few minutes. It causes respiratory stimulation, cardiac acceleration and, frequently, coughing and vomiting. It is desirable to follow intravenous aminophylline with vigorous encouragement to cough. Terbutaline or salbutamol may be given, subcutaneously or intravenously, as an alternative to aminophylline.

The majority of patients admitted to hospital with a severe exacerbation of chronic bronchitis accompanied by airways obstruction will recover in response to the above measures.

It may be difficult to decide whether or not the patient suffers from chronic asthma. Where there is doubt in a severely ill individual, it is reasonable to start intravenous or oral steroid therapy. The relevance of steroid therapy can be critically reviewed during the convalescent phase.

Basic investigations

1 *Chest X-ray.* Obvious pneumonia will affect antibiotic policy. There may be evidence of pneumothorax, pleural effusion, malignant disease, etc., all of which may affect management from a quite early stage.
2 *Arterial blood gas analysis.* (See below.)
3 *Blood urea and serum electrolytes.* Elevation of blood urea will suggest dehydration (common) or renal failure related to severe cardiac failure. Elevation of plasma bicarbonate level will suggest well-established chronic ventilatory failure.
4 *Sputum culture.* This is particularly relevant when the patient is collapsed or pyrexial, or has already failed to respond to adequate antibiotic therapy.
5 *Detailed documentation of disability.* Particular care should be taken to obtain details of the extent and duration of the patient's respiratory disability (and his tolerance of it) by interrogating close relatives at the time of admission. The extent

to which the patient has been exposed to various forms of treatment should also be noted. If the patient deteriorates, a decision on whether or not artificial ventilation should be undertaken cannot be made without this information.

Management of respiratory failure

Respiratory failure is generally regarded as being present when the arterial oxygen tension is low (in round figures below 9 kPa or below 70 mmHg) and the arterial carbon dioxide tension is high (above 6.3 kPa or 47 mmHg). In exacerbations of chronic airways obstruction accompanying chronic bronchitis, some degree of respiratory failure is common. Arterial P_{CO_2} is elevated because of reduced alveolar ventilation and arterial P_{CO_2} is reduced, partly as a direct consequence of the reduced alveolar ventilation and partly because of regional underventilation (ventilation/perfusion imbalance, see Fig. 2.7(c) and consider Fig. 2.10). Hypoxia is potentially lethal; hypercapnia is intoxicating but not immediately lethal.

The problem of oxygen therapy

Oxygen should not be given to patients in presumed respiratory failure without a good deal of careful thought; most patients do not need it.

Patients with established respiratory failure, who have had a raised P_{CO_2} for some days, become unresponsive to the CO_2 stimulus to ventilation and rely increasingly on hypoxia to maintain the drive to breathe. If they are given oxygen to breathe, they breathe less; if they are given high concentrations of oxygen, they breathe very much less. This underbreathing results in increasing hypercapnia, which intoxicates and ultimately acts as a respiratory depressant. Oxygen should therefore logically be reserved for those patients with *severe hypoxia*. Unfortunately, patients with severe hypoxia are generally those with a high P_{CO_2} and CO_2 insensitivity so that:

1   patients who really need oxygen often cannot tolerate it;
and conversely,
2   patients who tolerate oxygen often do not really need it.

Who has severe hypoxia?

This may be difficult to decide. The severity of hypoxia depends largely upon:

Arterial oxygen content.
Cardiac output.
Distribution of the cardiac output (Fig. 31.1).

The following points are worth making.
1   Patients in respiratory failure with cor pulmonale generally tolerate arterial hypoxaemia quite well since the cardiac output is usually normal.
2   Cyanosis is *not* an indication of oxygen therapy.
3   Severe hypoxia can be assumed to be present if the P_{O_2} is less than 5.5 kPa (about 40 mmHg).
4   There is some evidence that profuse sweating, moaning and grunting may denote severe hypoxia.

Controlled oxygen therapy

If oxygen is required, it is required *continuously*. Intermittent oxygen is illogical and can be more dangerous than either continuous oxygen or no oxygen. The aim is to increase the Po_2 slightly, accepting that this may mean a slight rise in Pco_2 if there is underventilation. If a free flow of oxygen is used, then underventilation will be extreme before the hypoxic drive reappears.

One approach is to use a venturi type of mask and to deliver just 24% or perhaps 28% oxygen (see Chapter 31). This is fine whilst the mask is in place, but inevitably it is displaced or taken off to talk or eat. The advantage of using nasal cannulae is that they reliably stay in place. Initially, a low flow of 1 litre min^{-1} is appropriate and this can be adjusted according to blood gas measurement. Saturation measurements, using a finger or ear probe, are very useful in confirming that adequate oxygenation is being obtained. A saturation of at least 85% should be achieved (a Pao_2 of approximately 6.7 kPa (50 mmHg) if pH is near normal). If the clinical state suggests that the patient is wakeful and co-operative, the Pco_2 is unlikely to be rising far. If there is doubt, then arterial blood gas measurement is needed.

The likely response to oxygen therapy can be judged from:

1   *The level of Pco_2 before oxygen starts.* Above 9 kPa (or about 70 mmHg) underventilation will be a problem.

2   *The appearance of the patient.* Patients who appear to have a strong drive to breathe, probably have (Fig. 21.1). Underbreathing on oxygen can be evident within minutes or after hours; more commonly, it is revealed overnight. It can be combated by respiratory stimulation.

Respiratory stimulation

Doxapram is an effective, short-acting respiratory stimulant, given by continuous intravenous infusion; it can often control the underventilation induced by oxygen. It is useful in controlling the initial unstable state. It should not be required for more than a day or two, at the most.

Respiratory stimulation can be achieved by encouragement to cough and breathe by staff, relatives and friends. The patients will generally breathe more effectively sitting up in bed or seated in a chair, rather than lying recumbent—particularly if obese.

Signs of heart failure usually subside spontaneously once respiratory failure and, in particular, hypoxia are treated. Severe oedema and ascites are helped by a diuretic such as frusemide. There is evidence that frusemide exerts a respiratory stimulant effect in established respiratory failure.

Avoidance of selatives

Patients in severe respiratory failure with hypercapnia are frequently confused and very noisy. The temptation to use sedative drugs must be resisted. There is no sedative which does not aggravate hypoventilation.

Arrested improvement

Occasionally patients relapse after an initial period of improvement and they are found to have reached a state of equilibrium with a Pco_2 of about 10.5 kPa (80 mmHg or so). They are seen to be asleep much of the day, perhaps having intermittent oxygen and apparently remaining too ill to be got out of bed. In addition to reintroducing treatment with aminophylline or doxapram the following measures may prove helpful:

1   Administration of frusemide 80 mg twice daily.
2   Complete withdrawal of oxygen.
3   Venesection if the packed cell volume (PCV) is in excess of 53%.
4   Sitting the patient out of bed.
5   Administration of the carbonic anhydrase inhibitor dichlorphenamide 50 mg three times daily.

A proportion of patients will remain in chronic respiratory failure after recovery with a persistent elevation of P_{CO_2}. The patient will usually be able to say when he is back to his usual state or better and this end-point should be heeded.

Artificial ventilation

The use of intermittent positive pressure ventilation (IPPV) should be considered when measures described so far fail to prevent deterioration and:

1   it proves impossible to secure adequate oxygenation;
2   the patient is unable to cough up secretions through stupor or exhaustion.

Before embarking upon IPPV, it is usual to review the patient's previous condition. If he or she had been totally immobilized and is in misery, despite adequate trial of available treatments, it may not be kind to restore him or her temporarily to this existence. Once the decision has been taken to embark on IPPV, oxygen can be given continuously and endotracheal intubation carried out without undue delay by the most skilled person available. During IPPV, the patient is sedated and rested and maintained on oxygen sufficient to keep the arterial P_{O_2} at about 60 mmHg. Secretions are removed by endobronchial suction. Vigorous mechanical ventilation is avoided, because rapid lowering of the P_{CO_2} may lead to circulatory collapse. Large volumes of intravenous fluid and dextran are sometimes required at this stage to maintain adequate circulatory filling, as judged by central venous pressure measurement. Usually at least 24 hours of IPPV is necessary. Attempts to withdraw ventilatory assistance are made on each following morning. Occasionally tracheostomy is necessary, where recovery is slow and intermittent ventilatory assistance and tracheal suction continue to be required.

Domiciliary oxygen therapy

Patients who have undergone a severe life-threatening exacerbation of chronic ventilatory failure may be suitable for long-term near-continuous oxygen therapy.

Chapter 22
Ventilatory Failure and Sleep Apnoea

Respiratory failure—definitions

Respiratory failure is a convenient shorthand term, used to describe failure of the respiratory system, as a whole, to maintain arterial blood gases within certain limits. Conventionally the limits are:

Pa_{O_2} above 8.0 kPa (60 mmHg)
Pa_{CO_2} below 6.7 kPa (50 mmHg)

Types of respiratory failure

Type 1 respiratory failure = failure to maintain Pa_{O_2} only.
Type 2 respiratory failure = failure to maintain Pa_{O_2} and Pa_{CO_2}.

Type 1 respiratory failure

The Type 1 pattern can be produced by breathing a mixture of gases with reduced oxygen content—for example at high altitude, or accidentally during anaesthesia. Apart from these circumstances, hypoxaemia in the absence of hypercapnia is indicative of severe disturbance of ventilation/perfusion (V/Q) relationships in the lungs. In its most extreme form, there is effective partial bypassing of the lungs, as in congenital heart disease or where there are large arteriovenous malformations which shunt blood past the lung. Usually, the hypoxia results from a patchy V/Q mismatch, with parts of the lung suffering from underventilation where blood is poorly exposed to air and there is an overall shunt effect. Other parts of the lung compensate for CO_2 elimination by being relatively overventilated. This overventilation is, however, unable to compensate for hypoxaemia, because blood from the overventilated areas cannot carry extra oxygen once it is saturated (this is explained in Chapter 2). Conditions in which Type 1 respiratory failure is seen include: pulmonary oedema, bronchial asthma, pulmonary embolism, pneumonia, lung fibrosis, septicaemic shock and low cardiac output states.

Type 2 respiratory failure

The combination of reduced arterial oxygen tension and increased P_{CO_2} is indicative of alveolar hypoventilation. For example, during a breath-hold, Pa_{O_2} is progressively reduced and Pa_{CO_2} increased in the alveoli. Examples of Type 2 respiratory failure are given below under the heading of alveolar hypoventilation. The terms ventilatory failure and alveolar hypoventilation are used synonymously here.

The extent of the hypoxaemia relative to the hypercapnia during alveolar hypoventilation is largely determined by the respiratory quotient. Very approximately the relationship is as follows:

$PA_{O_2} = PI_{O_2} - Pa_{CO_2}/R$

where PA_{O_2} is alveolar P_{O_2}, PI_{O_2} is the P_{O_2} of the humidified inspired air and R is the respiratory quotient (O_2 uptake divided by CO_2 production). In normal lungs, Pa_{O_2} should be close to PA_{O_2} (i.e. the alveolar–arterial oxygen difference should be small—not more than about 2 kPa). If hypoxaemia is more severe than can be explained by this, then a degree of abnormal V/Q mismatch must be present in addition to alveolar hypoventilation. The combination is common in clinical medicine.

Primary alveolar hypoventilation

Primary failure of central respiratory drive is a great rarity. It may be present at birth, presenting in the first few days with cyanotic episodes, especially during sleep. Treatment is difficult and mortality high.

Adult patients may occasionally be suspected of primary failure, but nearly always this is found, on close investigation, to be due to central nervous system disease, neuromuscular disorder or unrecognized chronic lung disease.

Secondary alveolar hypoventilation

Alveolar hypoventilation can occur from disorder anywhere along the chain of processes that connect the central drive to breathe with the eventual movement of air at the mouth and nose. Depending on the process involved, its speed of onset and severity, the resulting ventilatory failure can take the form of acute asphyxia or of chronic ventilatory failure with slow evolution of cor pulmonale—or of an intermediate form.

Some examples of disorders causing ventilatory failure are show in Fig. 22.1.

Respiratory failure due to lung disease such as COPD and fibrosing alveolitis is dealt with in the relevant chapters.

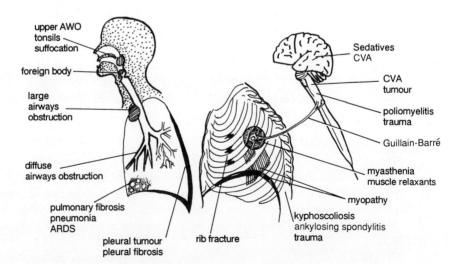

Fig. 22.1. Ventilatory failure (Type 2 respiration failure). Examples of processes which can lead to ventilatory failure (especially when they occur in combination)—extending (from right to left) from central nervous system to the upper airway. CVA, cerebrovascular accident; ARDS, adult respiratory distress syndrome.

Muscle and chest wall disorders

Progressive alveolar ventilation can occur in conditions affecting the strength of the respiratory muscles. This can lead to daytime somnolence, impaired sleep, oedema, headache, abdominal distension and all of the features of cor pulmonale seen in advanced COPD.

The same effect can be produced by severe chest wall deformity. The two forms most commonly responsible are: firstly, severe **kyphoscoliosis** and secondly, the consequences of **thoracoplasty**—an obsolete operation for tuberculosis carried out up to about 35 years ago, in which several upper ribs are removed and the underlying pleural cavity collapsed, sometimes with upper lobectomy. Decades later, patients present with features of chronic ventilatory failure.

Effect of associated airways obstruction
The normal compensation for the development of airways obstruction is to breath at a higher lung volume—a very effective means of bringing relief and reducing the effects. Patients with muscular weakness or chest wall deformity are unable to compensate in this way. If they develop airways obstruction associated with asthma or COPD, the labour or breathing is enormously greater and they may fail to breathe enough. During a respiratory infection, when airways obstruction worsens, patients with muscle and chest wall disorders may deteriorate very rapidly and even become unconscious with respiratory failure, with little warning.

Patients with chronic ventilatory failure due to muscle and chest wall disorders show severe underventilation and hypoxia at night. It has been found that if artificial ventilation is used at night to sustain ventilation, many patients can maintain adequate ventilation during the day, and the features of respiratory failure can be abolished. It is not clear whether this effect is due to resting the exhausted respiratory muscles during the night, or to resetting of the respiratory thermostat (e.g. by fall in plasma bicarbonate, so that a higher level of ventilation is required to achieve control of pH).

Domiciliary assisted nocturnal ventilation

So far this has only been introduced on a relatively small scale and most patients are from the group with neuromuscular or chest wall disorders.

Intermittent positive pressure ventilation by tracheal intubation
Intermittent positive pressure ventilation (IPPV) by cuffed tracheostomy tube is very occasionally undertaken at home, in severely disabled individuals. Generally, these patients have special problems, or require continuous ventilation and are not considered further here.

Negative pressure ventilation by cuirasse
In this method, the chest is covered by a firm shell and a plastic sheet. A large mechanical pump intermittently generates a negative pressure in the shell, or cuirasse, drawing air into the patient's chest. This method was first used decades ago, but fell into disuse until recently. Now it is being overtaken by nasal ventilation (see below). The cuirasse method is related to another negative pressure method—the iron lung or tank ventilator. This is a chamber in which the patient

lies with the head protruding through an air tight seal. Iron lungs were in wide-spread use 40 years ago during poliomyelitis epidemics.

Nasal positive pressure ventilation

This is a relatively new and expensive technique, in which a simple ventilator delivers positive pressure breaths to the patient, who wears a well-fitting nasal mask.

Sleep apnoea syndromes

Definition

This is conventionally defined as episodes of complete cessation of airflow for at least 10 seconds, with at least 40 episodes in a night of 7 hours sleep.

Normal breathing in sleep

Some people have markedly periodic breathing during sleep, with brief apnoeas. Severe hypoxia and arousal do not occur. In patients with severe COPD, more exaggerated intermittent underventilation of this sort occurs and is accompanied by much more severe hypoxia. This is not considered further here. Normal sleep is characterized by regular deep breathing during periods of rapid eye movement (REM) sleep. Snoring is a common and, arguably, normal phenomenon (see below) which does not normally cause impaired sleep quality, or arousal (at least for the snorer).

There are two principal types of sleep apnoea—central and obstructive.

Central sleep apnoea

This is much less common than obstructive sleep apnoea. Here there is failure of respiratory drive, intermittently, at night. It seems to be related to the normal intermittency of breathing, but exaggerated to the point where apnoeas are sufficiently long to induce hypoxia, arousal and poor sleep quality. Sometimes there is evidence of associated central nervous disease such as previous brain stem ischaemia or Parkinson's disease.

Obstructive sleep apnoea (OSA)

Mechanism

During sleep, relaxation of the musculature of the upper airway, particularly the palate and pharynx, allows the airway to fall in and obstruct breathing, particularly when the patient lies supine. Breathing movements continue, but airflow is obstructed. During the apnoea, arterial Po_2 falls and Pco_2 rises. The hypoxia eventually causes brief arousal and the patient moves restlessly and overcomes the obstruction, often with noisy snoring and grunting.

Aggravating factors

The most important factor is usually obesity, followed by alcohol, smoking and narrow upper airway, from congenital or acquired disorders such as tonsillar enlargement or partial nasal obstruction. It is rarely seen before middle age.

Clinical features

The complaints are mainly of daytime sleepiness. This may be severe and there is a serious risk of driving accidents. The sleepiness is partly countered by stimulation and interest. Patients may complain of headache, undue irritability, reduced work performance, depression and impotence. The patient's partner may describe the typical night time disturbances. Examination may reveal features of alcohol intake, obesity, a short neck, micrognathia, or other factors reducing pharyngeal size and, sometimes, associated nasal obstruction.

Investigation

There may be polycythaemia or a raised plasma bicarbonate level. Daytime blood gas measurements may be normal. The diagnosis can be confirmed most simply by the use of a finger oxygen saturation meter with a recording facility. The next most informative investigation is simply to observe sleep. This can be done conveniently by videorecording. Evidence of obstruction can be detected, by the experienced observer, by sight and sound. Full documentation of sleep apnoea may require polysomnography in a specialist sleep laboratory. This comprises: continuous multichannel recording of sleep quality and eye movements using an EEG; airflow at the mouth and nose using thermistors; chest wall and abdominal movement measurement by impedance plethysmography; ECG and oxygen saturation. The paradoxical breathing movements in the absence of airflow confirm obstructive sleep apnoea.

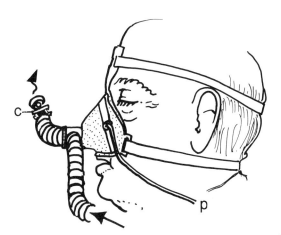

Fig. 22.2. Nasal CPAP. A continuous high flow of air (arrows) is delivered from a pump to a well-fitting nasal mask. The pressure at the nose is variable, by adjusting the escape of air from the open end with a screw clip (c). The pressure in the mask can be checked on a manometer connected to a separate pressure line (p). The effect is to maintain a positive pressure bias within the upper airway, which prevents collapse on inspiration.

Treatment

Mild cases
In mild cases, simple measures may suffice. Weight loss and the avoidance of alcohol are the most important. Other sedatives should be avoided. Partial nasal obstruction should be treated. Patients can sometimes be persuaded to avoid sleeping on the back. Some benefit has been shown in sleep apnoeas of both types with the use of protryptyline.

Nasal CPAP
Collapse of the upper airway can be prevented by applying a continuous positive airways pressure (CPAP) to the nose by means of a high flow air-pump and a special close-fitting and comfortable mask (Fig. 22.2). This treatment requires expert assessment and application. It is effective in relieving distressing symptoms and, once patients realize this, it is surprisingly well accepted.

Surgery
Obstruction of the pharynx may be successfully discouraged by surgical trimming of the soft palate, uvula and pharyngeal walls (uvulopalatopharyngoplasty). Treatment failure is, however, common and the procedure can cause distressing incompetence of the nasopharyngeal sphincter, with effects on speech and swallowing.

Chapter 23
Carcinoma of the Bronchus

Incidence

About 35 000 people die from carcinoma of the bronchus in England and Wales each year. Half of these deaths occur before the age of 65. The incidence has increased about tenfold from the beginning of the century, the increase being attributable to the increase in smoking. It is now about three times more common in men than women. The overall incidence in men has now levelled off and in younger men it is falling (Fig. 23.1). A cohort of older men appears to be moving through the population, who had heavy, unfiltered smoke exposure and are experiencing very high rates of bronchial carcinoma. The fall in incidence amongst younger men is more than is accounted for by the fall in cigarette comsumption and may reflect a lower carcinogenic effect from filtered cigarettes which now dominate the market. The incidence of bronchial carcinoma in women is still increasing rapidly, probably because, as a group, they took up smoking later in the century than men and the highly exposed group is only now showing the enhancing effect of age on carcinogenesis.

Aetiology

Smoking

There is now an overwhelming body of evidence which indicates that cigarette smoking is the major cause of bronchial carcinoma.

1 The rise in deaths from carcinoma of the bronchus has reflected increasing exposure to cigarette smoking over the past 50 years, particularly when the two sexes are studied separately.

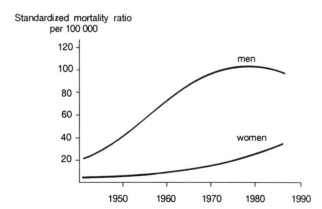

Fig. 23.1. Mortality from carcinoma of the bronchus. Standardized mortality ratios for men and women in England and Wales.

2   The risk of death from bronchial carcinoma increases by a factor roughly equal to the number of cigarettes smoked per day. That is to say that an individual smoking 25 cigarettes daily has about 25 times greater chance of dying from the disease than a non-smoker of the same age and sex. For some subgroups, the relative risk is even higher; for example, in men smoking unfiltered cigarettes, the risk of smoking between 30 and 40 cigarettes daily is about 80 times that of a non-smoker.

3   The risk of bronchial carcinoma is greatest in those who inhale cigarette smoke.

4   The risk of dying from bronchial carcinoma falls off dramatically if cigarette smoking stops. (The excess risk is approximately halved every 5 years after stopping smoking). Pipe and cigar smokers have a slightly increased risk of bronchial carcinoma, which is very much smaller than that of cigarette smokers.

Other factors

The strength of the association between cigarette smoking and bronchial carcinoma tends to swamp other factors.

Urbanization

The incidence of bronchial carcinoma is greater in urban than in rural areas, even when cigarette smoking is allowed for. Atmospheric pollution is regarded as the most likely explanation of this difference but the relationship is poorly defined. A linked relationship to occupation may explain part of the difference.

Occupational factors

Occupational factors appear to play a relatively small part in the causation of the disease, but there is nevertheless good evidence that industrial exposure to asbestos, chromates, haematite, nickel, carbonyl, arsenic, coal gas and radioactive gases is associated with an increased risk of bronchial carcinoma. Rates of carcinoma in smokers with established asbestosis are very high indeed.

Pathology

Cell types

Four main types of carcinoma may be distinguished (Fig. 23.2). Sometimes histological classification proves difficult. The cell type has some relationship to the pattern of growth and response to treatment. Probably the most important histological distinction is into two groups: small cell carcinoma and non-small cell carcinoma.

Small cell carcinoma

This develops from the Kulchitsky cells of the bronchial wall. These have endocrinological potential which is sometimes manifest clinically. The tumours develop rapidly and become generalized very early in their course, so that surgery is almost never curative. Untreated, small cell carcinomas have a very short median survival of 2–3 months, but they have been shown to be importantly susceptible to chemotherapy. The treatment of choice in virtually all small cell carcinomas is thus

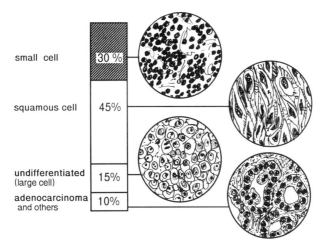

small cell   30 %

squamous cell   45%

undifferentiated (large cell)   15%

adenocarcinoma and others   10%

Fig. 23.2. Histological types of bronchial carcinoma. Small cell tumours are generally distinctive in their histological appearance. Well-differentiated squamous cell tumours have whorl-like orientation of cells and intercellular bridges (prickles). Well-differentiated adenocarcinomas have a perceptible glandular structure. Poorly-differentiated variants of these two tumour types are difficult to classify and they contribute to the group of poorly-differentiated (large cell) tumours. The percentages are approximate.

combination chemotherapy, whereas in other forms of bronchial carcinoma, chemotherapy plays a rather minor role.

Non-small cell carcinoma
This group comprises all other types including, principally, squamous cell carcinoma and adenocarcinoma. The treatment of choice in this group is surgical removal whenever practicable. A proportion of squamous cell carcinomas tend to grow more slowly and metastasize later than the other varieties. Adenocarcinomas appear not to be related to smoking exposure.

Tumour growth

From the time of origin, most of the life history of the tumour takes place before symptoms develop. The different rates of tumour growth can be expressed using estimates of the time taken to achieve a doubling of tumour volume. The length of time between origin and diagnosis is related to the length of time between diagnosis and death.

The rates of growth of different types of tumour can be expressed using estimates of the time taken to achieve a doubling of volume. Lung tumours are rarely diagnosed before they have a diameter of 1 cm and it has been calculated that by this stage at least 30 tumour volume doublings have occurred from the moment of malignant mutation. The implications for prognosis, early diagnosis, etc. are explored diagrammatically in Fig. 23.3.

Site of origin and spread

The majority of carcinomas originate in the larger bronchi; about two-thirds are visible on bronchoscopy. The tumours spread by direct invasion of the lung,

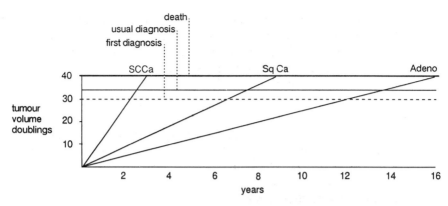

Fig. 23.3. Tumour growth. It has been estimated that when a tumour reaches a diameter of about 1 cm (when it might first be evident on a chest X-ray), about 30 volume doublings have taken place. Diagnosis is more usually made when the tumour is larger than this. By 40 doublings a theoretical diameter of about 10 cm is reached, by which stage death will usually have occurred. As a rough approximation, small cell carcinomas are thought to double monthly, squamous cell tumours 3 monthly and some adenocarcinomas 6 monthly. Some consequences of these estimates are: (1) most of the tumour's life history is subclinical; (2) some tumours have very long time-courses, despite relatively short life-expectancy after diagnosis; (3) untreated survival from diagnosis is related to tumour type; (4) early diagnosis by chest X-ray makes little impact on the total life history of the tumour; (5) early diagnosis by regular X-ray screening would be expected to be impracticable, as it would advance diagnosis by less than a year in most instances and accordingly would have to be performed more frequently than annually. In practice, screening has been found to have no effect on lung cancer mortality.

chest wall and mediastinal structures and particularly by metastasis to the hilar and the mediastinal lymph nodes.

Blood-borne distant metastasis is common, liver, adrenal gland and brain being particularly favoured organs. At death metastases are present in the great majority of cases.

Diagnosis

Clinical features

Bronchial carcinoma presents in a wide variety of ways. Commonly there are symptoms and clinical features relating to the chest, but the disease may present with metastatic complications or non-metastatic neuro-endocrine syndromes or because of non-specific symptoms such as malaise and weight loss.

Chest symptoms

Cough. Chronic bronchitis is usually present anyway, but a persistent aggrava-tion of cough may be the first features of carcinoma.

Dyspnoea. Usually this is a late symptom due to collapse of an obstructed lobe or lung, pleural effusion or extensive lymphatic infiltration of the lung.

Haemoptysis is common at any stage of the disease and occasionally massive.

Chest pain. Very common. Sometimes diffuse and poorly localized but tending to be constant. Sometimes well localized and related to chest wall involvement. Central chest pain may be related to mediastinal gland enlargement.

Hoarseness when it is persistent may be due to involvement of the left recurrent laryngeal nerve by hilar extension of the tumour. (Sometimes unilateral laryngeal paralysis is asymptomatic.)

Chest signs

Commonly there may be no physical signs on examination of the chest.

Lymph node enlargement may be apparent, particularly nodes behind the medial ends of the clavicles.

Signs of collapse (p. 51).

Signs of consolidation (p. 50).

Signs of pleural effusion (p. 51).

Stridor (p. 44) usually reflects extensive involvement of a main bronchus or the trachea. Where the tumour arises in the trachea or a main bronchus, the resulting dyspnoea may occasionally be confused with that due to diffuse airways narrowing—particularly if the chest X-ray is not obviously abnormal (see pp. 46 and 63).

Clinical situations

Carcinoma is strongly suspected in cases of unresolved pneumonia or recurrent pneumonia and pleural effusion (especially if large, recurrent or bloodstained). There is an increased incidence of bronchial carcinoma in conditions causing diffuse pulmonary fibrosis.

Metastatic complications

The range of syndromes encountered is large and includes cerebral tumour, paraplegia, painful hepatomegaly, obstructive jaundice, pathological fractures and bone pain, skin nodules, etc. Some syndromes deserve particular mention.

Superior vena caval obstruction (SVCO)

This causes venous engorgement of the upper part of the body, with facial congestion, oedema and headache, particularly in the morning. Examination shows a suffused face with peri-orbital oedema. The jugular veins are engorged and *pulseless*. There are distended veins over the chest and upper limbs. Fine veins around the chest, just above the costal margin, are prominent and major collateral veins may be seen running down the axillae. Superior vena caval obstruction is particularly likely to accompany small cell carcinoma and other tumours involving the upper part of the right hilum. The tumour is always inoperable but SVCO can usually be relieved by chemotherapy, in the case of small cell carcinoma, or radiotherapy, in the case of other tumours.

Pancoast's tumour

This term refers to carcinoma which extends upwards from the apex of the lung to invade the structures of the axilla. The lower part of the brachial plexus is particularly likely to be involved and this produces distressing pain down the inner surface of the arm. Involvement of the sympathetic ganglia or the thoracic sympathetic fibres may result in the production of Horner's syndrome.

Non-metastatic extrapulmonary manifestations
With the exception of clubbing, these manifestations are uncommon.
Clubbing occurs in about 25% of cases and is most common in squamous cell tumours.

Endocrine disturbances
These are most frequently associated with small cell carcinomas. They include the following:
Hypercalcaemia. Of obscure causation; causes polyuria and confusion.
Inappropriate ADH secretion. This usually presents with stupor, acute confusion or psychosis, sometimes accompanied by epilpsy. The feature may fluctuate. Some patients are misdiagnosed as suffering from intracranial metastases. A cardinal feature is the very low serum sodium level.
Cushing's disease. Bronchial carcinomas may be the site of inappropriate ACTH secretion.
Melanosis.
Gynaecomastia.

Neurological disturbances
Diffuse encephalopathy.
Cerebellar degeneration.
Myelitis.
Peripheral neuritis.
Myasthenic syndrome (Eaton–Lambert syndrome).
Polymyositis, producing proximal weakness and wasting, particularly of the trunk muscles.
Dermatomyositis comprising polymyositis with a violaceous telangectatic skin eruption.
These neurological features sometimes appear a year or so before there is any evidence of the bronchial carcinoma. They may regress after removal of the tumour.

Thrombophlebitis migrans
Bronchial carcinoma may present, like other malignancies, with repeated multiple peripheral venous thrombosis. Thrombosis in an upper limb is always suspicious.

Hypertrophic pulmonary osteoarthropathy
This is a rare complication. It presents with dull aching and sometimes swelling of the wrists or ankles. X-rays of the ends of the radius or tibia reveal subperiosteal new bone formation, in the form of linear opacities parallel to the outer surface of the bone. Usually it is associated with advanced clubbing. Other disorders which cause clubbing may rarely cause hypertrophic pulmonary osteoarthropathy.

Investigation
In most cases investigation is indicated, to confirm the diagnosis as a prelude to considering treatment, and as a means of excluding other treatable alternative

diagnoses. In older patients who have little or nothing in the way of symptoms, however, investigation may often be irrelevant to management. If it is clear that because of age or frailty only palliative treatment would be given (and if there are no symptoms this will not be needed), confirmation of the diagnosis may, with benefit, be deferred until such time as the gravity of the position is starting to become obvious. This may allow the patient some months of normal life unencumbered by premature hopelessness and foreboding. Sometimes, however, worry and uncertainty about the diagnosis are themselves the most disabling consequences of the disease; here investigation and frank discussion of the position may be helpful, even if therapeutic potential is limited.

Radiological features

The chest X-ray usually provides the most compelling early evidence of bronchial carcinoma. A wide range of appearances is encountered.

Rounded shadow

This is the most common X-ray finding at the time of presentation. Occasionally the carcinoma is a tiny nodule when first seen. Usually it is already in excess of 2 cm in diameter and may have a fluffy or spiked appearance at its border, or there may be radially-arranged shadows, indicating infiltration, or patchy collapse peripheral to the mass. Where there is evidence that a carcinoma is slow-growing or where there is cavitation, adenocarcinoma or squamous cell carcinoma become more probable. Slower growing squamous carcinomas may have a relatively smooth contour. Cavitation within the rounded shadow is common.

Collapse of a lobe or lung

In smoking adults, this finding is most usually due to carcinoma of the bronchus, although there are of course many other possible causes.

Hilar or mediastinal enlargement

These changes are usually the result of lymph node metastases. Where there is evidence of prominent and very rapid growth of lymph node metastases, a small cell carcinoma becomes more probable.

Pleural effusion

Particularly if it is large, or accompanied by other features outlined above, a pleural effusion always raises the possibility of bronchial carcinoma.

Lymphangitis carcinomatosa

This term refers to diffuse spread of carcinoma through the lymphatic channels of the lungs. Carcinomas of various types, particularly adenocarcinomata of stomach and breast, may present this picture, especially after mediastinal involvement. There is usually fairly severe dyspnoea. The X-ray appearances are of streaky micronodular mottling which is generally radially arranged and which may be very widespread. The diagnosis may be made by peripheral transbronchial biopsy (Fig. 23.7). When bronchial carcinoma is the cause, the shadow is usually asymmetrical and there may be a solid lesion. Localized streaky shadowing suggestive of lymphatic obstruction or infiltration is common in the immediate neighbour-hood of bronchial carcinomata.

No abnormality

The chest X-ray is found to be normal in only a small proportion of patients. In these the lesion is sometimes very tiny (in cases presenting, perhaps, with remote metastatic syndromes) or situated proximally in main bronchus or trachea. A tumour may lie posteriorly and medially and be obscured by the heart or hilar shadows.

Tomography

Sometimes better visualization of a doubtful lesion is possible with this technique. Narrowing of the trachea or main bronchus may be revealed. Tomography is expensive, rarely furthers the diagnosis appreciably and it should not be regarded as obligatory when a localized abnormality is detected on plain films.

Computerized tomography (CT)

This occasionally reveals small tumours, perhaps suspected on neuro-endocrinological grounds (see above), which are undetectable by other means. The main indication for CT imaging is in the assessment of operability.

Bronchography

This may occasionally be useful, particularly in localizing tumours prior to surgery.

Histological–cytological confirmation

The diagnosis may be near-certain from clinical and radiological features alone, but an attempt should normally be made to obtain histological or cytological confirmation.

Sputum cytology

The diagnostic yield from cytological examination depends upon the experience and interest of the pathology service and upon the provision of adequate fresh specimens of true sputum. In about half of patients with advanced bronchial carcinoma, diagnostic appearances are evident if at least three good specimens are examined. The yield in small peripheral lesions is very low.

Bronchoscopy

Bronchoscopy is usually indicated in suspected bronchial carcinoma. The aim is: (1) to obtain histological confirmation of the diagnosis; and (2) to assess operability.

More than two-thirds of tumours can be seen using fibre-optic bronchoscopy and diagnostic material obtained either in the form of a biopsy, or as brushings which are prepared for cytological examination. Bronchoscopy may be omitted in cases where the diagnosis is supported by sputum cytology or other evidence. The yield of bronchoscopy is low in malignant pleural effusion. Bronchoscopy may be irrelevant in terminal cases, where there is no possibility of specific treatment.

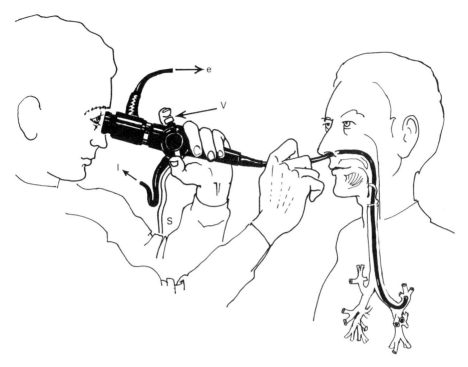

Fig. 23.4. Bronchoscopy using the flexible (fibre-optic) bronchoscope. The diagram shows the arrangement for transnasal examination in the conscious subject. The distal tip of the instrument is controlled by a lever which is moved with the left thumb. It can be moved through an arc of about 180° in one plane. The range of movement is extended by rotating the instrument as a whole. The section nearest to the operator's eye is a beam-splitting attachment (Lecturescope, Olympus Optical), which allows a second observer to view the bronchial tree via an additional eye piece (e). The bronchial tree is illuminated by light conducted to the instrument from a mercury vapour light source (l) by fibre bundles which continue to the tip. All but the smallest calibre instruments have a hollow channel. This connects to a suction line (s) by a valve (v) which operates the suction when the finger is applied. Small biopsy forceps and brushes for cytological sampling may also be passed through the channel (see also Fig. 23.7).

Fibre-optic bronchoscopy (Fig. 23.4)

This is most often used in diagnosis. It is usually performed transnasally in the conscious seated patient using topical anaesthesia. It is convenient, causes minimal upset to the patient and permits good visualization.

Rigid bronchoscopy

This is generally carried out under general anaesthesia with intravenous agents and muscle relexants (Fig. 23.5). Ventilation is maintained by venturi entrainment of air, with a nozzle injecting high pressure oxygen, at intervals, into the open end of the bronchoscope. Rigid bronchoscopy is often used immediately before surgery and is an important technique in the removal of foreign bodies, the management of profuse haemoptysis and the removal of tumour by laser therapy, cautery, etc.

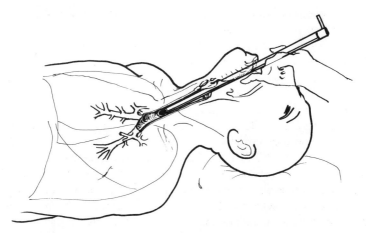

Fig. 23.5. Bronchoscopy using a rigid bronchoscope. Depending upon its size, the instrument can be passed most of the way down the main bronchi. Views of the orifices or the segmental bronchi are obtained (with the aid of angled telescopes in the case of the upper lobes). Rather less of the bronchial tree than is shown in the diagram is available for inspection.

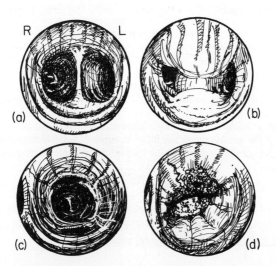

Fig. 23.6. Bronchoscopic appearance in carcinoma of the bronchus. (a) Sketch of normal appearances at the lower end of the trachea, showing sharp carina with a view down the right main bronchus and of the origin of the left main bronchus. (b) The appearances of mediastinal involvement by tumour in the subcarinal and related lymph nodes, with widening of the carina, bulging posteriorly and anteriorly and narrowing of both main bronchi. (c) Sketch of normal right intermediate bronchus. (d) Typical appearances of narrowing caused by tumour encircling the bronchus; there is also tumour occluding the narrowed lumen and invasion of the mucosa posteriorly. R, right; L, left.

The following features suggest that the tumour is inoperable:

1   Vocal cord paralysis (see above).
2   Involvement of the proximal part of a main bronchus.
3   Widening of the carina (Fig. 23.6) or tracheal compression from mediastinal lymph nodes.

Peripheral transbronchial biopsy

This technique is used for obtaining specimens of lung parenchyma, by means of very small biopsy forceps which are passed to the lung periphery through a flexible bronchoscope (Fig. 23.7). It may be useful in the diagnosis of diffuse lung involvement by bronchial carcinoma, alveolar cell carcinoma and by lymphangitis carcinomatosa. Histological material may sometimes be obtained in more localized parenchymal involvement. The technique is useful in the diagnosis of non-malignant diffuse infiltrations and infections of the lung.

Needle biopsy

Larger peripheral lesions can be biopsied using a Tru-cut needle, which removes a small core of tissue. Small lesions in the lung, even where these are close to the hilum, may be sampled by fine needle aspiration (FNA) biopsy. The needle is directed under fluoroscopic, or sometimes CT, control and produces positive confirmation of malignancy in about 85% of malignant nodules. Its capacity to confirm a non-malignant diagnosis is limited, although, in some circumstances, useful. Depending on clinical priorities, there may be no need to persist with attempts to obtain cytological or histological diagnosis, because an early thorac-

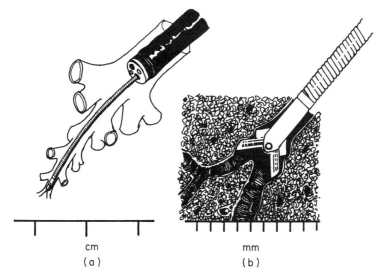

cm   mm
(a)   (b)

Fig. 23.7. Peripheral transbronchial biopsy. A small specimen of lung parenchyma is obtained by passing a long biopsy forceps through a flexible bronchoscope and beyond visual range into the lung periphery until it wedges (a). It is then withdrawn slightly and opened (b). The sample comprises the small tongue of lung tissue between two limbs of a branching small bronchus or bronchiole and it is obtained by closing the forceps as the patient breathes out.

otomy is usually indicated to produce secure diagnosis and treatment. Carcinoma is the most common cause of small rounded shadows and this group has the best chance of successful surgical treatment.

Pleural aspiration

The diagnosis of malignancy can be obtained by cytological or cytogenetic examination of pleural fluid. If stereotyped chromosomal abnormalities are identified, then the diagnosis of malignancy is virtually certain. Pleural biopsy should always be carried out if pleural aspiration is being undertaken for diagnostic purposes.

Pleural biopsy

The usual technique employs the Abrams punch (Fig. 23.8). This is introduced into the pleural space under local anaesthetic. Where the pleura ia greatly thickened, good specimens may be obtained with the air-driven trephine.

Mediastinoscopy and scalene-node biopsy

Mediastinoscopy comprises inspection of mediastinal structures, particularly lymph nodes, by blunt dissection downwards from the suprasternal notch, sometimes using a modified laryngoscope. Biopsy of mediastinal nodes may provide confirmation of the diagnosis (and of inoperability), prior to radiotherapy or chemotherapy, particularly when bronchoscopy is negative despite obvious mediastinal

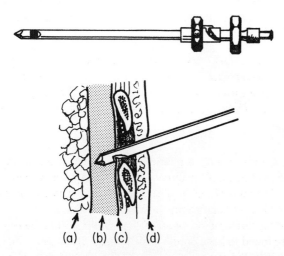

(a) (b) (c)   (d)

Fig. 23.8. Pleural biopsy using the Abrams punch. The instrument is in two parts. The outer pointed sheath has a notch near the tip and carries a spiral groove at the proximal end. The inner cylinder has a sharp cutting edge at its distal end and a lateral peg at its proximal end, which fits into the spiral groove. When the parts of the instrument are rotated relative to each other, the spiral groove causes the inner cylinder to close the notch, cutting off any tissue engaged in its mouth.

Below, the instrument is shown in position for obtaining a pleural biopsy. After aspirating fluid the instrument is withdrawn until the notch snags on the pleural surface. The cutting edge is then rotated into the closed position and the instrument withdrawn. (a) lung; (b) pleural fluid; (c) parietal pleura; (d) skin surface.

or hilar enlargement. Scalene-node biopsy may be performed with the same aim. These techniques are useful when lymphoma, or occasionally sarcoidosis, are likely alternative diagnoses.

Liver biopsy

Where there is liver enlargement or jaundice, liver biopsy may provide histological confirmation. The yield from this investigation can be improved by carrying out a liver scan and directing the biopsy needle to any accessible 'cold area' which is revealed.

Thoracotomy

In some cases the diagnosis may not be confirmed until thoracotomy is performed. Where all the evidence points to an operable bronchial carcinoma and there are no major contraindications, thoracotomy should not be unneccesarily delayed as the danger of metastasis increases with every day which passes.

Treatment

The options comprise:
1 Radical surgery.
2 Palliative surgery.
3 Radical radiotherapy.
4 Palliative radiotherapy.
5 Chemotherapy.
6 Palliative medical and nursing measures.
7 No treatment.

Each case will require careful individual consideration and the choice of treatment will be affected by such considerations as extent and type of the tumour, the age of the patient and presence of other (especially cardiopulmonary) diseases, the nature of the symptoms and also upon the patient's wishes.

Radical surgery

This offers the best chance of long-term survival in non-small cell carcinoma, where the tumour is apparently well localized to a lobe or lung and the patient can tolerate the excision. Unfortunately, 60% of patients with bronchial carcinoma are unsuitable for resection because of obvious spread to the mediastinum or beyond, or because of co-existent cardiopulmonary disability. Of those who are operated upon, one-quarter are found to have unresectable disease. Of those in whom the tumour is apparently resected at operation, about 25% are still alive at 5 years (Fig. 23.9). The operative mortality is generally 10% or less depending upon how aggressive the selection policy is.

Pre-operative functional assessment

Chronic bronchitis and associated airways obstruction frequently accompany bronchial carcinoma; the latter may make resection impossible. No single test permits prediction of feasibility of pneumonectomy and the decision depends on the balance of clinical and laboratory evidence, taken in conjunction with the

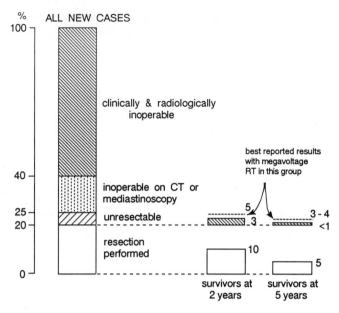

Fig. 23.9. Operability and survival in carcinoma of the bronchus. The figures are approximate and take no account of histological type. About 60% of cases are judged inoperable on clinical and radiological ground; a further 15% inoperable on CT imaging or mediastinoscopy; 5% are found unresectable at surgery. Thus only about 20% of all cases have the tumour resected. RT = radiotherapy; numbers indicate percentages of all cases of carcinoma.

likelihood of successful removal of tumour. Greater risks are justified in the case of a small squamous cell carcinoma.

The following features are associated with a high mortality and intolerable disability after pneumonectomy: an FEV_1 of less than half the predicted value; single-breath transfer factor of less than half the predicted value; evidence of chronic respiratory failure (elevated P_{CO_2}); exercise dyspnoea of Grade 2 or worse.

Palliative surgery

This is rarely carried out, but it may be useful in Pancoast's tumour, where severe pain results from involvement of the brachial plexus, or in the management of broncho-pleural fistula, severe haemoptysis, etc. Laser treatment has a limited place in the palliative treatment of tumourous narrowing of the main bronchi or trachea. Various neurosurgical procedures such as tractotomy and thalamectomy may be occasionally indicated for terrible pain from other areas.

Radical radiotherapy

Megavoltage techniques allow larger doses to be given in shorter time and with relatively less unwanted tissue damage: various techniques exist. Radical radiotherapy has found its principal application in patients who are in good general condition, but who have inoperable disease which is nevertheless relatively well localized within the thorax. Mean 3 year survival in this group is about 15% in squamous carcinoma and adenocarcinoma and 4% in the case of anaplastic tumours.

Palliative radiotherapy

This is undertaken for the relief of symptoms. Superior vena caval obstruction generally subsides dramatically after a few days and usually does not recur as the disease progresses. Pain due to chest wall invasion, lymph node enlargement or bone metastases may be susceptible to radiotherapy. Haemoptysis may be controlled.

Non-radical radiotherapy *does not extend survival*. There is thus no reason to subject patients to radiotherapy merely because of the presence of a carcinoma. When the diagnosis is known, however, some patients and their doctors find inaction unbearable and speculative 'palliative' radiotherapy is sometimes prescribed as a result.

Chemotherapy

Chemotherapy is the treatment of choice in small cell carcinoma and is offered to all except the elderly and debilitated. It is fairly demanding and requires full understanding and co-operation on the part of the patient. Three or four drugs are always used together. Those most frequently included are: cisplatin, cyclophosphamide, vincristine, doxorubicin, VP-16 (etoposide) and methotrexate. Treatment is given in pulses, at intervals of about 3 weeks, and is usually continued for at least 4 months. A variety of schedules have been evolved; all seem to have rather similar rates for the induction of remission. A process of refinement, through controlled clinical trial, is in progress. Some schedules incorporate radiotherapy to the primary and some include cerebral radiotherapy because of the high incidence of cerebral secondaries in patients who survive the initial phase of chemotherapy. The treatment produces nausea, malaise, alopecia and weight loss together with variable marrow depression.

About 80% of patients show clear evidence of tumour response which, initially at least, is often associated with gratifying improvement in tumour symptoms. Where the tumour is limited to one hemithorax and associated cervical glands (limited disease), about 40% of patients will achieve apparent disease-free remission. Where the tumour has spread beyond these bounds (extensive disease), half as many achieve apparent complete remission.

The overall impact of chemotherapy on prognosis in small cell carcinoma is illustrated in Fig. 23.10. The main effect has been to increase the proportion surviving 6–9 months. The best predictors of survival are activity index, serum albumin, alkaline phosphatase and sodium. The activity index (Karnofsky score) is a simple measure of the patient's well-being and degree of independence on a 10 point scale. Long survival, to 5 years, is rare except where these predictors show normal results.

Palliative medical and nursing measures

Pleural effusion

Rapidly recurring pleural effusion can be satisfactorily treated in about three-quarters of patients by one treatment with a pleural sclerosing agent. Three

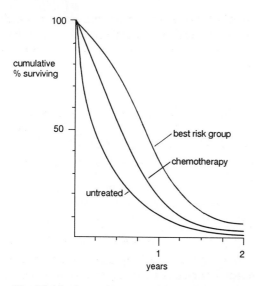

Fig. 23.10. Survival in small cell carcinoma. Representative curves illustrating survival in untreated cases; usual survival in a series of cases treated with combination chemotherapy and survival in a 'best risk' group of patients with normal activity index and normal serum sodium, albumin and alkaline phosphatase levels.

methods are in general use, involving instillation of either tetracycline, bleomycin or *Corynebacterium parvum*. The purpose in each case is to generate an inflammatory pleurisy. Results are similar in all three methods and are improved if particular efforts are made to aspirate the chest to dryness. A variable degree of temporary pain and malaise may be produced.

Hypercalcaemia

The acute effects of hypercalcaemia in an ill patient are controlled by rehydration and sometimes the use of mithramycin or calcitonin. Oral diphosphonates are useful in less florid illness and in continuation treatment.

General

The patient's principal need from his medical and nursing attendants is their time. Many patients want to talk about what is happening to them and to know more about the way ahead, but it may be an impossible topic for discussion unless unhurried opportunities are created.

There is great scope for alert symptomatic management in the later stages of bronchial carcinoma. Distressing cough usually responds to methadone linctus, if necessary in large doses. Pain commonly requires regular long-acting morphine, orally in 8 hourly doses, which is usually effective if the dose is increased sufficiently. The sedative effect is usually tolerable and diminishes with time. Additional treatment to control nausea and constipation is usually needed and patients need proper warning of these effects so that they are not discouraged at the start of treatment. Associated breathlessness and anxiety are greatly helped by morphine. Rarely, severe pain requires the use of transcutaneous nerve stimulation (TENS), nerve block or even nerve section or tractotomy.

Severe anorexia can distress patient and family alike and often responds to oral corticosteroid treatment.

No treatment

In very old patients with few symptoms, the discovery of a bronchial carcinoma does not usually demand any treatment. Some other symptom-free patients with inoperable disease, who are interested to seek a full display of the probabilities of survival after the available modes of treatment, opt to have no treatment, at least until palliable symptoms develop.

Alveolar cell carcinoma

This rather uncommon tumour arises from alveolar or bronchiolar epithelium and spreads along the alveolar and bronchiolar surfaces. The affected areas tend to become filled with whorls of tumour cells, but the essential architecture of the lung parenchyma is preserved in the early stages at least. The tumour shows some resemblance to adenocarcinomas and may be difficult to differentiate from metastatic adenocarcinoma from stomach, pancreas, etc. The tumour presents with cough, haemoptysis or non-specific symptoms. Some tumours produce a large amount of mucin and, at an advanced stage, the patient may report increasing production of large volumes of glary sputum. The chest X-ray may show irregular rounded or shaggy shawdows, which are unevenly distributed in one lobe or lung. The tumour sometimes appears to be disseminated or perhaps multi-focal in origin. Misdiagnosis is common (most usually as tuberculosis); the correct diagnosis may only become apparent by means of peripheral transbronchial lung biopsy, or after thoracotomy. Cytological examination of the sputum is sometimes helpful. The tumour is sometimes slow growing and in localized tumours the results of surgery are appreciably better than for bronchial carcinoma. Some patients may survive for over 5 years with relatively localized disease. Diffuse tumours do not respond to radiotherapy and are always fatal.

Bronchial adenoma

These uncommon tumours normally present with haemoptysis, cough and sputum; sometimes there is bronchial obstruction with distal collapse. Half may be biopsied at bronchoscopy. The great majority are bronchial carcinoids which are slow growing, locally invasive and which only rarely metastasize. Clinical evidence of secretory activity—the carcinoid syndrome—is rare and suggests the presence of metastases. The majority of the remaining tumours are cylindromata. These tumours are also slow growing and locally invasive, but at least 10% show malignant features. The overall mortality amongst patients with bronchial adenoma is of the order of 10%. If there are no metastases evident at the time of the operation and histological examination reveals no atypical features, long-term survival is the rule.

Mesothelioma

See Chapter 29.

Chapter 24
Pulmonary Embolism and Pulmonary Hypertension

PULMONARY EMBOLISM

Pulmonary embolism is important in that it is potentially fatal, often preventable and sometimes treatable. The mode of presentation depends to a large extent on the size of embolus (Fig. 24.1).

Source

Thrombosis—the systemic veins and occasionally the right side of the heart are the usual source of emboli.

Venous thrombosis

A number of factors predispose to venous thrombosis:

1 *Damage to vein wall.* Due to local trauma or inflammation.

2 *Slowing of the circulation.* Immobility, local pressure, venous obstruction, varicose veins, congestive cardiac failure, shock, dehydration, hypovolaemia, etc.

3 *Hypercoagulability of the blood.* Associated with recent trauma, childbirth or operations, thrombocythaemia, oral contraceptives, malignant disease, anti-thrombin III deficiency, etc.

Clinical evidence of venous thrombosis

Thrombosis in deep veins of the legs, pelvis or abdomen may be completely silent and be unsuspected until pulmonary embolism ensues (phlebothrombosis). The relative lack of local inflammatory reaction in the vessel wall may result in the clot being only loosely attached. Where there is more local inflammation of the vein (thrombophlebitis), the characteristic features of local *warmth*, tenderness, oedema and superficial venous dilation are more evident and the clot may be more securely adherent. *The severity of the local signs is a relatively poor indication of the risk of pulmonary embolism.*

Confirmatory tests of venous thrombosis

Ultrasonic probe. Occlusion of major leg veins may be revealed by this means. An ultrasonic probe is placed over a major vein (popliteal or iliofemoral) and the calf or thigh distal to the probe is compressed. The probe will produce a signal if blood accelerates through the vein beneath and absence of the signal (generally an audible one) suggests venous occlusion. The test is crude but rapid and atraumatic.

Venography. Radio-opaque contrast material is injected into a vein on the foot and films taken as it traverses the veins higher in the leg. This technique gives good evidence of major venous occlusion but is time-consuming, expensive and moderately uncomfortable.

I^{125} *fibrinogen.* The isotope is injected intravenously and the uptake in the legs compared with the uptake in other regions of the body. Preferential uptake

(a)

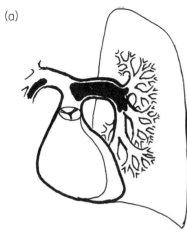

Massive pulmonary embolism
Acute:
>50% occlusion of circulation.
Sudden circulatory collapse. Cyanosis.
Central chest pain.
Hyperventilation. Engorged neck veins.
ECG: sometimes S1, Q3, T3 pattern.
CXR: usually unhelpful.
Angiography: shows filling defects and poor perfusion.
Scan: usually not done.

Subacute:
>50% occlusion of circulation.
Progressive severe dyspnoea over few weeks without
   obvious cause. Dyspnoea even at rest.
Raised jugular vein pulse, sometimes loud P2.
ECG: may show right ventricular hypertrophy (RVH).
CXR: may show infarcts.
Angiography and scan: always severe perfusion defects.

(b)

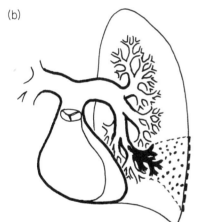

Acute minor pulmonary embolism
With infarction:
Pleural pain haemoptysis, effusion, fever, hyperventilation.
CXR: Segmental collapse/consolidation.

Without infarction:
May be 'silent'.
? Dyspnoea, hyperventilation.
? Fever.
CXR: may be normal.
ECG: unhelpful.
Angiography: usually shows obstruction if early.
Scan: shows perfusion defects.

(c)

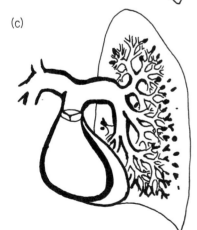

Chronic thromboembolic pulmonary hypertension
(repeated small emboli)
Progressive breathlessness, hyperventilation.
? Effort syncope.
Clinical features of pulmonary hypertension.
ECG: right ventricular hypertrophy and axis deviation.
CXR: prominent pulmonary artery.
Angiography: may be normal or show slow circulation
   or peripheral 'pruning'.
Scan: expected to show patchy irregularity of perfusion.

Fig. 24.1. Synopsis of pulmonary embolism.

suggests the incorporation of the fibrinogen into fresh thrombus. The test is very sensitive. Most postoperative patients show some uptake. Large proximal thromboses may be missed.

Clinical features, diagnosis and management

The consequences of pulmonary embolism depend very much upon the **size** of the emboli. Massive pulmonary embolism presents with circulatory collapse. Medium-sized pulmonary emboli tend to cause pulmonary infarction and a 'pneumonic' picture; multiple very small emboli cause gradual obstruction of the circulation and pulmonary hypertension, leading to gradually progressive dyspnoea and right heart failure.

These broad categories will be discussed separately.

Acute massive pulmonary embolism

Clinical features

Acute massive pulmonary embolism causes its effects by suddenly plugging up the pulmonary circulation, producing catastrophic drop in cardiac output. It presents with sudden collapse—the patient becomes shocked, pale and sweaty and usually strikingly tachypnoeic. Consciousness may be lost, usually transiently, and there may be fitting. The pulse is feeble and rapid and the blood pressure low; a third or fourth heart sound may be audible. The periphery becomes pale and cold and there may be mottled cyanosis especially in dependent areas. The cyanosis is generally central and may be unresponsive to oxygen administration. Where consciousness is preserved, severe crushing chest pain may be present. The neck veins are usually strikingly engorged.

When the circulation is more or less completely arrested, death ensues rapidly, and the picture is that of a 'cardiac arrest' and ventricular fibrillation may in fact be present. In this desperate situation, there is a notably poor response to external cardiac massage, even when promptly applied.

Diagnosis

This is commonly obvious from the circumstances (e.g. associated with postoperative venous thrombosis). The other conditions which often have to be considered are:

1 *Myocardial infarction.* Distinction may be difficult, especially in the early stages (when typical ECG changes of infarction might not have developed). Acute right bundle branch block and T-wave depression in $V_1–V_4$ suggest embolism but *the ECG is often normal*. Excessive dyspnoea without signs of pulmonary oedema may suggest embolism.

2 *Acute internal blood loss.* The most helpful distinguishing feature is the state of the neck veins, which will be barely filled, even in the recumbent patient, if blood loss is the explanation for profound collapse and well-filled-in acute massive embolism.

3 *Acute bacteraemic shock or pancreatitis.* Onset is generally less rapid, there may be evidence of the primary cause and central venous pressure will be low.

4 *Cardiac tamponade.* Tamponade due to pericardial effusion will generally

appear more gradually, there may be paradoxical variation of venous (up in in-spiration) and arterial (down in inspiration) pressures. Haemopericardium may be due to ruptured myocardial infarction, cardiac surgery, trauma, pericarditis (es-pecially on anticoagulants) and involvement of the pericardium by bronchial car-cinoma. Diagnosis of sudden tamponade may be difficult. The size of the heart shadow on a chest X-ray may be helpful. Echocardiography can provide firm evidence of the presence of pericardial fluid.

5   *Dissecting aortic aneurysm* may mimic pulmonary embolism. Sometimes the chest X-ray shows widening of the aorta.

6   *Pneumothorax and massive collapse of a lung.* May produce sudden shock, but will normally be identifiable by careful examination of the chest and by chest X-ray.

Where sudden death is averted, there is usually some improvement in the patient's condition over minutes or hours, attributable to movement of the clot further into one or both lungs.

Confirmatory tests

The most satisfactory investigation is pulmonary arteriography, which will usually demonstrate the obstructed zone. Lung scanning may be indicated if the patient's condition is good and there is serious doubt about the diagnosis. It is not normally carried out in this situation. A normal lung scan excludes significant embolism. In massive acute pulmonary embolism, hypoxia is almost invariable and hypocapnia usual; normal blood gases make significant acute massive embolism very unlikely.

Treatment

1   *Emergency treatment* comprises the administration of oxygen; there is very little else that can be done.

2   *Fibrinolytic therapy.* Where the patient's condition continues to give cause for concern, but he or she is considered likely to survive at least 24 hours, fibrinolytic therapy is indicated. Streptokinase or urokinase is administered intravenously and an infusion continued for up to 48 hours. This treatment greatly accelerates clear-ing of clot.

3   *Embolectomy* is now rarely carried out, but may be necessary where the peripheral circulation fails to be restored after a few hours and hypotension per-sists. Angiography may be of some assistance in highlighting those individuals who require surgical treatment. Thrombolytic therapy has made embolectomy a rather rare, high risk measure.

4   *Anticoagulant treatment.* This is instituted after fibrinolytic therapy is com-plete.

Prognosis

The short-term prognosis is very variable, but about 30% of truly massive emboli prove fatal. The outlook is usually clear within a few hours of the onset and is obviously related to the rapidity of recovery. Commonly, an acute massive embolus occurs on a background of several preceding emboli, which may have blocked off much of the remaining pulmonary circulation. Anticoagulation reduces the risk of further embolism to about half.

Long-term anticoagulation is not necessary after complete recovery from acute massive infarction. Recurrence of this form of embolism is rare. Long-term outlook is good.

Subacute massive pulmonary embolism

Major pulmonary embolism sometimes develops in a stepwise fashion over some weeks. There may be no pain, only breathlessness, which is severe and unexplained by the usual causes. Sometimes there may be complaints of faintness or episodes of collapse, which pass. These may be due to emboli passing through the heart, causing temporary interruption to flow, or arrhythmias, or they may reflect reduced cardiac output because of the pulmonary circulatory obstruction. As there has been more time, the right heart may show features of hypertrophy on ECG and it may be able to sustain increased pulmonary artery pressures (not seen in acute massive embolism).

The diagnosis is made on suspicion, because there is no obvious other cause. The chest X-ray may show major areas of underperfusion with few vascular marks, or may show some irregular collapse. It may be normal. The lung scan and pulmonary angiography always show grossly abnormal perfusion, sometimes with only a few zones receiving all of the cardiac output.

The condition is a serious one, which may proceed to severe right heart failure, or to circulatory collapse or sudden death from further embolism.

Acute minor pulmonary embolism

This is the most common form of pulmonary embolism presenting clinically. The usual first symptom is pleural pain, perhaps accompanied by breathlessness, haemoptysis and mild fever. There may be signs of pleural effusion or a pleural rub, or evidence of localized consolidation. Repeated medium-sized embolization may occur relatively silently in recumbent ill patients, particularly in the elderly. The only clinical feature may be tachypnoea.

The diagnosis depends upon thinking of pulmonary emboli whenever 'pneumonia' is the preliminary diagnosis. Aspiration of the pleural effusion usually yields a modest amount of blood-tinged fluid, but sometimes the fluid is clear.

Investigations

The chest X-ray commonly shows elevation of the diaphragm with linear areas of atelectasis in the basal zones, but may show no abnormality. The appearances of bilateral basal shadowing in a breathless patient should always suggest pulmonary embolism, if no other cause is evident.

Pulmonary function tests

The patient is nearly always found to be hyperventilating and the P_{CO_2} is low. Other tests of pulmonary function are not very helpful—there may be increased deadspace ventilation but this is tedious to measure, the normal range is very wide and it is found to be increased in many forms of pulmonary disorder.

The lung scan (V/Q scan)

In essence, the lung scan involves the use of a gamma camera, which builds up a plot of the distribution of radioactivity within the lung, firstly whilst the patient

breathes a radiolabelled gas which emits gamma rays and, secondly, after injection of radiolabelled albumin which displays the distribution of pulmonary perfusion.
1   *Ventilation images.* Radiolabelled xenon is added to the breathing circuit of a closed-circuit spirometer. As the patient breathes from this apparatus, the gamma emission from well-ventilated zones of the lungs builds up rapidly. Any less well-ventilated zones show a more gradual increase in radioactivity (slow 'wash-in'). At equilibrium, the camera image shows the distribution of aerated lung. When the patient breathes in from the room once more, there is a wash-out phase which can also reflect the speed of regional ventilation. Very elegant studies can be undertaken using radioactive krypton, which has a very short half-life, enabling rapid appreciation of regional ventilation; it is also possible to obtain images in many different projections. In practice it adds little to information obtained with xenon.
2   *Perfusion images.* Macroaggregated particles or microspheres of human albumin are labelled with a gamma-emitting radioisotope (generally technetium 99^m) and a dose is injected intravenously, with the patient lying down so as to minimize the effect of gravity. The particles of the preparation are of such a size that they impact in pulmonary capillaries. (Only about 1 in 1000 capillaries are obstructed and no detectable harm results. The albumin particles are broken down after a few hours.) The patient is seated in front of the gamma camera and an image is built up which reflects the distribution of pulmonary perfusion. Anterior, posterior and oblique images are usually obtained. In the normal individual, the lateral images will show a preponderance of perfusion, inferiorly and posteriorly, as a consequence of the influence of gravity on the normal pulmonary blood flow in the supine position.

Interpretation. 'Cold areas' are evident on the scan wherever there is a large area of defective blood flow; this is obviously useful in supporting a diagnosis of pulmonary embolism. Patchy cold areas are common in severe airways obstruction—especially in asthma, where they may change hour by hour without any accompanying clinical or radiological changes. Other localized conditions of the lung, such as pneumonia or carcinoma, are associated with localized defects of perfusion. The lung scan does not differentiate between embolism and other causes of defective perfusion, associated with obvious radiological abnormality. It is, however, very useful:
1   If it shows definite multiple areas of defective perfusion, which are not the site of obvious collapse or consolidation on the chest X-ray (Fig. 24.2), or of reduced ventilation as judged from the ventilation images. This is strong evidence to support pulmonary embolism.
2   If it shows completely normal distribution of pulmonary perfusion—this is strong evidence against the presence of pulmonary embolism.
Theoretically, it might be expected that a ventilation scan would always show striking diminution of perfusion relative to ventilation in the case of embolism and impairment of both ventilation and perfusion in other lung disease. In practice, the disinction remains difficult; pulmonary embolism may be accompanied by local reduction of both ventilation and perfusion.

In summary, the evidence which lung scans produce, concerning distribution of perfusion, must be interpreted in the light of the chest X-ray appearances and the clinical circumstances.

CXR   V̇   Q̇

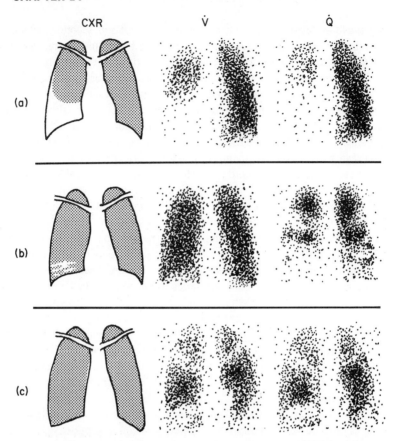

(a)

(b)

(c)

Fig. 24.2. Diagrammatic representation of the chest X-ray (CXR) appearance, together with ventilation (V̇) and perfusion (Q̇) images obtained with a gamma camera in three patients.

Only anterior projections are shown. In practice posterior, lateral and oblique projections would be obtained for perfusion images (and, less commonly, ventilation images). In the diagram, ventilation images are shown at a stage before complete equilibrium is established.

(a) *Large right pleural effusion.* Ventilation is reduced on the right as expected. Perfusion is also reduced as expected. Even though perfusion seems proportionately more reduced than ventilation, the diversion of blood flow is in keeping with that commonly seen in pleural effusion and the overall distribution of perfusion resembles that of ventilation—there is a 'matching defect'.

(b) *Pulmonary embolism.* In this particular case, the chest X-ray shows only trivial changes at the right base. Ventilation is uniformly distributed but there are several major defects in the distribution of perfusion. These are 'non-matching defects'. Such defects are typical of pulmonary embolism and the appearances shown are diagnostic of multiple pulmonary embolism. Radiological shadowing in the lung fields, of whatever cause, is almost inevitably accompanied by abnormality of ventilation and/or perfusion at that site. The interest, as in case (b), then centres on the other radiologically normal areas of lung.

(c) *Severe airways obstruction.* It is common for quite marked regional defects of ventilation and perfusion to accompany severe airways obstruction. The chest X-ray may show only overinflation. Usually the distribution of perfusion and that of ventilation are broadly similar (matching defects) as in (c).

Pulmonary angiography

If performed within a few days, pulmonary angiography will usually demonstrate embolized zones, if they are large enough.

The extent to which these investigations are employed depends upon the extent to which the diagnosis is in doubt, the condition of the patient and whether there are relative contraindications to anticoagulation.

Treatment

Immediate

Measures to relieve pain are required in the early stage when pleurisy may be extremely distressing. Opiate drugs are most useful. Anticoagulation is usually obligatory. If the patient is breathless and there are signs of extensive embolism, fibrinolytic therapy may be employed before anticoagulation.

Long term—how long should anticoagulants be continued?

Where embolism occurs in the postoperative period, or in association with an acute thrombophlebitis, an arbitrary period of 2–3 months is usually sufficient. Where there is repeated embolism with either long-established venous disorder, or with no obvious primary site for thrombosis, it may be necessary to continue anticoagulant indefinitely.

Prognosis

Anticoagulant therapy is generally effective in preventing new thrombus formation, but further embolism from existing clot is always possible for several days after starting treatment. Usually healing of the lung is near-complete, the affected areas re-expand or contract to linear scars. Sometimes pleural adhesions produce lingering painful tethering of the chest and the vital capacity may be slightly reduced. Haemoptysis sometimes continues for a week or more.

Chronic thromboembolic pulmonary hypertension

Clinical features

Very small emboli (microemboli) will go unnoticed until a large part of the pulmonary circulation has become impacted. If repeated embolization continues over weeks or months, pulmonary hypertension develops. The outstanding symptom is dyspnoea on exercise, which is generally an easy, panting dyspnoea resembling that seen in cardiac disease. Severe pulmonary hypertension is eventually accompanied by clinical ECG and radiological evidence of right ventricular hypertrophy (Fig. 24.3). Tiredness, syncope on effort and angina reflect a critically limited cardiac output. Usually there is no obvious peripheral source of emboli, although many of the patients with this disorder are found to have extensive varicose veins. A proportion of the remainder may follow pregnancy or use of oral contraceptive agents. Rarely, tumour emboli (e.g. trophoblastic tumours or carcinoma of the breast) may lead to the appearance of pulmonary hypertension.

Investigations

Electrocardiogram

This will generally show clear evidence of right ventricular hypertrophy (Fig. 24.3).

Chest X-ray

This will generally reveal prominence of the pulmonary arterial conus and proximal pulmonary arteries; there may be a suggestion of undervascularization of the peripheral lung fields.

Pulmonary angiography

This is generally unhelpful and merely shows dilated proximal pulmonary arteries and a rather slow pulmonary circulation.

Lung scanning

This is similarly unhelpful. There may be relatively poor perfusion of the bases, but by the time severe symptoms are present the whole of the pulmonary circulation is involved and regional underperfusion is not seen.

Cardiac catheterization

This is important: (1) the presence of pulmonary hypertension is confirmed; (2) by measuring wedge pressure, left heart disease (particularly unsuspected mitral

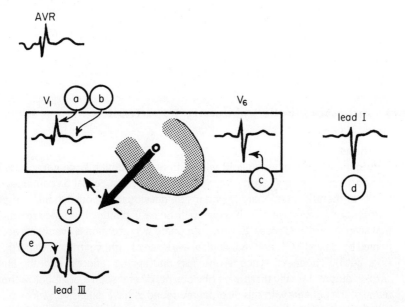

Fig. 24.3. ECG changes in right ventricular hypertrophy. The solid arrow represents the mean QRS vector in the frontal plane; it is deflected to the right as indicated by the interrupted arrow. See text for description.

stenosis) is excluded, (3) by measuring the oxygen content of blood in the right heart, a left to right shunt may be excluded.

Treatment

Long-term anticoagulant treatment is the only really important treatment apart from anti-failure measures where they are necessary.

Prognosis

The outlook depends upon severity and duration, but is generally poor. Once established, pulmonary hypertension is usually progressive. Patients who lack an obvious source for pulmonary emboli fall into the group labelled idiopathic primary pulmonary hypertension.

Footnote

Post-mortem studies have shown that failure to diagnose pulmonary embolism is common. A substantial proportion of patients who die from potentially treatable pulmonary embolism, which has not been diagnosed in life, have been thought at some stage of the illness to have a psychogenic cause for their breathlessness. The lack of a clear cause for breathlessness in terms of obvious cardiac or pulmonary disorder, together with normal simple pulmonary function tests, should lead to the suspicion of pulmonary embolism until this is excluded, for example by lung scan.

IDIOPATHIC PRIMARY PULMONARY HYPERTENSION

This rare disorder presents in precisely the same manner as microthromboembolic pulmonary hypertension; usually the cause is unknown. From 1957 to 1959, a large number of cases appeared in central Europe which seemed to be related to consumption of aminorex fumarate—an anorectic agent used to assist weight loss.

The course is almost always progressive and the disease is fatal within a few months or years. Heart–lung transplantation offers the only prospect of longer survival. Death either occurs suddenly, probably from syncope, or gradually with intractable heart failure. Anticoagulants are generally used because it is virtually impossible to exclude microthromboembolism. Vasodilators, such as tolazoline, may provide some relief and dipyrimadole may help, perhaps by exerting an effect upon platelet function.

COR PULMONALE

Some confusion arises from the differing ways in which this term is employed. Essentially it means heart disease, secondary to primary disease of the lungs. Some (particularly American) clinicians use the term to indicate any cardiac change—especially ECG evidence of right ventricular hypertrophy. Others reserve the term to describe episodes of overt heart failure, especially those which accompany chronic airways obstruction with respiratory failure. Pulmonary embolism is not usually included in the group labelled cor pulmonale.

In practice, persons who develop right-sided heart disease have chronic hypoxia. In persons with airways obstruction, cor pulmonale (however defined) is almost always confined to individuals who are chronically hypoventilating and have elevated levels of arterial P_{CO_2} as well as hypoxia. In diffuse parenchymal disorders, such as fibrosing alveolitis, cor pulmonale develops at a late stage when there is chronic hypoxia. In this instance the patient is usually not underventilating and the $P\text{co}_2$ is normal or low, until terminally.

Hypoxia is, of course, a potent cause of pulmonary arteriolar constriction.

Evidence of right ventricular hypertrophy

Clinical

1 In the absence of airways obstruction, the signs comprise: a prominent parasternal heave, a loud pulmonary second sound (the last component of a split-second sound on inspiration) and sometimes a right atrial protodiastolic gallop. In very severe pulmonary hypertension, pulmonary valve incompetence and tricuspid incompetence may supervene.

2 Where pulmonary hypertension is secondary to obstructive airways disease, right ventricular hypertrophy is difficult to diagnose clinically, because over-inflation of the chest almost invariably obscures the physical signs.

ECG

The best evidence is provided by the chest leads—other features merely provide helpful support. Letters in brackets refer to Fig. 24.3.

Leads V_1–V_2
The appearance of a QR complex or an RSR′ complex, in which the upward (R or R′) deflection is dominant, constitutes strong evidence of right ventricular hypertrophy (a). Widening of the QRS complex is also suggestive; the T wave is commonly inverted (b).

Lateral chest leads (V_5–V_6)
Deep S waves suggest right ventricular hypertrophy (c). Usually this is accompanied by 'clockwise rotation' with the QRS complex becoming mainly positive only in V_5 or V_6 (V_3 or V_4 in the normal).

Other supporting evidence
This may take the form of *right axis deviation* (a mean QRS vector in the frontal plane of greater than 100°—crudely detected by observing the dominant QRS to be directed downwards in lead I and upwards in lead III (d) 'pointing towards each other'). ST depression and T-wave inversion may be present in the inferior leads (II, III, VF). Right atrial hypertrophy may be reflected by *P. pulmonale*—tall peaked P waves with a vertical axis best seen in inferior leads (e).

Treatment

Heart failure

This comprises use of diuretics for severe oedema and improved oxygenation to relieve pulmonary artery pressure. Digoxin is used for the control of atrial fibrillation.

Ventilatory failure

Where the cor pulmonale is a consequence of chronic ventilatory failure associated with airways construction, there may be limited scope for improvement in some cases. Where failure of ventilation is primarily due to muscular weakness or to deformity of the thorax (for example in severe kyphoscoliosis or following thoracoplasty), long-term ventilatory support, particularly at night, may be indicated (see Chapter 31).

Hypoxia

Reversal of hypoxia is important in the management of overt heart failure; where this arises in the setting of chronic ventilatory failure, it is usually necessary to use low inspired concentrations of oxygen, together with infusion of a respiratory stimulant such as doxapram. Patients with respiratory failure who have suffered an episode of oedema, and particularly those who have recurrent or resistant heart failure, should be assessed for treatment with long-term (near-continuous) domiciliary oxygen treatment.

SOME UNCOMMON CONDITIONS AFFECTING PULMONARY VASCULATURE

Pulmonary arteriovenous aneurysm (arteriovenous fistula)

The lesion takes the form of a lobulated swelling connecting pulmonary artery and pulmonary vein. Small or medium-sized fistulae produce no symptoms and tend to be found on routine chest X-ray. Large fistulae may cause arterial desaturation and be associated with telangiectasia elsewhere (e.g. nose, causing epistaxis). There is a risk of embolism and cerebral abscess. Lesions may be obliterated by selective embolization.

Polyarteritis nodosa

This condition is characterized by arteritic lesions in many organs, due to deposition of antigen–antibody complexes in the walls of small vessels. The pulmonary circulation may be involved, leading to the development of multiple nodular infarcts which may be evident on the chest X-ray. Polyarteritis is sometimes associated with asthma. The diagnosis becomes evident by virtue of associated arteritic lesions in the skin, kidney or nervous tissue. The ESR is always high and there may be blood eosinophilia. Treatment with corticosteroids is indicated.

Wegener's granuloma

This rare condition is generally regarded as a variant of polyarteritis nodosa. The principal features are: (1) nasal or aural granulomata, causing ulceration, crusting, pain and bone erosion; (2) pulmonary nodules 0.5–3 cm in diameter; (3) renal involvement. The diagnosis may be made from the features described and supported by biopsy. The condition was formerly invariably fatal, but prolonged survival is now usually achieved with prednisolone and cyclophosphamide.

Goodpasture's syndrome

The combination of glomerulonephritis and intra-alveolar haemorrhage is called Goodpasture's syndrome. Haemoptysis may be stricking or slight and mottling is generally evident on the chest X-ray. Transfer factor may be increased because of the increase in intrapulmonary haemoglobin. The pulmonary lesion may precede the onset of nephritis. Differentiation from polyarteritis nodosa depends on whether there is evidence of arteritis in other areas apart from the kidneys. The distinction may be artificial. The associated glomerulonephritis is generally very severe. Antiglomerular basement membrane antibody may be present in the serum.

Idiopathic pulmonary haemosiderosis

This rare condition is characterized by treated intra-alveolar capillary haemorrhage of obscure cause. It presents in childhood or young adult life with either anaemia or haemoptysis. The chest X-ray generally shows a miliary mottling pattern. The diagnosis may be confirmed by lung biopsy or by bronchoalveolar lavage, both of which may reveal the presence of large numbers of iron-laden alveolar macrophages. Treatment with corticosteroids is generally tried, but may have little effect. Death may follow a massive haemoptysis.

Chapter 25
Pulmonary Oedema

In its simplest terms, pulmonary oedema may be regarded as an increase in the fluid content of the extravascular tissues of the lung. By far the most common cause of pulmonary oedema is increased capillary pressure, usually due to impaired performance of the left heart. Pulmonary oedema may also result from increased alveolar capillary permeability, due to a physical or chemical insult to the lung (see p. 267) or as part of the adult respiratory distress syndrome (ARDS).

PULMONARY OEDEMA WITH RAISED CAPILLARY PRESSURE

Primitive view of pulmonary oedema

Until fairly recently, the prevailing view of pulmonary oedema was that increased capillary filtration led immediately to fluid entering the alveoli, and that this fluid then caused bubbling sounds (crackles). This simple model ignores the important effects of the interstitial space and the function of lymphatic channels.

Interstitial oedema

Electron microscopy has shown that a very thin continuous space exists between the alveolar cells and capillary endothelium, and that this space is continuous with the interstitial connective tissue surrounding airways and larger blood vessels in the lungs. The osmotic pressure exerted by plasma proteins drains any fluid from the space, so that the space is of negligible size. In the normal situation, hydrostatic, osmotic and tissue time pressures are nicely balanced (Fig. 25.1a). Increase in capillary pressure may cause increased filtration and interstitial oedema which may initially be limited to lymphatic drainage. Further increase in filtration may lead to substantial oedema of the interstitial space. The interstitial oedema extends in the form of a 'cuff' around small airways and blood vessels (Fig. 25.2). This produces important local changes in ventilation and perfusion.

1 Small airways become narrowed by interstitial oedema.

2 The lung tissue becomes firm and non-compliant—less air enters the zone on inspiration; during expiration closure of the airways occurs early leading to wheezing.

3 On inspiration, when the airways eventually open they do so with a click—producing crackles.

4 Reduced ventilation of the firm non-compliant zone leads to local hypoxic and reflex arteriolar constriction; in addition, the accumulated interstitial oedema may compress vessels, resulting in reduced perfusion to the zone (blood is directed to less affected areas—an appropriate compensation).

5 Defective perfusion may lead to defective local production of surfactant.

6 Distortion of the cuffed bronchiolar/vascular bundles in the lung may cause irritation of vagal sensory endings (J receptors), leading to reflex stimulation of ventilation.

259

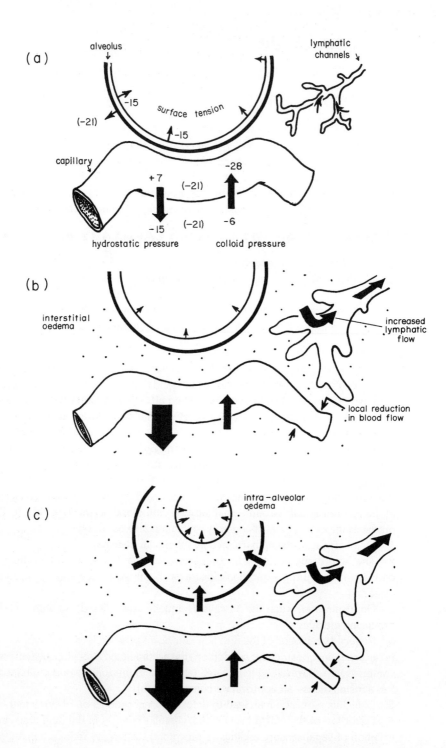

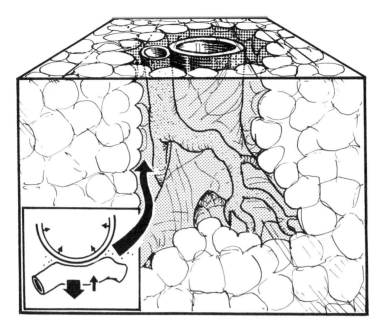

Fig. 25.2. Diagrammatic representation of the formation of interstitial oedema extending in the form of a 'cuff' around the bronchovascular bundle.

Because of the effect of gravity, capillary filtration is always greatest in the lower zones and interstitial oedema, cuffing, crepitations, etc. are all more marked at the base of the lungs. Ventilation and perfusion become directed increasingly to the upper zones.

Alveolar oedema

Further increase in interstitial oedema, which overloads the capacity of the lymphatics to preserve a state of balance, may lead to alveolar oedema. The surface tension of the lung layer draws fluid into the alveoli (Fig. 25.1c). In doing so, the diameter of the alveolar bubble becomes reduced and surface tension increases. The effect of surface tension is to some extent counteracted by the surfactant layer, but this may become defective with reduced blood flow. When imbalance becomes

---

Fig. 25.1. (*Opposite*) Pulmonary oedema. Diagram of an alveolus and pulmonary capillary.
(a) *Normal situation:* approximate values for hydrostatic and colloid pressures in mmHg. These forces are in equilibrium or slightly in favour of fluid reabsorption so that the interstitial space is negligible at alveolar level.
(b) *Pulmonary oedema.* Increase in pulmonary pressure leads to increased transudation of fluid. Increase in lymphatic fluid transport. At this stage interstitial oedema involves mainly the bronchovascular connective tissue (Fig. 25.2).
(c) *Severe pulmonary oedema.* There is now separation of the fluid film from the alveolar surface and intra-alveolar oedema.

severe, fluid may pour into the alveoli and accumulate in the airways. In florid pulmonary oedema, pink fluid and foam are coughed up in large quantities.

Symptoms of pulmonary oedema

Shortness of breath is the principal symptom. This may be accompanied by:

Exercise dyspnoea.
Tachypnoea.
Cough.
Orthopnoea and paroxysmal nocturnal dyspnoea.
Cheyne–Stokes respiration.
Finally, extreme dyspnoea, cyanosis, coughing up of foaming sputum, haemoptysis.

Mild pulmonary oedema may cause no symptoms at rest, but exercise dyspnoea is inevitable. More severe oedema causes breathlessness at rest and often an irritating cough.

Orthopnoea

Typically orthopnoea is present (but also occurs in other forms of dyspnoea).

Paroxysmal nocturnal dyspnoea (PND)

This may occur—the patient characteristically wakes in the early hours with wheezy cough and severe dyspnoea. This episode may sometimes be indistinguishable from nocturnal attacks of bronchial asthma. One of the most helpful distinguishing features is the complaint of morning tightness, cough and dyspnoea by the asthmatic patient; this is lacking in the patient with PND due to pulmonary oedema.

The precise mechanism of production of orthopnoea and PND is debatable, and probably complex, but one important factor may be the effect of gravity causing spread of basal pulmonary oedema to relatively oedema-free areas of the lung when the patient reclines, without important improvement in the bases.

Cheyne–Stokes respiration

This is waxing and waning ventilation generally with periods of apnoea. Cyclical breathing is commonly present in pulmonary oedema, but is rarely sufficiently striking to be remarked upon. It is an expression of unstable ventilatory control due to a slowed circulation time, increased ventilatory drive and hypoxia. Fulminant pulmonary oedema is characterized by extreme respiratory distress, with wheezing and commonly a rattling sound on breathing.

Cyanosis and the coughing up of foamy pink sputum

In this situation, ventilation may be impeded and the $P\text{co}_2$ may rise.

Signs

The character of the breathing may be laboured and wheezing, or rapid and panting, sometimes with a fine rattling sound audible. In mild pulmonary oedema, the only sign may be fine crackles at the bases. Generally, these are mainly mid- or end-inspiratory in timing (p. 49). In some cases, widespread fine rhonchi are audible.

There may be obvious signs of the cause of the oedema—particularly mitral or aortic valvular heart disease, or cardiac enlargment with the characteristic sustained impulse of left ventricular enlargement. A third or fourth heart sound (or gallop) is a particularly valuable sign when the cause of the dyspnoea is in doubt.

X–ray changes

The heart may be enlarged and pulmonary vessels may appear to be prominent, particularly those to the upper lobes. Mild pulmonary oedema may cause no radiological features. Kerley 'B' lines are very useful evidence of established pulmonary oedema (Fig. 25.3). These comprise short horizontal linear opacities, which are found next to the pleural surfaces in the costophrenic angles. They are probably caused by dilated lymphatic channels in interlobular septa. Blotchy lung shadowing is common in severe pulmonary oedema. Very striking perihilar oedema may be somewhat fancifully referred to as a 'bat's wing' pattern; it is not of any special significance. A fine mottling is occasionally seen in persistent pulmonary oedema.

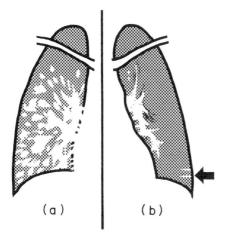

(a)   (b)

Fig. 25.3. Radiographic appearances in pulmonary oedema. (a) Severe pulmonary oedema. (b) Early pulmonary oedema. The arrow indicates the appearance of Kerley 'B' lines. The vascular shadows passing up to the upper zones are more prominant than in the normal resting erect individual.

Functional disturbance

Spirometry usually reveals a restrictive pattern of ventilatory impairment but prolonged expiratory time and reduced FEV_1/VC fraction are common. Hyperventilation is usual and the P_{CO_2} is low in all but the most severe cases.

Arterial P_{O_2} is almost always reduced—sometimes to critically low levels—but the reduction is often modest when the radiological extent of the pulmonary oedema is considered (a testimony to the efficiency of the redistribution of the pulmonary circulation away from oedematous underventilated areas).

Treatment

Primary disturbance

Where pulmonary oedema results from valvular heart disease, renal failure, hypertension or other obvious primary disturbance, special measures will be required.

Oxygen

Oxygen should be given in as high a concentration as practicable (see p. 297).

Diuretic

Intravenous frusemide (40–80 mg) is generally very effective within a few hours. Sometimes improvement is dramatic; evident within 15 minutes, before any notable increase in urine formation by the kidneys—an effect attributable to a peripheral effect of frusemide causing increased venous capacitance.

Vasodilators

Peripheral resistance and cardiac output can be increased by vasodilator treatment, provided hypotension is not already too severe. Useful agents include isosorbide dinitrate, either sublingually or by slow infusion, hydralazine and nitroprusside in emergencies. Angiotensin converting enzyme (ACE) inhibitors and calcium channel blockers are useful, in addition, in more established forms of left heart failure.

Digitalization

This may be helpful when failing left ventricular function is important, particularly when atrial fibrillation is present with a fast ventricular rate.

Opiates

Morphine is particularly useful; opiates perhaps act by reducing fear, ventilatory drive and possibly also by inducing relaxation of sympathetically–mediated peripheral vasconstriction.

Exceptional measures

Inotropic agents such as salbutamol or dopamine may be relevant in overwhelming heart failure.

Venous cuffs applied to the arms and legs may improve the situation for a short time in the critically ill patient.

IPPV. In patients overwhelmed by fulminating pulmonary oedema, IPPV is occasionally life-saving. The principal benefits which follow are: (1) improved clearing of foam and secretions by bronchial suction; (2) the ability to administer really high concentrations of oxygen continuously if necessary; (3) the relief of exhaustion and terror by the use of powerful sedation. Some authorities support the use of high inflation pressures throughout the breathing cycle with the aim of 'pushing' fluid back into the pulmonary capillaries. Such measures can, however, cause embarrassment of the circulation, as the increased airway pressure is transmitted directly to the pulmonary capillaries (and especially to those in the less oedematous areas).

Less common forms of pulmonary oedema

Pulmonary oedema which is not due to left-sided heart disease is uncommon. It is sometimes helpful to demonstrate that the oedema is not due to raised pulmonary capillary pressure, by measuring the pressure recorded by a catheter in the pulmonary artery advanced into the lung until it wedges. It is not always necessary to make this measurement, because the nature of the pulmonary oedema may be evident from the preceding circumstances or from features of associated illness.

Lowered plasma oncotic pressure

Pulmonary oedema may develop when the oncotic pressure of plasma is severely reduced due to hypoproteinaemia (e.g. in nephrotic syndrome), but this is unusual without some co-existing increase in pulmonary capillary pressure.

Altitude pulmonary oedema

Acute pulmonary oedema may develop in unacclimatized individuals soon after arrival at altitudes in excess of 9000 ft (2740 m). It is uncommon, but can be life-threatening. The mechanism is poorly understood, but it may be due to severe pulmonary arteriolar constriction, due to hypoxia, occurring with a patchy incomplete distribution, so that an excessive fraction of the cardiac output is forced through a small proportion of scattered unconstricted areas. Pulmonary capillary pressure may be elevated.

Lymphatic obstruction

Obstruction of the lymphatic drainage of all or part of the lung may produce a degree of local or generalized pulmonary oedema as part of the disturbance.

Increased capillary permeability

Increased permeability of the capillary endothelial and alveolar lining layers may be produced by the direct effect of toxic agents, or by other complex indirect effects in the course of overwhelming illness or major trauma (see ARDS, Chapter 26).

Chapter 26
Adult Respiratory Distress Syndrome

Definition

The term adult respiratory distress syndrome (ARDS) is used to describe severe respiratory inadequacy, developing in the course of severe illness or after trauma. The diagnosis is made when there is:

1 A catastrophic infective, toxic or traumatic illness.
2 Respiratory distress (laboured, rapid breathing).
3 Hypoxia, despite oxygen administration. ($Pa_{O_2} < 6.6$ kPa (50 mmHg) despite an inspired concentration of 60% or more.)
4 Bilateral lung shadowing sparing the costophrenic and cardiophrenic angles and without venous congestion.
5 Absence of pulmonary disease to explain the appearances; absence of left heart failure and absence of raised pulmonary wedge pressure (that is pressure measured by a catheter wedged in the peripheral pulmonary arterial circulation, which reflects pulmonary venous pressure).

There is usually an imminent or actual need for IPPV.

Cause

The evolution and cause of the condition are poorly understood. A central feature is protein-rich exudation into the alveoli, due to abnormal alveolar capillary permeability. Neutrophils are present in the lungs in abnormal numbers and may release mediators and oxygen radicals, which affect the capillaries. Evidence of complement activation is often present in patients with ARDS. Other mediators such as histamine, platelet activating factor and bradykinin have been suggested as contributing to the increase in permeability.

Pathology

The alveolar spaces become filled with protein-rich exudate containing inflammatory cells, especially neutrophils; patches of relatively aerated lung lie adjacent to solid areas, and air spaces show a crescent-shaped rim of proteinaceous material—the hyaline membrane, which resembles that seen in respiratory distress of the newborn. The capillaries may contain fibrin or platelet thrombi.

Precipitating circumstances

Major trauma with multi-organ failure was the first setting to be recognized as a cause of ARDS. Overwhelming septicaemic infections, severe pneumonia, burns or pancreatitis are other relatively common examples. Aspiration of gastric contents, oxygen toxicity, transfusion reactions, effects of cardiopulmonary bypass, direct lung trauma or inhalation of toxic fumes may all cause, or play a part in, the syndrome.

Management

There is no treatment which has been shown to reverse the abnormal capillary permeability. Treatment is directed to preserving adequate oxygenation and compensating for the multi-organ failure which usually supervenes in severe ARDS.

Oxygen

Oxygenation is improved by enriching inspired air, but minimum concentrations of oxygen are used because of the risk of aggravating lung damage due to oxygen toxicity (p. 302).

Positive end-expiratory pressure

In patients on IPPV, the addition of a continuous positive end-expiratory pressure (PEEP) throughout the respiratory cycle may tend to bias fluid movement inwards and keep poorly compliant lungs inflated. Very high pressures interfere with cardiac output.

Fluid balance

Diuretics are used to lower pulmonary wedge pressure to about 5–10 mmHg, to reduce leakage. This may aggravate renal failure. Inotropic support may be needed if cardiac output is reduced by PEEP and diuretic treatment. A delicate balancing act is attempted.

Prognosis

In established ARDS, which shows no improvement, the outlook is grave. Mortality is about 40–60%. Poor prognostic indicators are failure of oxygenation to improve after starting PEEP and a lung biopsy appearance showing most alveoli filled with exudate and few areas of persisting aeration.

Exceptionally, heart–lung transplantation has been used to rescue the patient.

NON-CARDIOGENIC PULMONARY OEDEMA

Some causes of non-cardiogenic pulmonary oedema are:

Toxic chemical agents

Amongst these, the most common is acid gastric fluid. A florid form of pulmonary oedema may develop after inhalation of what may seem to be quite a modest amount of fluid. This is sometimes referred to as Mendelson's syndrome. Other harmful agents include smoke, in those severely affected in fires, and certain metal fumes. Harmful exposure to oxides of nitrogen may occur in welders working in extremely confined spaces and in silo-fillers, encountering gases given off by stored grain or silage. In all of these forms, the oedema may be delayed for some hours after the exposure.

Bacterial toxins

Some forms of acute septicaemia (e.g. due to Gram-negative organisms) may be accompanied by pulmonary oedema. This is particularly likely to occur when there has been severe shock (see shock lung and ARDS).

Viral infection

A severe infection by influenza A virus may occasionally present as acute pulmonary oedema.

Near–drowning

Pulmonary oedema—sometimes delayed—may develop during resuscitation from near-drowning.

Lung re-expansion

Pulmonary oedema may develop in a lung soon after relief of a large pleural effusion or pneumothorax. This is most likely to occur when a large amount of fluid or air has been removed and when the lung has been collapsed for more than a few days.

Neurogenic pulmonary oedema

This is a rare complication of serious intracranial disease (usually cerebral tumour or haemorrhage). The mechanism is unclear, but it is known to be mediated via the nerve supply to the lungs. Pulmonary capillary pressure may be elevated.

Narcotic overdosage

This generally arises as the result of miscalculation by a drug addict and may be produced by heroin or any other member of the opiate group of drugs. Onset may be abrupt or delayed and death may ensue. The mechanism is obscure.

Other drugs

A number of drugs may produce pulmonary oedema, usually in a subacute form. They include bleomycin, salicylates in overdosage, nitrofurantoin and cyclophosphamide.

Chapter 27
Pneumothorax and Pleural Effusion

PNEUMOTHORAX

Air may enter the pleural space from the lung, or rarely from the outside as in the case of major chest trauma or thoracotomy. The intrapleural pressure is normally negative, owing to the retractive force of lung elastic recoil, so that once a communication is established between atmosphere and the pleural space, the lung tends to deflate.

Spontaneous pneumothorax

The most common form of pneumothorax occurs spontaneously, usually in previously healthy young males. The source of the air leak is usually a tiny bleb on the surface of the lung near the apex.

The condition usually presents with the development of sudden unilateral pain, which may be pleuritic and severe and accompanied by pallor, tachycardia and sweating. Breathlessness may follow if the pneumothorax is large or under tension (see below).

Physical signs

The principal physical sign is **diminution of breath sounds on the affected side**; in the absence of dullness to percussion, this is usually most apparent anteriorly in the semi-recumbent position. Hyperresonance is usually unimpressive. Small left-sided pneumothoraces may give rise to a sticky clicking sound, in time with the heart.

Chest X-ray

The diagnosis is confirmed by chest X-ray. When the pneumothorax is small, a fine crescentic line is found, almost parallel to the chest wall, outside which no lung markings are seen.

Tension pneumothorax

Tension pneumothorax constitutes something of a medical emergency. It arises in a small proportion of spontaneous pneumothoraces in which the communication between lung and pleural space acts as a valve, permitting air to enter the pleural space during inspiration, but closing during expiration. This results in more and more air accumulating in the pleural space, which compresses the affected lung to about the size of a hand. The pressure within the pleural space may become positive throughout almost all the breathing cycle. The mediastinum becomes pushed to the opposite side and expansion of the opposite lung becomes impeded. The high mean thoracic pressure begins to impede return of blood to the heart and shock develops. Death may ensue from the combined effects of acute ventilatory and circulatory failure.

Signs

The signs of tension pneumothorax are: increasing respiratory distress; tachypnoea and tachycardia; evidence of mediastinal shift, as judged by movement of the trachea or cardiac apex.

Treatment

No treatment is required for very small pneumothoraces. There is no need to hospitalize such patients, provided they are intelligent and able to return rapidly for attention if worsening symptoms develop. Pneumothoraces in which the lung is less than 2 cm from the chest wall resolve in about 2 weeks.

Usually the pneumothorax occupies more than half of the chest and in this case active treatment is preferable, as resolution is otherwise very protracted. Moderate pneumothoraces without tension and without features suggesting significant underlying lung disease can be dealt with satisfactorily by simple aspiration using a fine plastic 'intravenous' cannula, although a proportion prove impossible to aspirate, or recur immediately. The technique is enjoying a return to popularity at present, but intercostal drainage is still the most usual form of treatment.

Tension pneumothorax demands immediate treatment. An intercostal catheter of rubber or plastic is introduced in the mid clavicular line in the 3rd interspace, or in the axilla in the 4th or 5th interspace, and connected to an underwater seal (Fig. 27.1). (Some clinicians favour the use of a rubber and plastic flutter valve, which is equally satisfactory and permits the patient to be mobile.) Air bubbles out at each expiration or cough and, if the lung perforation has sealed, bubbles soon stop. The fluid level is then seen to swing with each breath from about -3 to -10 cmH$_2$O. If there is no further bubbling after 24 hours, and the chest X-ray shows complete re-expansion of the lung, the tube may be removed.

Indications for surgical treatment

In a few cases, bubbling continues for several days. If it continues, surgery is required to remove and oversew the lung perforation. About 1 in 5 spontaneous pneumothoraces recur, usually within the first year. If there are further recurrences, or if an individual pneumothorax on the other side develops, it is usual to recommend pleurodesis.

Pleurodesis

A pleural reaction is then generated, with a view to producing fibrous obliteration of the pleural space. Some surgeons favour the use of talc and others favour stripping of part of the parietal pleural. Both methods give reliable security against subsequent pneumothorax.

Pneumothorax accompanying other lung disease

In the older age group, pneumothorax most often results from rupture of an emphysematous bulla in an individual with established chronic airways obstruction. In this situation, an already disabled patient may be rendered critically ill by a relatively small pneumothorax. Treatment by intercostal drainage is generally

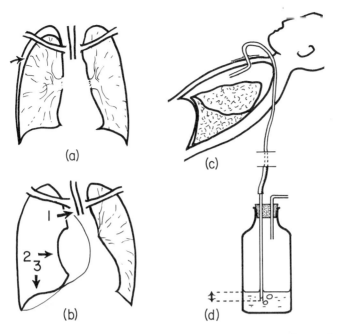

Fig. 27.1. Pneumothorax. (a) Radiographic appearances of a small right pneumothorax. (b) Radiographic appearances of a large tension pneumothorax on the right: (1) the trachea and mediastinum are displaced to the left; (2) the right lung has collapsed completely; (3) the diaphragm is depressed. (c) Intercostal tube in place. An anterior position of the chest drain is commonly used in treatment of pneumothorax, but a mid-axillary line site is increasingly favoured. Drainage of any associated pleural fluid is assisted and trauma due to introduction is less likely to be important. (d) Underwater seal. The end of the tube is 2–3 cm below the level of the water in the bottle. If intrapleural pressure rises above 2–3 cmH$_2$O, air will bubble out. If intrapleural pressure becomes negative, water rises up the tube, only to fall again when the intrapleural pressure falls towards atmospheric. The system operates as a simple one-way valve. When the pneumothorax has resolved, the water level will generally be slightly negative throughout the respiratory cycle, reflecting the normal fluctuations in intrapleural pressure, and when the patient coughs air will no longer bubble out.

satisfactory, but a greater proportion continue to leak air for many days and eventually come to require thoracotomy and excision of the bullae.

A pneumothorax may result from rupture of lung cysts associated with advanced fibrosing alveolitis, other forms of lung fibrosis, eosinophilic granuloma, etc. A lung abscess or carcinoma may break down and lead to the development of a bronchopleural fistula. In this situation a pyopneumothorax is generally present and there is a well established persistent communication with the bronchial tree. Surgical treatment is always necessary.

Bronchopleural fistula

This term merely indicates that there is a persistent communication between the airways and the pleural space, via a relatively large hole in the lung tissue. The communication may be with the pleural cavity as a whole, as in a straightforward pneumothorax, or with a loculated section of an abnormal pleural cavity, as in some empyemata. If a chest drain is inserted, the size and permanence of the communication is evident from voluminous and persistent bubbling of the underwater seal. Surgical closure of the leak is almost always necessary.

Hydropneumothorax

This term is used to describe the presence of fluid and air together in the pleural space. The chest X-ray shows a pneumothorax, bounded below by the horizontal surface of the pleural fluid. The air may have entered the pleural space from a break in the visceral pleura (e.g. a ruptured bleb or lung abscess), or may have been introduced inadvertently during chest aspiration. A rare cause of gas and fluid occurring together in the pleural space is infection by anaerobic gas-forming organisms, especially *Clostridium welchii*. The gas is usually present in small loculated collections.

Pyopneumothorax

This term describes the same situation as in hydropneumothorax except that there is pus, instead of pleural fluid, present together with air in the pleural cavity.

PLEURAL EFFUSION

Fluid dynamics

The two pleural surfaces are normally in close contact and the potential space between the two membranes contains only a very thin layer of fluid. Dryness of the pleural cavity is maintained principally by the osmotic pressure exerted by albumin in the intravascular space. Some forces influencing fluid movement within the pleural space are represented in Fig. 27.2. The oncotic pressure of plasma amounts to about 34 cmH$_2$O. Against this, the small amount of protein in the pleural fluid exerts an osmotic pressure of about 8 cmH$_2$O. The hydrostatic pres-

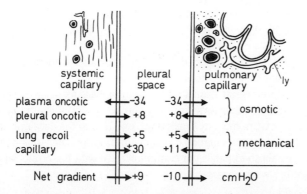

Fig. 27.2. Fluid equilibrium in the pleural space. Pressures influencing the movement of fluid are shown in cmH$_2$O. Positive values indicate forces encouraging entry of fluid into the space (and negative values the opposite effect). All values are crude approximations. Capillaries are profuse in the pulmonary subpleural layers and there is also a rich lymphatic drainage (ly); by contrast the parietal pleura is less vascular and less well supplied by lymphatics.

sure within capillaries tends to contribute water to the space. In the case of the pulmonary capillaries, this pressure varies from the top to the bottom of the lung and with pulmonary artery and pulmonary venous pressure, but it is effectively about 11 cmH_2O. In the case of systemic capillaries of the parietal pleura, the mean pressure is probably of the order of 30 cmH_2O. Elastic recoil of the lungs makes the intrapleural pressure subatmospheric most of the time. The intrapleural pressure is influenced by a number of factors, such as gravity and breathing pattern, but a mean value of $-5\ cmH_2O$ is usually accepted as an approximation in normals. In Fig. 27.2 it can be seen that the resultant gradients at the parietal and visceral surfaces are such that there tends to be contribution of fluid from the parietal surface and absorption of fluid by the visceral surface. In life, other influences probably operate. The drying influence of pulmonary capillaries is probably the dominant effect, because of the profusion and superficial distribution of these capillaries compared with those of the parietal pleura. The subpleural layer is very richly supplied with lymphatic channels which exert an active fluid-extracting effect.

This analysis is a crude oversimplification of the operative factors, but it does allow an appreciation of the manner in which pleural effusion may accompany certain disturbances. For example:

1   Increased pulmonary capillary pressure, secondary to raised pulmonary venous pressure.
2   Obstruction to the lymphatic drainage of a lung—for example, by malignant tumour.
3   Hypoproteinaemia.
4   Increased parietal pleural vascularity accompanying neoplasia.

The discovery of pleural fluid is always important and demands explanation. Pleural effusion may complicate a wide variety of pulmonary conditions, but discussion will be limited here to pleural effusion apparently occurring in isolation.

Signs
Features indicating pleural effusion are outlined on p. 51.

Radiological features
Features apparent in radiology are outlined on p. 82.

Pleural aspiration
Useful information relating to the cause of the effusion can be obtained from pleural aspiration. Heavily-bloodstained fluid suggests pulmonary malignancy, unless there is strong suspicion of pulmonary embolism and infarction. Pleural effusions fall into two main groups: transudates, which as a rule accompany generalized oedematous states, and exudates, which are derived from inflammation of the pleural membrane and adjacent tissues. It is not possible to discriminate between these groups completely, but fluid with a high protein content (above about half of the serum protein value) is likely to be an exudate.

A pleural fluid lactic dehydrogenase (LDH) level of greater than 200 IU, or more than 60% of the serum LDH level, is also characteristic of an exudate.

Cytological examination of the fluid is valuable if expertise is locally available. The patient should be tipped into various positions immediately before aspiration, because cells tend to sediment into the dependent part of the pleural space and may not be sampled on aspiration. A large volume of fluid should be obtained and centrifuged and a smear of the sediment examined.

Cytogenetic. If the cause of the effusion is unknown, cytogenetic study is probably the most discriminating procedure for the diagnosis of underlying malignancy. If examination of the fluid reveals dividing cells with an abnormal number of chromosomes, abnormal chromosomes, or abnormal banding patterns on the chromosomes, malignancy is very likely. If the abnormality is seen in stereotyped form in a number of cells, then an abnormal clone of cells is clearly present and malignancy is virtually certain. Failure to find cytogenetic abnormalities in dividing cells from a pleural effusion is weak evidence in support of a non-malignant cause.

Bacteriological examination is important in the presence of fever after pneumonia or in suspected tuberculosis.

Pleural biopsy . A pleural biopsy should be performed whenever a diagnostic pleural aspiration is undertaken (Fig. 23.4). This technique is particularly effective in the diagnosis of tuberculous and malignant pleural effusions.

Causes (see Table 27.1)

There are be difficulty in differentiating between exudates and transudates in practice.

Table 27.1. Causes of pleural effusion.

Transudates (hydrostatic, osmotic)	Exudates (inflammatory, neoplastic)

Cardiovascular
  congestive failure
  constrictive pericarditis
  SVC obstruction
	Malignant
	  bronchial carcinoma
	  metastatic disease
	  mesothelioma

	Pulmonary embolism

Hypoalbuminaemia
  cirrhosis
  nephrotic syndrome
  malnutrition
	Infective
	  tuberculosis
	  post-pneumonic
	  empyema and lung abscess

From peritoneal cavity (right-sided effusions)
  cirrhosis
  peritoneal dialysis
	Inflammatory
	  rheumatoid arthritis
	  collagen vascular diseases

	Trauma
	  haemothorax
	  chlyothorax
	  ruptured oesophagus

	Subdiaphragmatic
	  subdiaphragmatic abscess
	  pancreatitis (left-sided)

Although it is convenient for purposes of classification, the division into transudates and exudates is not a rigid one. Measurement of fluid protein content plays little part in diagnosis.

Pleural transudates

Pleural effusions are common in florid right heart failure and in constrictive pericarditis. They may less commonly accompany other generalized oedematous states; for example, renal failure or hypoproteinaemic states such as nephrotic syndrome or chronic hepatic failure. Right-sided pleural effusion may sometimes be due to ascitic fluid which may pass through congenital transdiaphragmatic communications on the right side. An ovarian fibroma may cause such a combination of ascites and pleural effusion (Meigs' syndrome). Peritoneal dialysis fluid may produce a right-sided pleural effusion.

Pleural exudates

These are most commonly due to pulmonary malignant disease or infection. In the developed world, the vast majority of very large effusions, resulting in a radiological 'white out' of one hemithorax, are due to underlying malignancy. Pulmonary tuberculosis may cause pleural effusion in the early post-primary phase but this presentation of tuberculosis is now rather rare. The effusion is generally large, has a high protein content and contains mainly lymphocytes. Pleural effusion may develop after almost any form of bacterial or viral pneumonia, but is not usually massive. The cells may be largely either polymorphs or lymphocytes and the fluid is usually extensive. Persistent recurrence of effusion suggests that a neoplasm may have been the cause of the original pneumonia. Pleural effusion may accompany pulmonary embolism. It is sometimes haemorrhagic; the protein content may suggest exudate or transudate. Acute pancreatitis may be associated with a left-sided effusion. The fluid contains a high level of amylase and the effusion may be in fistulous communication with a pancreatic pseudocyst. A subdiaphragmatic abscess may sometimes result in the development of a 'sympathetic' pleural effusion, without fistulous communication.

Pleural effusion is not uncommon amongst patients with rheumatoid arthritis. The effusion is usually small and sometimes asymptomatic. It usually resolves after some months. The diagnosis rests on clinical features of RA and on positive rheumatoid factor. Pleuritic pain, and sometimes pleural effusion, is one of the more common features of systemic lupus erythematosus (SLE) in relapse. There may occasionally be underlying irregular lung infiltrations evident on the chest X-ray at this time. The diagnosis rests on other characteristic features of SLE, particularly skin rashes and arthritis, and on the finding of antinuclear factor and LE cells in the blood.

Treatment

The management of pleural effusion naturally depends upon treatment of the primary cause. Malignant pleural effusion may be very distressing and demoralizing; treatment is discussed on p. 243.

Empyema

This term signifies the presence of pus in the pleural cavity. Usually it arises after severe pneumonia, rupture of a lung abscess or after thoracic surgery. Rupture of the oesophagus may lead to a left-sided empyema, particularly when it is due to invasion by a malignant tumour. Actinomycosis is a rare cause of empyema. Sometimes it progresses to form a discharging chest wall sinus.

Empyema may complicate pulmonary tuberculosis. Whatever their origin, empyemata become the seat of anaerobic infection by a variety of organisms, often occurring together.

The patient generally has a high swinging fever and is profoundly ill with high leucocytosis. The collection of fluid is often loculated and difficult to aspirate. The radiological appearances may vary from the usual appearance of an effusion, because of fibrous adhesions and loculation.

The management of empyema depends upon antibiotic treatment, drainage and attention to the primary cause. Sometimes decortication (operative stripping of the pleura and pus-filled cavities) is necessary.

Haemothorax

Bleeding into the pleural cavity may complicate:
1   chest injury—especially with rib fracture;
2   rupture of pleural adhesions;
3   pulmonary infarction (usually not massive);
4   anticoagulant therapy especially with (1) or (2).

If massive intrapleural bleeding occurs and the patient becomes shocked, blood transfusion and even emergency surgical exploration to arrest bleeding may occasionally be required.

If repeated aspiration fails to remove the blood clot, a fibrinous rind may develop, which may become organized, lead to fibrosis and cause permanently restricted movement of the chest. In this situation, a thoracotomy may be required for removal of the fibrinous rind.

Chylothorax

A rare phenomenon characterized by the accumulation of lymph in the pleural cavity. It is caused by leakage from the thoracic duct or other major lymphatic channel, as a consequence of surgical trauma, other injury or malignant invasion. The chylous effusion re-accumulates rapidly after aspiration. Repeated aspiration leads to protein and lymphocyte depletion. Surgical treatment is required if it persists. Tying of the thoracic duct is generally effective.

Dry pleurisy

Pleurisy is a term used merely to indicate inflammation of the pleura and the characteristic pain that this causes. Any of the conditions which give rise to an exudative pleural effusion may cause dry pleurisy.

Bornholm disease (epidemic myalgia)

This uncommon condition is characterized by an extremely severe, immobilizing, pleuritic type of chest pain and sometimes abdominal pain, variable symptoms of fever and sometimes sore throat. The pain probably arises in the chest wall musculature, rather than the pleura. The condition persists for several days before spontaneously resolving. It is due to infection with Coxsackie B virus and the diagnosis may be confirmed by isolation of the virus from the throat or stool or, retrospectively, by observing a rising titre of specific antibody in the serum.

Chapter 28
Trauma and the Lungs

Penetrating wounds of the chest

Stabbing and similar penetrating injuries commonly cause a pneumothorax from lung perforation, or sucking wound, and may also result in intrathoracic haemorrhage. The management comprises: infusion of blood and plasma; drainage of the pneumothorax and, if there is evidence of continued bleeding, emergency thoracotomy. Gaping sucking wounds of the chest may rapidly cause ventilatory failure.

Pneumothorax

See p. 269 for discussion of this topic.

Haemothorax

See p. 276 for discussion of this topic.

Rib fracture

Fracture of ribs is usually due to a fall or direct trauma to the chest, but ribs may be fractured by strenuous coughing. The cardinal sign is exquisite local tenderness.

Traumatic fracture

Fracture of ribs is usually due to a fall or direct trauma to the chest. The trauma may be slight in elderly or osteoporotic individuals.

Cough fracture

Fracture of a rib sometimes develops, apparently spontaneously, without a history of trauma. Usually there is an association with vigorous or repetitive coughing, due to acute tracheobronchitis or an exacerbation of underlying lung disease. Cough fractures are most common in young women and middle-aged men, and are particularly likely to occur in those who are obese, muscular, or have severe intractible asthma requiring long-term systemic corticosteroid therapy. The fracture is usually of the 7th rib, or a near neighbour, and situated laterally or at the angle of the rib.

Pathological fracture

This may be due to a local deposit of malignant disease, which may or may not be painful and is sometimes associated with a palpable swelling. Local rib erosion is generally evident on X-ray. Rib fractures due to osteomalacia or osteoporosis are sometimes referred to as 'pathological'; there are usually other clues of bone disease or of the underlying disease causing it.

Diagnosis

The presence of a rib fracture may be revealed during examination of a patient with obscure pleuritic chest pain, by compressing the chest laterally (tentatively to start with, and never with more force than is required to produce slight movement). This will produce a sharp pain which can then be pursued by a careful search along the likely ribs. The cardinal sign is exquisite and reproducible local tenderness; occasionally—and undesirably—crepitus is elicited.

Acute fracture can be impossible to see on a chest X-ray if there is no displacement—even if special oblique views are taken. The diagnosis is primarily a clinical one. After a few weeks, the development of callus at the site provides confirmation.

Complications

Distressing pain may lead to suppression of coughing and retention of bronchial secretions with subsequent pneumonia. Pain causes splinting of the affected side; progressive lung collapse may occur due to failure to take occasional deeper breaths. Rib fracture is a serious event in the elderly and those with advanced chronic obstructive lung disease. Pneumothorax and haemothorax may complicate rib fracture.

Management

A combination of adequate analgesia (sometimes with the help of intercostal block), antibiotic therapy and encouragement to cough and take occasional deep breaths may be all that is required, but occasionally tracheostomy, with or without IPPV, is necessary. Pneumothorax and haemothorax may require drainage.

Multiple rib fractures—flail chest

Massive blunt injury to the chest occurs in car crashes and some industrial accidents and constitutes an immediate emergency. If more than two or three ribs are fractured in two places, a substantial segment of the chest wall loses its rigidity and may flap in and out during breathing—this results in very inefficient ventilation and may be enough to cause acute respiratory failure with hypercapnia and hypoxia. Intermittent positive pressure ventilation is essential in this situation and, as it is required for a few weeks to ensure splinting of the chest whilst the ribs unite, it is usual to perform an elective tracheostomy at an early stage. In the early hours or days, heavy sedation and muscle relaxants may be necessary to prevent respiratory distress and excessive displacement of the fracture ribs.

Vertebral fracture (crush fracture)

Occasionally this is the result of severe trauma—usually a fall, landing on the feet (e.g. in parachuting). After a short period of rest, recovery is usually rapid in this group.

More commonly, vertebral fracture occurs in elderly patients with senile osteoporosis, or in patients on long-term corticosteroid treatment. In these groups management can be difficult, particularly if there is accompanying lung disease. Pain is severe and impedes breathing and coughing. The diagnosis is confirmed by evidence of new wedging of the vertebrae—almost always in the mid-thoracic region. Regular opiates may be needed for a week or two, despite the risk of respiratory depression. Careful nursing in bed, over a month or more, is often required. Corsets and braces are useless. Eventually the spine settles into a new shape and pain lessens. Prophylactic treatment should be explored (calcium supplements, hormone replacement therapy, etidronate?).

Rupture of the diaphragm

Severe injury to the lower chest or upper abdomen may lead to diaphragmatic rupture, which is nearly always left-sided. Diagnosis is sometimes difficult and centres on the radiological findings.

Injury to trachea and bronchi

Severe deceleration injury may cause rupture of the lower trachea or a major bronchus. The features which draw attention to the injury are surgical emphysema and perhaps pneumothorax, haemoptysis and lung or lobar collapse. Pneumomediastinum may be detected radiographically. The rupture may be confirmed by bronchoscopy. Large tears require early surgical repair.

Surgical emphysema

This term refers to the presence of air in the connective tissues. Air may enter from a surgical wound—particularly one in the chest and most commonly from an intercostal tube draining a pneumothorax. Sometimes it accompanies a tension pneumothorax, when it is presumed air enters from a flaw in the parietal pleura. The phenomenon is sometimes seen in severe asthma (especially in small children) and occasionally during treatment with IPPV. In these circumstances, the leak is thought to occur in some overdistended distal air-space with air tracking back along the bronchovascular connective tissue to the mediastinum. Air may also reach the mediastinum from rupture of the oesophagus.

Surgical emphysema is usually trivial, being detected by a peculiar downy, crackling sensation on light palpation and also visible radiographically as air-defined fascial places. Occasionally it reaches alarming proportions, with distension of the whole upper trunk, neck and face.

Rupture of the oesophagus

This usually results from trauma caused during intubation, bouginage or endoscopy and is occasionally due to a sharp swallowed object or vigorous vomiting. Rupture is particularly likely to occur if the oesophagus is involved by carcinoma. The rupture may communicate with the left pleural cavity, leading to hydropneumothorax, or it may communicate with the loose connective tissue of the mediastinum. One consequence of this may be acute mediastinitis, which is a serious condition characterized by collapse, high fever and substernal pain, sometimes with cyanosis and dyspnoea. Sometimes infection can be controlled by antibiotic treatment and interruption of oral feeding. Occasionally, a mediastinal abscess or abscesses may form, being recognized by unremitting swinging fever, leucocytosis and radiological displacement and widening of the mediastinum. This requires surgical drainage.

Crush injury to the lung

Blunt crushing injuries to the chest, with or without rib fractures, can cause profound pulmonary disturbance over the course of the first few days after injury. Widespread fluffy shadowing on the chest X-ray reflects alveolar haemorrhage and oedema and there is progressive dyspnoea and cyanosis. This sometimes proves fatal despite IPPV and oxygen.

Secondary effects of major trauma—ARDS

In major trauma, not necessarily affecting the chest, there may be severe pulmonary effects due to:

Thromboembolism;
Fat embolism (from fractured longbones);
Aspiration;
Resuscitative measures.

Adult respiratory distress syndrome

This is dealt with in Chapter 26. Characteristically, there is a 12–24-hour delay between the trauma and the development of respiratory distress, radiological lung shadowing and progressive hypoxia, despite oxygen therapy. The mechanism is unclear and probably involves multiple factors including those listed above.

Chapter 29
Occupational Lung Disease

The term pneumoconiosis is reserved for a group of occupational lung diseases, characterized by a parenchymal reaction (which is usually fibrosis) to inhaled mineral dust. Although this group is the best-known form of occupational lung disease, a variety of other reactions to dusts, gases, fumes and vapours are encountered. The character of the lung reaction depends upon the chemical nature of the substance, its physical form and the intensity and duration of exposure; it may also be influenced by the presence of pre-existing lung disease. The clinical features of occupational lung disease are, in the main, non-specific and the diagnosis depends to a large extent on obtaining a comprehensive occupational history.

Penetration, deposition and clearance of particles within the lung

The distance to which inhaled particles penetrate the respiratory tract depends principally upon their size. Particles smaller than 3 μm are most likely to penetrate as far as the alveoli and those of the order of 1 μm are most likely to be deposited there (see Fig. 4.1). Clearance of these particles is effected by alveolar macrophages. These cells are phagocytic and mobile; they engulf deposited particles and transport them to the terminal bronchiole from where they are carried on the 'mucociliary escalator', eventually to be swallowed or expectorated in the sputum. Some particles are toxic to macrophages, in which case transport to the terminal bronchiole is impaired. The particles tend to be liberated and re-engulfed repeatedly by macrophages; particles may accumulate in respiratory bronchioles. A proportion gain entry to the interstitial tissue of the lung and may ultimately be transported proximally via lymphatic channels (Fig. 29.1).

Fibrogenesis is poorly understood, but may be related to the death of overloaded macrophages and liberation of particles, or to loss of coating from certain types of particle. Fibrogenic potential varies with the shape and charge of particles.

Bronchial reactions

Acute tracheitis and bronchitis

These reactions are most likely to arise following rare accidental exposure to irritant fumes, gases, or aerosols of irritant liquids (especially ammonia, chlorine).

Chronic bronchitis may also be caused by prolonged exposure to dust and fumes, but disability due to chronic airways obstruction from this cause is unconfirmed in the case of most substances.

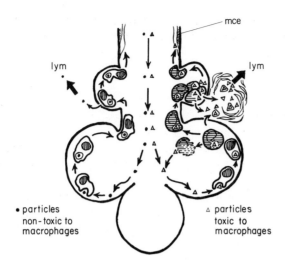

Fig. 29.1. Removal of inhaled particles. The arrows indicate the routes for disposal of inhaled particles within the lobule. Particles deposited in alveoli are ingested by phagocytic macrophages which migrate towards the terminal bronchiole. Most non-toxic particles (shown at the left) are successfully transported to the mucociliary escalator (mce). Some penetrate the alveolar wall, if the inhaled load is heavy, and are carried away by the lymphatics (lym). Particles (such as silica) which are toxic to macrophages may be liberated after death of the macrophage and be subsequently re-ingested. The particles may become covered with a proteinaceous coating. Damaged macrophages and particles tend to accumulate, particularly in respiratory bronchioles. Coated particles which penetrate the alveolar walls appear to be capable of exciting a fibrous reaction.

Occupational asthma

The term is usually reserved for asthma induced by hypersensitivity to an agent encountered at work. Atopic individuals are particularly likely to become hypersensitive but, with higher levels of exposure, non-atopics may become sensitized. A wide range of inhaled substances may cause asthmatic responses. The subject is a difficult once, since some irritant substances may cause obvious symptoms in individuals who already have hyperreactive airways because of asthma. In true occupational asthma, the hyperreactive state develops along with the development of specific hypersensitivity to the agent in question; the agent itself should be known to be capable of sensitization, and disappearance or reduction in the hyperreactive state can be expected in a high proportion of those who cease to be exposed.

Exposure to the agent in question may be followed by an immediate response or by a delayed response or by both (Fig. 17.3). Where there is an immediate response, the relationship to work and to a particular agent is usually obvious to everyone. Where delayed response is more prominent, the relationship may be more difficult to detect. Symptoms may then be worst when the subject is away from work; for example, during the night. Repeated delayed reactions induce a state of continuous asthmatic symptoms, in which morning and nocturnal aggravation are more remarkable than worsening at work. The relationship to the work environment may then only become clear when improvement is noted at weekends or during holidays.

Causes

Exposure to the following can cause occupational asthma:

Small laboratory animals—the sensitizing proteins are mainly in urine.

Locusts—highly antigenic to laboratory workers.

Proteolytic enzymes—manufacture of enzyme washing powders, brewing.

Grain, flour and contaminants—mites, weevils and mould may be the principal source of antigen.

Colophony—used as a flux for soft solder in the electronics industry.

Di-isocyanates—especially toluene di-isocyanate (TDI), used in manufacture of polyurethane foam, some spray paints which need an activator and in specialized printing, e.g. on plastic surfaces.

Acid anhydrides—used in special paints and adhesives.

Platinum salts—released in refining.

Drugs—manufacture of antibiotics, cimetidine, ispaghula ipecacuanha.

Wood dusts.

Azodicarbonamide—manufacture of polyvinyl type plastics, floor coverings.

All of the above are recognized as causes of occupational asthma under the UK Industrial Injuries Act; those affected are eligible for compensation for resulting physical disability and for hardship through termination of employment. There are numerous other causes of occupational asthma which are not yet included.

Diagnosis

The diagnosis rests on an accurate history and an informed assessment of the occupational exposure. The key questions are:

1   Is there improvement on days away from work?
2   Is there improvement on holiday?

Important supporting evidence can be obtained by the use of peak flow recordings at 2-hourly intervals throughout the day, if necessary for a prolonged period. This can be a very subtle method of determining the potentially quite complex nature of the relationship between asthma and working environment (see above). Other evidence may come from skin-testing and measurement of specific immunoglobulin concentrations. Here, interpretation rests on knowledge of the prevalence of positive results in other workers and the normal population. Only rarely will diagnosis depend on the result of inhalation challenge testing; this is difficult to do properly as control inhalations and prolonged observation and measurement are necessary.

Management

This is problematical. The simple solution of giving up the job may not be acceptable to the individual because of the economic consequences but, on the other hand, an employer may not be keen to accept responsibility for the long-term effects of continuing exposure. Suppression of the symptoms by treatment may be sought by the sufferer who wishes to remain at work, although the doctor will usually be unable to advise on the likelihood of long-term pulmonary damage from continued exposure, with or without treatment. Information on prognosis after stopping work is slender. Roughly half of sufferers can be expected to lose symptoms completely. Outlook may depend on duration of exposure.

Byssinosis

This disorder occurs in cotton workers employed in the card room, after many years of heavy exposure to cotton dust. It is characterized by tightness in the chest and cough occurring promptly on entering the mill, particularly after a few days' absence. The symptoms are particularly likely to develop in individuals who already have chronic bronchitis or asthma. There is no parenchymal lung involvement and no abnormalities are evident on the chest X-ray. There is some evidence to suggest that both Type I and Type III reactions may occur in the bronchi in response to an antigenic fraction of cotton dust.

Occupational causes of lung cancer

See p. 230 for discussion of this topic.

Alveolar reactions

Extrinsic allergic alveolitis

Most varieties of extrinsic allergic alveolitis arise as a consequence of heavy occupational exposure to allergenic dusts, e.g. farmer's lung. See p. 183 for further discussion of this topic.

Humidifier fever

This is due to microbial contamination of water used to humidify air-conditioning systems. Air tends to be recirculated, so as to conserve heat, and this, together with progressive accumulation of organic dust from the workplace, encourages build up of organisms. Affected individuals develop flu-like symptoms and may have mild fever. Usually, respiratory features are minor or absent. Symptoms typically begin 4–6 hours after starting work, but can abate despite continuing exposure. X-ray changes are not seen; serum precipitins in extracts of the humidifier water and usually present. It is not clear whether the reaction is an immunological reaction or the result of endotoxins produced by the organisms. The humidifier water contains a complex mixture of organisms including bacteria and unicellular organisms such as amoebae and fungi. Legionnaire's disease is another condition propagated by air-conditioning plants.

Pulmonary oedema

Acute pulmonary oedema may occur following inhalation of some toxic gases including sulphur dioxide, chlorine and ammonia. The reaction may be prompt or delayed.

Welding yields a variety of oxides of nitrogen and, if it is undertaken in very confined spaces, exposure to the gases may result in the development of acute pulmonary oedema with cough, tightness, dyspnoea, widespread crepitations and radiological shadowing. This may resolve slowly and reappear later, sometimes after an interval of some weeks. Fresh silage yields nitrogen dioxide; workers entering silo towers may develop similar pulmonary oedema, which may be delayed in appearance.

Metal fumes may cause pulmonary irritation and pulmonary oedema or pneumonia. Cadmium workers may develop severe reactions, with subsequent lung destruction. Lesser reactions follow exposure to magnesium, vanadium, zinc and tungsten fume. 'Metal fume fever' is a term used to describe generalized symptoms of malaise which may accompany exposure.

Pneumoconiosis

Coalworker's pneumoconiosis

The development of pneumoconiosis is directly related to the total exposure to dust. Dust exposure varies in different parts of the coal-mine and is heaviest at the coal face. Strenuous efforts have been made to reduce dust exposure during the last 20 years and there has been a reduction in the incidence of new cases. There is an important distinction to be made between the two major categories of coalworker's pneumoconiosis.

Simple pneumoconiosis

This term refers to the accumulation, within the lung tissue, of relatively small (up to 5 mm diameter) aggregations of coal particles, which are fairly uniformly dispersed and evident on the chest X-ray as a delicate micronodular mottling. A series of X-rays is published by the International Labour Office (ILO), which allows standardized categorization of the radiological appearances. Numerals (0, 1, 2, 3, 4) are used to indicate the profusion of opacities and letters to indicate size (p, q, r, for rounded opacities and s, t, u for irregular opacities). Examination of the lungs may show localized dilatation of the air-spaces immediately adjacent to the aggregations of coal (sometimes referred to as focal emphysema). **Simple pneumoconiosis causes no important symptoms, signs or physiological impairment.** There is to date no strong evidence that its presence influences subsequent health or life expectancy. The benign nature of simple pneumoconiosis is sometimes not appreciated; there is a widespread tendency to attribute almost any respiratory symptoms to pneumoconiosis, once simple pneumoconiosis has been recognized from the chest X-ray. An alternative explanation—usually in the shape of COPD, asthma or heart disease—should always be suspected.

Progressive massive fibrosis

In progressive massive fibrosis (PMF), larger opacities are evident on the chest X-ray. The ILO classifications A, B and C are used to indicate opacities of greater than 1 cm in diameter.

A = sum of diameters of opacities less than 5 cm.
B = sum of diameters of opacities more than 5 cm, but the opacities occupy less than one-third of the area of the right lung field.
C = greater than B.

Category C is more commonly accompanied by symptoms of breathlessness and detectable physiological impairment, in the form of a restrictive ventilatory defect and a variable reduction in transfer factor. On the other hand, extensive PMF may be present without notable symptoms or important physiological impairment. Categories B and C do carry a higher than expected risk of subsequent respiratory illness and premature death.

The lungs contain condensed masses of fibrous tissue, heavily infiltrated with collections of coal-dust particles. Sometimes the centres of these masses become softened and they rupture into the lung tissue. Large amounts of black material may be coughed up and part of the radiological shadowing may be found to have disappeared.

It is not clear why some coalworkers develop PMF, whilst others, equally exposed to coal-dust, do not. The condition is not closely related to the silica content of the workings or to pulmonary tuberculosis; it may perhaps depend on obscure individual differences in reticulo-endothelial function.

Caplan's syndrome (rheumatoid coal pneumoconiosis)

Coalworkers with rheumatoid arthritis may develop multiple nodular pulmonary opacities, usually about 0.5–2 cm in diameter, which may superficially resemble PMF. Usually, however, the nodules are accompanied by only very modest evidence of simple pneumoconiosis and there may be no background stippling at all. Sometimes the manifestations of rheumatoid arthritis are very slight, or even absent, but rheumatoid factor is always present in the serum. The radiological appearances may sometimes be misinterpreted as being due to multiple pulmonary metastases.

Silicosis

Silicosis is now uncommon because of widespread recognition and control of the hazards of respirable silicaceous dust. There is still a risk of harmful exposure in certain quarrying and mining operations, particularly in developing countries. Sandblasting of castings in foundries; the maintenance of the refractory lining of kilns and dry-grinding of ceramic products may carry a risk.

Simple nodular silicosis, like simple coalworker's pneumoconiosis, causes no symptoms and is an X-ray phenomenon. Advanced nodular silicosis with widespread fibrosis is disabling and may be progressive long after exposure ceases. Accidental, very heavy, short-term exposure can lead to an accelerated acute fibrotic reaction, leading to end-stage lung destruction in a few months.

Siderosis

Dust containing iron and its oxides is encountered in haematite mines, at various stages in the iron and steel industry and in welding. It gives rise to a simple pneumoconiosis (siderosis) which produces a striking mottled appearance on the chest X-ray because of high radiodensity of iron, but which is not accompanied by symptoms, signs or physiological defect. Other metals, such as antimony and tin, may produce a similar picture.

Asbestos

Asbestos is a collective term which refers to a number of naturally occurring fibrous mineral silicates which have found widespread use throughout the developcd world, on account of their ability to bind other materials together, and because of striking resistance to heat and corrosive agents. The most important forms of asbestos are:

Chrysotile (white asbestos)
This is a 'serpentine' form of asbestos; the fibres are wispy, flexible and often relatively long. Chrysotile accounts for most of the asbestos used. It appears as a bonding agent in asbestos–cement products—pipes, tiles, roofing materials, etc.— and is also included in asbestos–paper insulating materials and brake-linings.

The amphibole group
These forms have straighter, more brittle fibres. Crocidolite (blue asbestos), amosite and anthophyllite are the most important members of the group. Longer fibres can be carded, spun and made into heat-resistant fabric; shorter fibres tend to be used in other forms of insulation and as fillers and re-inforcing agents in a variety of plastic, rubber and paint products. Despite its universal presence, the great bulk of asbestos is safely bound within composite materials; important exposure is still largely confined to certain occupations in which actual dust is produced. Amongst those at risk are pipe-laggers and industrial plumbers who come into contact with asbestos insulation, and workers in the construction industries, who process asbestos–cement products, laminated asbestos materials used in fireproof partitions and sprayed wall coverings. In some industries (e.g. shipbuilding), heavy environmental contamination may result in significant exposure of workers not handling asbestos.

Consequences of heavy exposure

Asbestosis
The term 'asbestosis' is usually reserved for the description of diffuse parenchymal pulmonary fibrosis. This is only seen after heavy occupational exposure to asbestos; the worker will certainly have been handling asbestos as part of the job and exposure is generally over many (say 10) years; casual or short-term contact with asbestos does not lead to asbestosis.

Diffuse fibrosis may be evident on the chest X-ray as a fine basal haziness or mottling, sometimes accompanied by streaky shadows. Clinically, the disease presents with cough and slowly progressive dyspnoea, which may later be accompanied by cyanosis and clubbing. The earliest clinical sign is usually fine basal crackles. Tests of pulmonary function reveal reduction in vital capacity and lung compliance and a progressive impairment of gas transfer. The condition may progress even after exposure has ceased.

Bronchial carcinoma
A high proportion of individuals with established pulmonary asbestosis die from bronchial carcinoma. Carcinoma occurring in this situation qualifies for compensation under the Industrial Injuries Acts.

There appears to be an increased incidence of bronchial carcinoma amongst those exposed to asbestos, but without clinical asbestosis. Cigarette smoking appears to increase the risk of carcinoma by about the same factor as it increases risk in non-asbestos-exposed individuals. The risks are multiplicative.

Consequences of even trivial exposure

Pleural calcification

Calcified pleural plaques are very common in workers exposed to asbestos and are also found amongst members of their families and those who have had quite trivial exposure. The plaques are visible on the chest X-ray but are quite harmless. They serve as a 'marker' of asbestos exposure and may develop many years later. They are raised lesions, situated on the parietal pleura; the pleura is not adherent over them. They are most common over the diaphragm and interiorly projected over the mid-zones.

Pleural thickening

Localized or occasionally diffuse thickening of the pleura may be seen with or without notable calcification. Small areas are without effect. Diffuse involvement

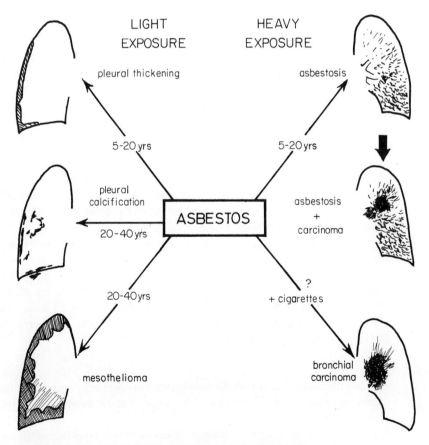

Fig. 29.2. Pulmonary diseases relating to exposure to asbestos.

may be associated with reduced exercise tolerance, or even a restrictive ventilatory defect. Sometimes there are strands of subpleural fibrosis extending into the lungs.

Disability from bilateral diffuse pleural thickening (but not pleural plaques alone) is compensatable under UK industrial injuries legislation.

Mesothelioma

This malignant pleural tumour is most commonly seen in occupationally-exposed individuals, but it is probable that only relatively light exposure is necessary. Mesothelioma generally develops some 20–40 years after exposure. The condition presents with pleurisy and perhaps a small pleural effusion. Progressive pleural thickening follows due to tumour extension and this may show a lobulated appearance on the chest X-ray (Fig. 29.2).

Progressive restriction of chest movement and severe persistent chest pain are features of the advanced disease and death follows within a year or two of diagnosis. Metastasis is rare, but surgery is generally useless because of diffuse chest wall and mediastinal invasion. No other treatment affects progress of the disease—only palliative measures are relevant.

Asbestos bodies

After deposition in the lungs, asbestos fibres become engulfed by macrophages, which deposit a proteinaceous material on their surface. Repeated ingestion, liberation and re-ingestion probably results in the production of asbestos bodies, with their characteristic bulbous ends. They may be present in the sputum and a small proportion may gain access to the interstitium. Asbestos bodies are thought to be produced from fibres of the amphibole group. They serve as another 'marker' of previous asbestos exposure but they are not essential to the diagnosis of the asbestos-related conditions. Asbestos bodies are found fairly commonly in the lungs and sputum, in industrial societies.

Chapter 30
Drug-induced Lung Disease

Adverse drug reactions affecting the lung are not common, but they are nevertheless important because they are generally avoidable, sometimes dangerous and they can cause diagnostic difficulty. The clinical features may be quite indistinguishable from those of naturally occurring disease if the possibility of a drug-induced effect is not considered.

Drug-induced bronchoconstriction

The most vigorous drug-induced bronchial effects are seen in asthma.

Protein preparations

Individuals may become sensitized to protein preparations and develop broncho-constriction as part of a response on re-exposure. The preparations responsible include:

Antisera—produced in animals.

Pituitary snuff—used in the treatment of diabetes insipidus (but now superseded).

Skin-testing solutions—used in the diagnosis of allergic disorders.

Solutions of antigens—used in desensitizing treatment of allergic disorders.

Blood and blood products in transfusion treatment.

Penicillin allergy

Acute 'asthmatic' reactions may form part of an anaphylactic response to penicillin; circulatory collapse is usually a more prominent feature. Anaphylactic reactions are rare but very dangerous. Penicillin allergy is much more common amongst asthmatic subjects than amongst others; the possibility of its existence should be constantly considered when treating infections in patients with asthma. All of the penicillins can provoke the reaction in a hypersensitive subject and there is commonly cross-reaction with the cephalosporins and erythromycin— these should also be avoided in severe penicillin allergy.

Dextran

Acute bronchospasm may accompany anaphylactic reactions due to dextran infusion.

Contrast media

Acute 'asthmatic' reactions to contrast media used in X-ray diagnosis are occasionally seen, particularly during intravenous cholangiography. Some authorities recommend pretreatment with hydrocortisone and antihistamines if contrast media are to be used in cases of severe asthma. Bronchography may cause serious aggravation of asthma.

Histamine

Bronchial hypersensitivity to histamine is one of the hallmarks of asthma, and occasional unintended severe reactions may be seen when histamine is used as a bronchial challenge test, or as a test of gastric acid secretion.

Cholinergic drugs

Carbachol and related drugs may be used in the management of urinary retention and can lead to aggravation of asthma and other forms of chronic airways obstruction. Cholinesterase inhibitors, such as pyridostigmine, used in myasthenia gravis, may also aggravate asthma.

Beta-blocking drugs

All beta-blockers can produce some increase in airways obstruction in asthma and should be avoided if possible. Even eyedrops for glaucoma can cause dangerous worsening. Of the currently widely used beta-blockers, atenolol and metoprolol have a relatively selective effect on cardiac receptors. Propranolol and oxprenolol are relatively unselective, and can cause important aggravation of asthma or other forms of chronic airways obstruction.

Prostaglandins

Prostaglandin $F_{2\alpha}$ has a bronchoconstrictor effect: subjects with asthma are generally very sensitive to its effect.

Aspirin sensitivity

A small proportion of asthmatic patients (but perhaps 15% of severe asthmatics) are extremely hypersensitive to aspirin, so that dangerous or even fatal attacks may follow ingestion of a small dose. Aspirin hypersensitivity may accompany any form of asthma at any age, but it is particularly seen in those with nasal polyposis and 'intrinsic' asthma and seems more common in middle-aged female subjects. Patients with these features who do not know themselves to be tolerant of aspirin, should be warned never to take aspirin (in any form) or any of the other antipyretic analgesic drugs.

The mechanism of the reaction seems to be related to the suppression of prostaglandin synthesis and it is possible that sensitive individuals are unduly dependent upon the bronchodilator effect of prostaglandins E_1 and E_2. Other non-steroid anti-inflammatory drugs (NSAIDs) provoke asthma in aspirin-sensitive patients. Their ability to provoke a reaction is in proportion to their effectiveness in suppressing prostaglandin synthesis.

Tartrazine sensitivity

Individuals who are sensitive to aspirin are commonly also sensitive to tartrazine and other agents used to provide a yellow colour in confectionery, cooking and drug manufacture. Aspirin-sensitive asthmatic patients should be advised to avoid all orange or yellow artificial colouring agents in food.

Anaesthesia

Wheezing which develops during anaesthesia is commonly due to the reflex effects of mechanical stimulation of the airways, particularly in individuals with airways obstruction. Rarely, a very severe bronchoconstrictive reaction may follow administration of thiopentone or succinylcholine. Sometimes the reaction takes the form of acute anaphylaxis with immediate shock and sometimes the bronchial obstruction itself leads to respiratory arrest and subsequent cardiac arrest. Severe or fatal reactions are almost confined to those with asthma, but there is no close relationship between the severity of the asthma preceding anaesthesia and predisposition to adverse reaction.

Hypotonic inhalations

Nebulized water causes bronchoconstriction in asthmatic subjects, but inhalation of nebulized isotonic saline does not. Hypotonic preparations for inhalation, or inappropriate dilution of preparations for inhalation, can provoke bronchoconstriction.

Drug effects on the pulmonary vasculature

Pulmonary thromboembolism

There is a small but significant increased risk of pulmonary thromboembolism amongst women taking oral contraceptive agents. There is no known means of forecasting this tendency.

Other forms of embolization

These include foreign material contaminating infusion fluids and certain forms of oily radiocontrast material, especially that used in lymphangiography.

Pulmonary oedema

Acute pulmonary oedema may be produced by:
1   Overtransfusion, or infusion of excessive quantities of intravenous fluid.
2   Hypersensitivity to transfused blood—usually to infused IgA, white cells or platelets.
3   Narcotic overdosage.
4   Rare reactions to phenylbutazone and hydrochlorothiazide.
5   Hypersensitivity to contrast media used in right-sided angiocardiography and pulmonary arteriography.
6   Reaction to bleomycin.

Drug-related opportunistic pulmonary infections
(see Chapter 12)

Corticosteroids, antineoplastic agents and other immunosuppressive drugs may dispose to pulmonary infection. This may take a variety of forms of which the following are noteworthy:
1   Pulmonary tuberculosis.
2   Infection by *Pseudomonas aeruginosa* and other Gram-negative bacteria.
3   Cytomegalovirus and other viruses such as varicella.
4   Infection by *Pneumocystis carinii*.

Pulmonary Infiltrations due to drugs

Systemic lupus erythematosus

Over 20 drugs have been recorded as causing this phenomenon, those most commonly to blame being hydralazine, procainamide, isoniazid and phenytoin. The pulmonary manifestations include cough, dyspnoea and sometimes pleuritic chest pain, associated with patchy pulmonary infiltration and sometimes pleural effusion. Systemic lupus erythematosus (SLE) follows a more favourable course when secondary to drug administration.

Pulmonary eosinophilia

Irregular or diffuse radiological shadowing in the lung fields, accompanied by a high blood eosinophil count, may be produced by reactions to sulphonamides (including salazopyrin and the sulphonyl urea oral hypoglycaemic agents), sodium *para*-aminosalicylate (PAS) and nitrofurantoin.

Reactions to methotrexate

This antineoplastic antimetabolite may produce a variety of pulmonary reactions, including pulmonary eosinophilia, diffuse pneumonia or patchy pulmonary consolidation.

Pulmonary infiltration leading to fibrosis

Some forms of diffuse drug-induced pulmonary infiltration are followed by fibrosis. Drugs which may cause this include:

Amiodarone—a very effective anti-arrhythmic agent.
Hexamethonium—a little-used ganglion blocker.
Busulphan—used in the treatment of chronic myeloid leukaemia.
Melphalan—used in the treatment of multiple myeloma.
Cyclophosphamide—widely used as an immunosuppressive and antimitotic agent.
Bleomycin—an antineoplastic antibiotic.

Fibrosis may complicate the pulmonary reaction in oxygen toxicity.

Pleural inflammation

Methysergide, a drug used in the treatment of intractible migraine, may produce a diffuse pleural thickening, with or without pleural effusion. Practalol has produced a similar phenomenon, but its long-term use has now been discontinued. Pleural effusion may accompany various pulmonary drug reactions, especially those of the SLE type. Haemothorax should be suspected in patients on anticoagulants who present with obscure pleural effusion, shock or anaemia.

Control of ventilation

Any sedative drug may produce depression of ventilation—this is particularly likely to occur in patients with pre-existing chronic ventilatory failure or hepatic failure. Sedative drugs predispose to inhalation of gastric contents in patients who vomit.

Muscular paralysis

Prolonged apnoea and hypoventilation due to muscular weakness may occur in certain individuals who receive succinylcholine and other muscle relaxants. Patients being treated with polymyxin antibiotics are especially vulnerable. The aminoglycoside antibiotics can also produce neuromuscular weakness, particularly where renal failure results in sustained high blood levels. Patients with myasthenia gravis are at increased risk of all the above effects.

Chapter 31
Hypoxia and Oxygen Therapy

Hypoxia

Hypoxia is ultimately a cellular phenomenon. Mitochondrial activity continues by aerobic metabolism, until very low intracellular oxygen tensions are reached (about 0.15 kPa or 1 mmHg P_{CO_2}), after which anaerobic metabolism appears. This is inefficient and leads to accumulation of lactic acid, a by-product.

Tissues vary greatly in their susceptibility to hypoxia. Broadly, those tissues with a high extraction rate are the most susceptible (brain, heart). Hypoxia becomes important when:

1 It causes reduction in function of the organ with remote adverse effects which could themselves worsen hypoxia (the positive-feedback situation).

2 It threatens to cause irreversible damage to the organ.

It is often difficult to estimate when these two situations exist. The diagnosis of hypoxia relies heavily on the overall assessment of the factors known to be important in determining the rate of oxygen delivery to the tissues. These factors are summarized in Fig. 31.1.

Arterial O_2 content

This is determined by:

1 Haemoglobin concentration.

2 Factors affecting the shape of the dissociation curve, such as pH and P_{CO_2}.

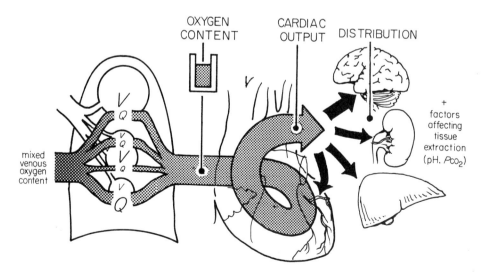

Fig. 31.1. Factors to be considered in the assessment of hypoxia. V, ventilation; Q, perfusion.

3 Ventilation/perfusion relationships within the lung. When these include an important shunt component, the mixed venous oxygen content influences arterial oxygen; venous content is itself determined by O_2 delivery to the tissues.

Cardiac output

O_2 delivery to the body (or O_2 flux) is determined by:

Arterial O_2 content $\times$ Cardiac output

Circulatory impairment is potentially a much more potent cause of hypoxia than pulmonary impairment.

Distribution

Local vasoconstriction or vasodilatation is determined by reflex and local metabolic factors, which can have a marked effect on O_2 delivery. The effect can be in the direction of aggravating hypoxia, or ameliorating it (for example, hypercapnia, hypoxia and hypotension all have a vasodilator effect in the cerebral circulation).

Other factors

Other factors which are of some importance include those affecting tissue O_2 extraction. Increase in H^+, P_{CO_2} and temperature all shift the dissociation curve to the right and facilitate the unloading of O_2.

From the foregoing discussion it should be evident that:
1   The arterial O_2 content is only one factor which determines the development and severity of hypoxia.
2   The only part of the O_2 delivery system which can readily be influenced by O_2 administration is the arterial O_2 content.

Oxygen therapy

Indications

The indications for oxygen therapy are difficult to define rigidly. Broadly speaking, O_2 should be given when arterial hypoxaemia is an important threat to the patient's security, provided that it is safe to do so.

Limiting factors
The two main considerations limiting the use of O_2 are:
1   The danger of inducing hypoventilation in patients with poor respiratory drive, who may be relying on the ventilatory stimulus of hypoxia.
2   The danger of O_2 toxicity which accompanies the administration of high concentrations.

Correction of arterial hypoxaemia
Arterial hypoxaemia arises as a consequence of underventilation of all or part of the circulating blood.

Alveolar hypoventilation
This results in hypoxaemia and reciprocal hypercapnia (p. 18). O_2 administration may completely reverse the hypoxaemia. The problem of underventilation remains.

Disturbed ventilation/perfusion relationships
O_2 administration may completely reverse the arterial hypoxaemia from this cause, as the blood perfusing underventilated areas then encounters adequate O_2 tensions.

Right–left shunts
Such shunts may be regarded as an extreme form of disturbed ventilation/perfusion relationships, except that the blood passing to the shunt is inaccessible to the increased O_2 tension.

Other indications
O_2 administration is desirable in situations where the cardiac output is seriously low, even if arterial O_2 saturation is normal. Very severe anaemia and carbon monoxide poisoning constitute further indications for O_2 administration. This is because a small amount of O_2 can be carried in the plasma of the blood traversing the lungs—about 2 ml per 100 ml for every 101 kPa (760 mmHg) Po_2—and this can be useful in the critically-placed patient.

Method of administration

100% O_2
Most of the masks in general use, although supplied by 100% O_2, in fact achieve much lower inspired concentrations. An inspired concentration of 100% O_2 can only be achieved with apparatus which provides a complete seal from the outside air and a non-return valve; in the clinical situation this only occurs in the context of artificial ventilation. One hundred per cent O_2 may be indicated in exceptional circumstances; prolonged use is attended by the risk of O_2 toxicity.

Masks delivering 40–60%
A variety of masks achieve inspired levels of this order: two are shown in Fig. 31.2. The actual inspired concentration depends upon a number of factors which include: rate of O_2 flow, breathing pattern (tidal volume, frequency and inspiratory flow rate) and the amount of rebreathing permitted by the mask. The effective concentration of O_2 is also influenced by the position of the mask on the face.

Application
Masks in this group are appropriate in patients with good respiratory drive—severe asthma, infiltrative lung disorders, pneumonia, pulmonary oedema, etc. They are suitable for relatively short-term supervised use during respiratory crises. They are inevitably removed from time to time and should be replaced by

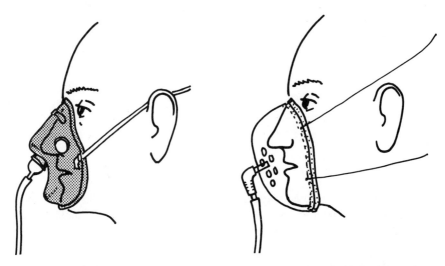

Fig. 31.2. High concentration masks. Two designs in common use. These are simple masks, in which the O_2 is supplied direct to the mask space. The masks are sometimes wrongly referred to as 100% masks. The effective concentration achieved depends upon the rate of O_2 flow and, to some extent, upon the breathing pattern adopted by the patient. It is commonly in the range 30%–60% with flows of 3–6 l min^{-1}. The reason is that during inspiration the patient may breathe in faster than the rate of O_2 supply, so that some air from the room is drawn into the mask. At low flows, some rebreathing of exhaled air is possible. In dire emergencies, where the highest possible concentration is required, a simple mask of this sort is used and the flow rate turned up as high as possible (e.g. 12 l min^{-1}).

O_2 cannulae for more reliable, longer term use, particularly at night. An oximeter is very useful in ensuring that conversion to cannulae is consistent with adequate oxygenation.

Masks delivering low O_2 concentrations

These masks produce a fast-flowing stream of fixed low O_2 concentration (Fig. 31.3). Air is entrained by a jet of O_2, exploiting the Venturi principle. The inspired O_2 concentration is independent of breathing pattern, no rebreathing occurs and the position of the mask is less critical than is the case with some other masks. The concentration delivered is also relatively independent of the O_2 flow rate, being determined by the geometry of the air entrainment mechanism. A selection of masks giving 24, 28 and 35% O_2 is available.

Note: although these masks limit the extent of hypoventilation accompanying O_2 administration, they do not necessarily prevent it altogether. Even with the lowest concentration mask (24%), the Pa_{CO_2} could drift upwards in some patients by about 2.5 kPa (19 mmHg) and with a 28% mask the increase could be over 5 kPa (38 mmHg).

Application

The only indication for the use of low concentration masks of this sort is an acute exacerbation of chronic ventilatory failure in which there is already serious underventilation (high Pa_{CO_2}) and a poor drive to breathe.

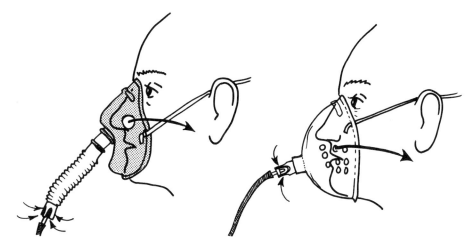

Fig. 31.3. Low concentration masks. Two designs using the Venturi principle. O_2 emerges from a pinhole orifice and the local negative pressure entrains room air (small arrows). The result is a high flow of low O_2 concentration. The concentration delivered is dependent upon the size of the pinhole and the design of the apertures which surround it, and is relatively independent of the O_2 flow within certain limits. The flow of low O_2 concentration (up to 70 litres min^{-1}) is sufficient to flush the mask space continuously, ensuring that virtually everything the patient breathes is this low concentration mixture (large arrows).

Venturi masks are noisy and often removed intermittently by the patient; it is usually preferable to give low flow O_2, using nasal cannulae at 1–2 litres min^{-1}, which provides the equivalent of 24–28%, depending on breathing pattern. The use of an oximeter or repeat blood gas measurement allows the flow to be regulated to the minimum necessary to achieve adequate oxygenation.

Nasal cannulae

The overriding advantage of nasal cannulae is that they are usually well tolerated and kept in place continuously. All other masks are intermittently removed in order to eat, or sometimes to speak, and rarely stay in place during sleep. Some patients dislike the feeling of the face being covered by a mask.

O_2 is administered by two short cannulae which fit in the anterior nares (Fig. 31.4). An even simpler method is to administer oxygen through a soft catheter reaching to the nasopharyynx.

Nasal cannulae are the only practical means of administering near-continuous long-term O_2 treatment (see below).

Other methods

Oxygen tents provide an O_2-rich environment, but it is extremely difficult to maintain a constant inspired oxygen concentration. Oxygen tents severely limit ease of access to the patient for nursing purposes. Their main application is in childhood; children do not tolerate masks well.

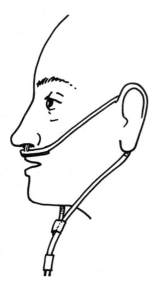

Fig. 31.4. Nasal cannulae. Lightweight transparent tubing carries O_2 to short, soft, backward-curving prongs which lie in the anterior nares. Some breathless patients do not tolerate their face being covered by a mask, but tolerate nasal cannulae. Cannulae are often the preferred means of O_2 administration, because treatment is not interrupted during speech, eating, drinking or sleep and they are cosmetically unobtrusive. Low concentration administration can be mimicked using low flows.

Masks incorporating a nebulizer

These masks, which are described in Figs. 17.13 and 17.14, also provide a useful means of administering larger doses of bronchodilator drug to individuals who are either too ill to use pressurized aerosols, or are unfamiliar with them. Used with O_2, these are effectively high concentration masks. They may be driven by compressed air in ventilatory failure, if the patient is intolerant of O_2, but this is rarely necessary, as nebulization only takes a few minutes and the patient can be stimulated by carers during this time.

Oxygen therapy in exacerbations of chronic bronchitis

See p. 220 for discussion of this topic.

Domiciliary oxygen therapy

There are a few instances in which oxygen therapy may be valuable at home.

To aid exercise in the home

Oxygen therapy can be used, for example, when climbing stairs, washing, or moving from room to room. The cylinder should be situated strategically and long lengths of low-pressure plastic tubing used to make oxygen available at a distance.

Portable O_2

In a few patients, exercise is much extended by use of O_2 and they may find it useful out of doors. It is very desirable to test a patient's response to O_2 under controlled conditions before supplying portable equipment; detailed instruction is required. In practice, most systems are too cumbersome and heavy and, although the idea of portable oxygen therapy appeals to disabled patients, it is found useful in only a few cases.

Long-term oxygen therapy

The long-term administration of O_2 in the home has a place in the management of patients with severe airways obstruction, accompanied by chronic hypoxia. Typically, the patient is of the 'blue bloater' type and there is an element of underventilation also present. The aim of this treatment is to give O_2 for as many hours of the day and night as is possible. This is not to say that treatment is required for minute-to-minute survival; the patient is able to interrupt treatment for modest periods to travel, visit shops and friends. It has been found, in controlled trials conducted in the UK by the Medical Research Council and in the USA by the National Institutes of Health, that survival is increased if at least 15 of the 24 hours are spent breathing O_2-enriched air. Furthermore, it seems that the results are proportionately better if more than 15 hours are spent breathing O_2, and best of all if O_2 is breathed more or less continuously. For the first year or so of treatment, mortality in most studies has been similar in treated and control groups, suggesting that there may be some patients who are so deteriorated that O_2 breathing will not materially extend life. After a year, treated and untreated mortality rates become increasingly different. With near-continuous O_2 it is probable that the untreated mortality of 70% at 5 years could be approximately halved.

Protection from severe nocturnal hypoxia and relief of severe pulmonary hypertension may be responsible for improved survival. Increased well-being, and improvement in sleep patterns and mood are also observed. Progressive CO_2 retention is not a problem in patients in a steady state, who are not in a severe exacerbation.

A number of practical problems must be overcome in order to achieve near-continuous O_2 breathing. The only practical form of O_2 delivery is the oxygen concentrator. This is an electrically powered instrument which compresses air and then releases it through a molecular filter which retains nitrogen. Continuous supply of about 90% O_2 is achieved at a flow rate of between 1 and 3 l min^{-1} by switching compression and release between twin sets of reservoirs and filters. Lightweight transparent nasal cannulae are used, together with long lengths of non-kinkable tubing which lead around the house. The patient uses oxygen throughout the night and throughout the day whilst ordinary quiet domestic activities are carried out.

Suitable patients should have documented daytime chronic hypoxaemia and severe airways obstruction (FEV_1 usually well below 1 litre), and they should have been shown (by two separate measurements of carboxyhaemoglobin or expired carbon monoxide concentration) to be current non-smokers. The treatment is expensive but much cheaper than the use of cylinders. It should only be invoked in the specific circumstances described. It is available on prescription through the National Health Service in the UK.

End-stage pulmonary infiltration or fibrosis
  Severe hypoxaemia may require continuous oxygen for symptomatic relief. A concentrator (or two) makes treatment easier.

Placebo effect
  All O_2 administration exerts a strong placebo effect. Where advanced disease is causing great anguish, the availability of oxygen may do much to relieve the worst moments, even if its use seems illogical. The hazards of inappropriate use may sometimes be acceptable under these circumstances.

Humidification
  Humidification is almost never necessary, except when O_2 is being administered directly by tracheostomy. The nose and mouth achieve adequate humidification under all ordinary conditions and the idea that secretions can be loosened by humidification is usually spurious.

Hazards of oxygen therapy

Hypoventilation (see above)

Withdrawal of O_2
  If O_2 is being given to a patient with severe hypoventilation it may be dangerous to withdraw it.
  The dotted line in Fig. 2.7 shows the relationship between alveolar Po_2 and Pco_2 when breathing air. The extent to which hypoventilation can progress is limited by hypoxia. For example, if the Pco_2 rises to 12 kPa (90 mmHg), the Po_2 falls to about 4.7 kPa (35 mmHg). Survival is unusual if the arterial Po_2 falls much below 25 mmHg. When O_2 is administered, much more severe hypoventilation can be tolerated. If O_2 is then withdrawn, the patient will be plunged into catastrophic hypoxia. Even if ventilation is then increased, the body reserves of accumulated CO_2 will ensure that the alveolar Pco_2 remains elevated for some time.
  If O_2 is being administered to a patient with severe hypoventilation of whatever cause, it must be administered **continuously** until ventilation has been improved.

Retrolental fibroplasia
  Administration of high concentrations of O_2 (sufficient to produce an arterial Po_2 of over 19 kPa or approximately 140 mmHg) may produce retrolental fibroplasia in the neonatal period, leading subsequently to variable degrees of blindness.

Pulmonary O_2 toxicity
  High concentrations of O_2 cause damage to the alveoli. The earliest changes are those of capillary proliferation followed by intra-alveolar haemorrhage and exudation and the formation of hyaline membranes. Areas of collapse develop, lung compliance falls and gas transfer becomes progressively impaired, leading ultimately to arterial hypoxaemia despite the high inspired concentration. Inhalation of 100% O_2 causes reversible symptoms in 48–72 hours, but changes may be

irreversible after exposure for many days. The rate of development of the pulmonary reaction is influenced by a number of metabolic and pharmacological factors, as well as by the inspired concentration. Prolonged exposure to concentrations in excess of 50% appears to be necessary. Interruption of the exposure by periods of breathing lower concentrations appears to have a protective effect. In practice, uninterrupted administration of really high concentrations of O_2 is mainly confined to patients with tracheostomies or endotracheal tubes, who are receiving artifical ventilation. Clinically overt O_2 toxicity is almost unheard of as a consequence of O_2 administration using conventional masks. Whenever patients require high concentrations of O_2, care must be taken to ensure that the inspired level is maintained at the lowest compatible with a safe arterial O_2 tension. Once the condition is established, no treatment, other than lowering of the O_2 concentration, is of any avail—and this may be impossible.

Fire

The hazard of fire should not be underestimated. Many materials which are normally relatively non-flammable burn furiously in an O_2-rich atmosphere. Naked flames and smoking must be absolutely forbidden in the vicinity of O_2 administration.

Further Information

The reader who needs more information on a subject may find it by access to:

Reference textbooks
> Some respiratory textbooks are listed below. Most will provide quite detailed information on specific topics and offer a reasonable selection of references. A good starting place for matters not likely to be affected by recent research findings.

Mainstream medical journals
> Respiratory topics are regularly covered in editorials or other review articles in the main journals, such as the *British Medical Journal, Lancet, New England Medical Journal*. Working back through the contents section (for leading article titles in unbound issues), or the indexes (for the subject title) of recently bound volumes is a good way of getting started when the topic is a common disorder or the matter is controversial and of general interest.

Specialist respiratory journals
> The same technique can be used with the specialist journals. The most useful are likely to be: *Thorax; British Journal of Diseases of the Chest* (after 1989 renamed *Respiratory Medicine*); *American Review of Respiratory Disease; Chest*.

Compiled reviews
> There are a number of volumes which appear either annually or less often, containing a collection of reviews. *Recent Advances in Respiratory Medicine* (referred to below) and the *Yearbook* series are examples.

Monographs
> Some areas of respiratory medicine are served by excellent monographs and a few are noted below. These will usually be hardback volumes, filed in the book section of the library. In libraries following the Dewey system, relevant monographs will be found under 616.2.

Index Medicus
> If the subject is a well-defined one, *Index Medicus* will be helpful for references over about 9 months old. Computer searches require a very specific well-defined target to be useful, otherwise too little or too much information is yielded.

The librarian

The early advice of an experienced medical librarian can save hours of frustration and wasted effort; if the reader's early efforts do not easily produce an expanding stream of relevant information, a librarian should be consulted.

Reference textbooks

Brewis R.A.L., Gibson G.J. & Geddes D.M. (eds) (1990) *Respiratory Medicine.* London: Baillière Tindall.
Comprehensive reference textbook containing sections on relevant basic science. Written by over 90 specialist authors (who are mainly British).

Fraser R.G., Paré J.A.P., Paré P.D., Fraser R.S. & Genereux G.P. (1988, 1989a, 1989b) *Diagnosis of Diseases of the Chest* (3 vols). Philadelphia: Saunders.
Enormous scholarly inventory of clinical and radiological information. Excellent radiology. No therapeutics.

Murray J.F. & Nadel J.A. (eds) (1989) *Textbook of Respiratory Medicine.* Philadelphia: Saunders.
Two volume collection of extensive specialist reviews, mainly by American authors. High quality source.

Seaton A. Seaton D. & Leitch A.G. (1989) *Crofton and Douglas's Respiratory Diseases,* 4th edn. Oxford: Blackwell Scientific Publications.
General textbook of respiratory disease with useful references, largely written by three authors.

Other selected sources

Physiology

Cotes J.E. (1979) *Lung Function*, 4th edn. Oxford: Blackwell Scientific Publications.
Standard reference work on laboratory investigation of pulmonary function and, in particular, as a source of normal values.

Gibson G.J. (1984) *Clinical Tests of Respiratory Function*. London: Macmillan.
Critical review of tests used in clinical practice and research. Lung mechanics well dealt with.

Nunn J.F. (1977) *Applied Respiratory Physiology, With Special Reference to Anaesthesia*, 2nd edn. London: Butterworth.
Clear and comprehensive. Relevant to respiratory medicine as well as to anaesthesia.

West J.B. (1990) *Ventilation/ Blood Flow and Gas Exchange*, 5th edn. Oxford: Blackwell Scientific Publications.
A classic. This small book provides lasting illumination of a central concept of lung function, which is usually poorly grasped.

Childhood respiratory disease

Phelan P.D., Landau L.I. & Olinsky A. (1990) *Respiratory Illness in Children*, 3rd edn. Oxford: Blackwell Scientific Publications.
Standard text on childhood respiratory disease. Clinical and readable.

rosis

...ild M.C. & Dodge J.A. (1985) *Cystic Fibrosis; Manual of diagnosis and Management*, 2nd edn. London: Baillière Tindall.

...ison M.E., Norman A. & Batten J.C. (eds) (1983) *Cystic Fibrosis*. London: Baillière Tindall.

Tuberculosis

Ross J.D. & Horne N.W. (1983) *Modern Drug Treatment in Tuberculosis*, 6th edn. London: Chest, Heart and Stroke Association.

Invaluable source of practical information on treatment, despite age.

Asthma

Barnes P.J., Rodger I.W. & Thomson N.C. (1988) *Asthma: Basic Mechanisms and Clinical Management*. London: Academic Press.

Particularly strong on basic mechanisms.

Clark T.J.H. & Godfrey S. (eds) (1983) *Asthma*, 2nd edn. London: Chapman and Hall.

Collection of useful reviews. Basic mechanisms now out of date, but much of the rest valuable.

Shneerson J. (1988) *Disorders of Ventilation*. Oxford: Blackwell Scientific Publications.

Deals with muscular and chest wall disorders leading to underventilation; their assessment and treatment.

Fibrosing alveolitis

Hay J.G. & Turner-Warwick M. (1986) Cryptogenic pulmonary fibrosis. In: Flenley D.C. & Petty T.L. (eds) *Recent Advances in Respiratory Medicine*, Vol. 4. Edinburgh: Churchill Livingstone.

Sarcoidosis

Scadding J.G. (1976) *Sarcoidosis*. London: Eyre and Spottiswoode.

Still a valuable clinical source.

Fanburg B.L. (ed) (1983) *Sarcoidosis and Other Granulomatous Diseases. Lung Biology in Health and Disease*, Vol 20. New York: Marcel Dekker.

Collection of 17 reviews of specialized aspects of the disease. High quality series of monographs.

Smoking

Golding J.F. (1990) Smoking. In: Brewis R.A.L., Gibson G.J. & Geddes D.M. (eds) *Respiratory Medicine*. London: Baillière Tindall.

Nath U.R. (1986) *Smoking; Third World Alert*. Oxford: Oxford University Press.

Wald N., Kiryluk S., Darby S., Doll R., Pike M. & Peto R. (1988) *UK Smoking Statistics*. Oxford: Oxford University Press.

Comprehensive data on tobacco sales and smoking in the community.

Chronic obstructive pulmonary disease

Fletcher C., Peto R., Tinker C. & Speizer F.E. (1976) *The Natural History of Chronic Bronchitis and Emphysema*. Oxford: Oxford University Press.

Detailed presentation of major longitudinal study. Important but not light reading.

Heard B.E. (1969) *Pathology of Chronic Bronchitis and Emphysema*. London: Churchill Livingstone.
Beautiful account of pathology; worth looking at if only for illustrations.

Carcinoma of the bronchus
Hansen H.H. & Rorth M. (1983) Small cell cancer of the lung. In: Flenley D.C. (ed) *Recent Advances in Respiratory Medicine*. Edinburgh: Churchill Livingstone.
Handle K.R. & Des Prez R.M. (1983) Non-small cell cancer of the lung. In: Flenley D.C. (ed) *Recent Advances in Respiratory Medicine*. Edinburgh: Churchill Livingstone.
Stradling P. (1986) *Diagnostic Bronchoscopy: a Teaching Manual*, 5th edn. London: Churchill Livingstone.
Worth looking at if only for illustrations.

Pulmonary embolism and pulmonary hypertension
Harris P. & Heath D. (1986) *The Human Pulmonary Circulation*, 3rd edn. Edinburgh: Churchill Livingstone.
Illustrated readable reference work.

Occupational lung disease
Cotes J.E. & Steel J. (1987) *Work-related Lung Disorders*. Oxford: Blackwell Scientific Publications.
Readable reference work. Good examples. Good discussion of problems of assessing environmental hazards at work.
Morgan W.K.C. & Seaton A. (1984) *Occupational Lung Diseases*, 2nd edn. Philadelphia: Saunders.
Comprehensive and well-referenced. Useful introduction and pathology.
Muir D.C.F. (ed) (1972) *Clinical Aspects of Inhaled Particles*. London: Heinemann.
Useful sections on deposition and clearance, also asbestos-induced diseases.
Parkes W.R. (1981) *Occupational Lung Disorders*, 2nd edn. London: Butterworth.
Definitive reference work, still valuable.

Index